Neuropsychological Assessment in the Age of Evidence-Based Practice

National Academy of Neuropsychology Series on Evidence-Based Practices

SERIES EDITOR

L. Stephen Miller

SERIES CONSULTING EDITORS

Glenn J. Larrabee
Martin L. Rohling

Civil Capacities in Clinical Neuropsychology
Edited by George J. Demakis

Secondary Influences on Neuropsychological Test Performance
Edited by Peter A. Arnett

Neuropsychological Aspects of Substance Use Disorders: Evidence-Based Perspectives
Edited by Daniel N. Allen and Steven Paul Woods

Neuropsychological Assessment in the Age of Evidence-Based Practice: Diagnostic and Treatment Evaluations
Edited by Stephen C. Bowden

Neuropsychological Assessment in the Age of Evidence-Based Practice

Diagnostic and Treatment Evaluations

Edited by Stephen C. Bowden

OXFORD
UNIVERSITY PRESS

OXFORD
UNIVERSITY PRESS

Oxford University Press is a department of the University of Oxford. It furthers the University's objective of excellence in research, scholarship, and education by publishing worldwide. Oxford is a registered trade mark of Oxford University Press in the UK and certain other countries.

Published in the United States of America by Oxford University Press
198 Madison Avenue, New York, NY 10016, United States of America.

Library of Congress Cataloging-in-Publication Data
Names: Bowden, Stephen, C., 1955– editor.
Title: Neuropsychological assessment in the age of evidence-based practice : diagnostic and treatment evaluations / edited by Stephen C. Bowden.
Description: New York, NY : Oxford University Press, 2017. |
Series: National Academy of Neuropsychology series on evidence-based practices |
Includes bibliographical references and index.
Identifiers: LCCN 2016033650 (print) | LCCN 2016042206 (ebook) |
ISBN 9780190464714 (hardcover : alk. paper) | ISBN 9780190464721 (UPDF) |
ISBN 9780190663773 (EPUB)
Subjects: LCSH: Neuropsychological tests. | Clinical neuropsychology. | Evidence-based psychology.
Classification: LCC RC386.6.N48 N477 2017 (print) | LCC RC386.6.N48 (ebook) |
DDC 616.8/0475—dc23
LC record available at https://lccn.loc.gov/2016033650

This book is dedicated to my four inspirations—Sylvia, Robyn, Jenny, and Claire. And to the memory of Fiona J. Bardenhagen, PhD, who introduced me to evidence-based practice.

Contents

Preface to the *National Academy of Neuropsychology Series on Evidence-Based Practices*

The field of clinical neuropsychology has advanced extensively and successfully in the worlds of psychology and neurology by following two major tenets. The first has been the constant focus on exploring and understanding the complex and intricate relationship between observed behavioral function and brain structure (and, of course, changes to that structure). From early observation of the relationship between injury and behavior to today's combination of psychometric testing, cognitive neuroscience, and structural and functional neuroimaging techniques, this focus has served the field extremely well. The second has been the rigorous adherence to careful, replicable scientific principles of questioning and theorizing, data collection, and use of sophisticated statistical analysis in testing, evaluating, and interpreting information about brain–behavior relationships. More than ever, this has been backed by greater and greater reliance on an evidence-based approach. It is in the spirit of this strong foundation of empirical evidence aimed at improving the quality of informed clinical decision making that the National Academy of Neuropsychology Series on Evidenced-Based Practices developed and continues.

For a significant amount of time, members of the neuropsychology community and, in particular, the membership of the National Academy of Neuropsychology (NAN) had voiced a desire for the development and availability of thorough and accurate resources that are directly applicable to the everyday needs and demands of clinical neuropsychology in a meaningful and accessible way, but provide the latest knowledge based on the most recent and rigorous scientific evidence within the field. The *National Academy of Neuropsychology Series on Evidence Based Practices* is meant to provide just such a series of resources.

At the Series' inception, it was important to first identify an excellent publisher with a history of publishing significant psychological and scientific volumes who would share this vision and provide significant support for a quality product. After lengthy research and discussions with multiple publishers, the venerable Oxford University Press (OUP), one of the most renowned and respected publishing companies in existence, was selected by the NAN Board of Directors. For their part, OUP has committed to the long-term development and support of the NAN Series and, as can be seen in the pages herein, has spared no effort or expense to provide the finest-quality venue for the success of the Series.

The Series is designed to be a dynamic and ever-growing set of resources for the science-based clinical neuropsychologist. As such, the volumes are intended to individually focus on specific, significant areas of neuropsychological inquiry in depth, and together over time to cover the majority of the contemporary and broad clinical areas of neuropsychology. This is a challenging endeavor, and one which relies on the foremost experts in the neuropsychological field to provide their insight, knowledge, and interpretation of the empirically supported evidence within each focused topic. It is our hope that the reader recognizes the many established scholars from our field who have taken on the task of volume editor and/or chapter author.

While each volume is intended to provide an exhaustive review of its particular topic, there are numerous constants across the volumes. Importantly, each volume editor and respective chapter authors have committed to constraining themselves to providing only evidence-based information that meets that definition. Second, each volume maintains a broad consistency in format, including an introductory chapter outlining the volume, and a final discussion chapter summarizing the state of the art within that topic area. Each volume provides a comprehensive index, and each chapter provides relevant references for the reader. Third, each volume is designed to provide information that is directly and readily usable, in both content and format, to the clinical neuropsychologist in everyday practice. As such, each volume and chapter within the volume is obliged to provide information in such a way as to make it accessible as a "pull off the shelf" resource. Finally, each volume is designed to work within a pedagogical strategy such that it educates and informs the knowledgeable neuropsychologist, giving a greater understanding of each particular volume focus, and provides meaningful (read "useful") information geared towards enhancing her/his empirical practice of neuropsychology. In keeping with the educational focus of the Series, a unique aspect is a collaboration of the Series contributors and the NAN Continuing Education Committee such that each series volume is available to be used as a formal continuing education text via the Continuing Education Units system of NAN.

It is my hope, and the hope of the consulting editors who provide their time, expertise, and guidance in the development of the NAN Series, that this will become an oft-used and ever-expanding set of efficient and efficacious resources for the clinical neuropsychologist and others working with the plethora of persons with brain disorders and dysfunction.

L. Stephen Miller
Editor-in-Chief
National Academy of Neuropsychology
Series on Evidence-Based Practices

Preface to the Fourth Volume in the *National Academy of Neuropsychology Series on Evidence-Based Practices*

An edited volume devoted to the contemporary as well as the aspirational understanding of neuropsychological test methods as a way to inform and direct the practitioner's selection, evaluation, use, and interpretation of assessment tools might be seen as a daunting task. In truth, it is a difficult undertaking, but one that is so very important to our field, that NAN and the editors of this ongoing Series felt it was worth the challenge. The field of neuropsychology has maintained a long history of following best practices of test psychometrics and using that knowledge in the design and interpretation of assessment tools, and has been a leader in the larger field of clinical assessment. However, advances in our analysis of the influence of test-associated factors on our test results has provided opportunities for much greater rigor and precision in the use of these clinical tools. This opportunity comes with a responsibility to expand our skills and understanding of the ways in which we evaluate the reliability and validity of our tools, their sensitivity and specificity as related to our clients, and the best ways in which to present and use this information for the betterment of our clients. This results in a need to develop these skills as new advances occur.

Even within the ranks of psychometric-savvy neuropsychologists, however, there remains a gap between the current state of recognized best practices in assessment-tool evaluation and the everyday use of these practices within those same ranks, and in applying that information to those everyday practices with the clients seen. Much of this can be found to be the result of few, if any, approachable and readable materials to help in the understanding of these best evaluation practices, combined with the intimidating prospect of learning new statistical methods. Hence, the thrust of this volume and its main objectives are the presentation of the current state-of-the-art best evaluation practices in neuropsychological assessment, directly addressing the major issues and skills needed to appropriately integrate statistical best practices into our understanding and evaluation of our assessment tools, and real-world examples on how to do so.

Here, in this fourth volume of the *National Academy of Neuropsychology's Series on Evidence-Based Practices—Neuropsychological Assessment in the Era of Evidence-Based Practice: Diagnostic and Treatment Evaluations*—Dr. Stephen

C. Bowden has taken on the formidable task of assembling international experts across a diverse landscape of the most important issues associated with a best-practices approach that is truly evidence-based, yet provides methods applicable to the real world of the practicing clinical neuropsychologist. This important volume provides an empirically derived set of methods to evaluate our measures, from selection to use through interpretation, that can and should be adopted at the individual-patient level. This will inform researchers and practitioners alike, and make available the latest science examining these relationships.

Dr. Bowden is Professor of Psychology at the Melbourne School of Psychological Sciences in Melbourne, Australia. He is a member of NAN and a Fellow of the Australian Psychological Society. He is also Co-Editor-in-Chief of the prestigious journal *Neuropsychology Review.* Dr. Bowden is a prolific researcher of neuropsychological methodology and evaluation, receiving multiple extramural grants and publishing in the best journals of our field. He has been a standard-bearer in advocating for greater evidence-based support for the tools we use, has been a leader in the development of critically appraised topics (CATs) in neuropsychology, and has written extensively on a host of issues concerning the reliability, validity, and interpretability of tests and test findings. Additionally, as an academic full professor, he has a long history of teaching complex neuropsychological and statistical theory. Thus, he is the perfect choice for providing this platform for evidence-based methods of neuropsychological practice.

This volume covers the major thematic issues in evidence-based neuropsychological assessment, including evaluation of the quality of test research, current approaches to understanding assessment tools, evaluating reliability and validity specific to neuropsychological tests, and even what we mean by "evidence-based neuropsychological practice." Additionally, the great group of chapter authors provides specific skills and knowledge of critical areas to consider, including test-reliability levels, test-score change criteria, neuroimaging data, and evaluating performance validity tests. Importantly, these chapters all aim to provide this information in practical and approachable methods, with practical and concrete examples throughout.

As with the earlier volumes in the NAN Series, this volume is aimed primarily at neuropsychologists, but it should also be useful to a multitude of professionals who are interested in understanding how issues of reliability and validity, and their evaluation and interpretation, influence what we can and cannot say about our neuropsychological data. It is my hope that this volume provides the much-needed base on which all empirically driven neuropsychologists can rely.

L. Stephen Miller
Editor-in-Chief
National Academy of Neuropsychology
Series on Evidence-Based Practices

Editor's Preface

Welcome to *Neuropsychological Assessment in the Age of Evidence-Based Practice: Diagnostic and Treatment Evaluations*. With heartfelt thanks to the excellent group of contributing authors herein, and the support of the National Academy of Neuropsychology for allowing a work of this type to be brought to fruition, I hope that this volume will provide a welcome and timely addition for clinical neuropsychologists. Appropriate methods of evidence-based neuropsychology practice can provide skills that are critically needed and easily learned, and provide information of direct relevance to clinical decisions, yet these have not always been readily available for clinicians. This volume is meant to help fill this void.

In this volume, two key elements of evidence-based practice that facilitate clear thinking about the validity of clinical judgements are emphasized. Firstly, learning to understand the most important elements of research design so as to quickly identify published research studies of high quality, and avoid over-reliance on studies of low quality. Secondly, developing a better understanding of the rules of evidence, so that statistically significant research findings derived from higher-quality studies can be turned into patient-relevant information.

The contributing authors and I have worked to insure that these methods of evidence-based assessment are clearly described for neuropsychologists. The key elements of research design are described, including the relevance of study design, reporting guidelines, and methods of critical appraisal. The aim is to provide everything necessary for a clinician to understand how to identify and evaluate high-quality scientific research methods, how to incorporate this evaluation into our everyday practice, how to communicate the relevance of study results to our work with patients, and how to do this in an approachable and user-friendly manner.

Although the concept of evidence-based practice is familiar to many clinical neuropsychologists, the term has nevertheless gained many meanings. For some clinicians, the term evidence-based practice refers to little more than the practice of consulting the literature on a regular basis to ensure that there are statistically significant research findings supporting established or newer assessment or intervention techniques. Or clinicians consider that they are engaging in evidence-based practice by generating statistically significant research findings.

However, as several authors in this volume show, evidence-based practice conveys much more meaning than a general scientific disposition to clinical practice. Instead, evidence-based practice enables a clinician to subject published research, and established or authoritative opinion, to careful scrutiny to discern the scientific rigor and practical value for any aspect of clinical activity. Clinicians adopting the methods of evidence-based practice described in this volume, can be confident that they are adopting methods that are subject to some of the most rigorous peer-review and widely-debated scientific evaluation in the history of health-care.

I would like to extend my appreciation to Joan Bossert at Oxford University Press for her continuing support of this series, and to the National Academy of Neuropsychology book series committee of Steve Miller, Glenn Larrabee, and Martin Rohling for their invitation and assistance with the production of this volume. A particular word of thanks goes to Steve Miller for his sustained support and advocacy throughout the compilation of this volume. I thank Lib Yin Wong and Simon J. Scalzo for assistance with manuscript preparation. Finally, I would like to thank the many graduate students and colleagues who have helped me better understand evidence-based practice. I hope this volume will prove a useful addition to any clinician's skill-set.

Sincerely,
Stephen C. Bowden
Editor

Contributors

David T. R. Berry
Department of Psychology
University of Kentucky
Lexington, Kentucky, United States
dtrb85@gmail.com

Erin D. Bigler
Department of Psychology and Neuroscience Center
Brigham Young University
Provo, Utah, United States
erinb@cortex.byu.edu

Stephen C. Bowden
Melbourne School of Psychological Sciences
University of Melbourne
Melbourne, Victoria, Australia
sbowden@unimeb.edu.au

Martin Bunnage
Institute of Clinical Neuroscience
North Bristol NHS Trust
Bristol, United Kingdom
mbunnage@npsych.co.uk

Gordon J. Chelune
Department of Neurology
University of Utah School of Medicine
Salt Lake City, Utah, United States
Gordon.Chelune@hsc.utah.edu

Hannah L. Combs
College of Arts and Sciences
Department of Psychology
University of Kentucky
Lexington, Kentucky, United States
hannah.combs@uky.edu

Heather A. Davis
College of Arts and Sciences
Department of Psychology
University of Kentucky
Lexington, Kentucky, United States
h.davis@uky.edu

Sue Finch
Statistical Consulting Centre
University of Melbourne
Melbourne, Victoria, Australia
sfinch@unimelb.edu.au

Jordan P. Harp
Department of Psychology
University of Kentucky
Lexington, Kentucky, United States
jordanharp@gmail.com

Anton D. Hinton-Bayre
School of Surgery
Ear Sciences Centre
The University of Western Australia
Perth, Western Australia, Australia
anton.hb@hotmail.com

Christopher J. Hopwood
Department of Psychology
Michigan State University
East Lansing, Michigan, United States
hopwood2@msu.edu

Paul A. Jewsbury
Melbourne School of Psychological Sciences
University of Melbourne
Melbourne, Victoria, Australia
jewsbury@unimelb.edu.au

Lisa Mason Koehl
Department of Psychology
University of Kentucky
Lexington, Kentucky, United States
lisa.mason13@gmail.com

Karleigh J. Kwapil
Department of Psychology
Princess Alexandra Hospital
Brisbane, Queensland, Australia
karleighk@gmail.com

Tayla T. C. Lee
Department of Psychological Science
Ball State University
Muncie, Indiana, United States
ttlee@bsu.edu

Justin B. Miller
Cleveland Clinic Lou Ruvo Center for Brain Health
Las Vegas, Nevada, United States
millerj4@ccf.org

Katie E. Osborn
Vanderbilt Memory & Alzheimer's Center
Department of Neurology
Vanderbilt University Medical Center
Nashville, Tennessee, United States
katie.osborn@vanderbilt.edu

Elizabeth N. Riley
College of Arts and Sciences
Department of Psychology
University of Kentucky
Lexington, Kentucky, United States
enriley1231@gmail.com

Mike Schoenberg
Department of Neurosurgery and Brain Repair
University of Southern Florida, Morsani College of Medicine
Tampa, Florida, United States
mschoenb@health.usf.edu

Martin Sellbom
Department of Psychology
University of Otago
Dunedin, New Zealand
msellbom@psy.otago.ac.nz

Gregory T. Smith
College of Arts and Sciences
Department of Psychology
University of Kentucky
Lexington, Kentucky, United States
gsmith@uky.edu

Jason R. Soble
South Texas Veterans Healthcare System
San Antonio, Texas, United States
Jason.Soble@va.gov

Neuropsychological Assessment in the Age of Evidence-Based Practice

1

Why Do We Need Evidence-Based Neuropsychological Practice?

STEPHEN C. BOWDEN

Paul Meehl argued that knowledge gained through clinical experience in professional practice was inevitably a mixture of truths, half-truths, and myth (Meehl, 1997). The possibility that learning through clinical experience gives rise to knowledge that is not valid, or is based on myth, creates challenges for any discipline that claims scientific credentials. These challenges have an impact on educational practices, the development of scientific thinking in graduate students, and on methods of professional development for mature professionals. As is well known, scientifically unfounded practices have been described throughout the history of clinical psychology, including the use of tests without established validity and reliance on clinical decision-making methods that preclude scientific evaluation (Garb, 1988; Wood, Nezworski, Lilienfeld, & Garb, 2003). And clinical neuropsychology is not free from a history of myth, mostly arising from a neglect of scientific methods. Instead, we need methods that allow students, young professionals, and mature professionals alike to identify clinical knowledge that is based on good evidence and so limit the potentially misleading effects of unscientific thinking. Unscientific thinking risks wasting patients' time, misusing scarce health-care resources, and may be potentially harmful (Chelmsford Royal Commission, 1990; Wood et al., 2003).

As Meehl (1997) argued, scientific methods are the only way to distinguish valid clinical knowledge from myth. Many older professional colleagues were trained in an era when scientific methods for the refinement of professional knowledge were less well taught. As a consequence, many colleagues developed their approach to professional practice in an era when scientific methods to guide clinical practice were less valued or less accessible (Grove & Meehl, 1996; Lilienfeld, Ritschel, Lynn, Cautin, & Latzman, 2013; Wood et al., 2003). One effect of the less rigorous scientific training in the past has been to encourage clinicians to believe that a reliance on "clinical experience" is a valid source of knowledge, without the need for explicit evaluation of knowledge claims (Arkes,

1981; Garb, 2005; Meehl, 1973). Younger colleagues trained in clinical neuropsychology at the present time, and critically, older colleagues who choose to engage in effective professional development, have access to scientific methods to refine clinical thinking that were relatively little known just two to three decades ago. Using resources that are readily available on the Internet, professionals of any age can train in methods for the scientific evaluation of clinical knowledge that are widely adopted across health care disciplines (see www.cebm.net/; www.equator-network.org/). These are the methods of evidence-based practice (see Chelune, this volume).

In fact, methods of evidence-based practice are not new, but they have often been neglected (Faust, 2012; Garb, 2005; Lilienfeld et al., 2013; Meehl, 1973). The methods provide a refinement of scientific thinking that has been at the center of scientific psychology for many years (Matarazzo, 1990; Meehl & Rosen, 1955; Paul, 2007; Schoenberg & Scott, 2011; Strauss & Smith, 2009). However, in contrast to many conventional approaches to evaluating validity in psychology, the methods of evidence-based practice provide skills that are quickly learned, easily retained if practiced (Coomarasamy, Taylor, & Khan, 2003), and provide information of more direct relevance to clinical decisions than the broad principles of test validity and research methods typically taught to most graduate psychologists. While good research-methods training is critical for development of the scientific foundations of practice, evidence-based practice builds on, and brings into sharp clinical focus, the relevance of a strong foundation of scientific education. As Shlonsky and Gibbs (2004) have observed, "Evidence-based practitioners may be able to integrate research into their daily practice as never before" (p. 152). Ironically, however, "evidence-based practice" is in danger of becoming a catchphrase for anything that is done with clients that can somehow be linked to an empirical study, regardless of the quality of the study or its theoretical rationale, any competing evidence, or consideration of clients' needs (Shlonsky & Gibbs, 2004, p. 137).

CLINICAL VALIDITY HAS MANY LEVELS OF QUALITY

The two key elements of evidence-based practice that facilitate clear-thinking about the validity of clinical judgements are (i) understanding the most important elements of *research design* to quickly identify published research studies of higher quality, so avoiding over-reliance on studies of lower quality, and (ii) understanding *rules of evidence*, so that statistically significant research findings derived from higher-quality studies can be turned into patient-relevant information (Sackett, 1995; Straus, Richardson, Glasziou, & Haynes, 2011). These methods of evidence-based practice are described for neuropsychologists throughout this volume and show that "validity" is not an all-or-none condition, but varies widely across a range of quality (Gates & March, 2016). Key elements of research design are described in the chapters that explain the relevance of study design and reporting guidelines and ways to grade the quality of methods used in any particular study (see chapters by Chelune and Schoenberg, this volume). Rules of evidence are described in detail in chapters by Berry and Miller, where methods of critical appraisal are illustrated. The methods of critical appraisal are designed to allow practitioners to quickly evaluate the quality in a published study and so to grade the level of validity from weaker to stronger (www.cebm.net/; www.equator-network.org/). As these chapters show, it is not necessary to be an active researcher to be a sophisticated consumer of research and a provider of high-quality evidence-based practice (Straus et al., 2011). Rather, a clinician needs to understand how to identify high-quality scientific research methods and how to communicate the relevance of study results to patients. The latter techniques are facilitated by the methods of critical appraisal described by Berry and Miller herein.

As Meehl (1997) also argued, the adoption of careful scientific scrutiny to guide clinical practice is not merely the best way to refine scientific understanding, but is also a fundamental ethical stance. We owe our patients accurate guidance regarding which of our practices rest on good evidence and which of our practices rely on less certain evidence or unfounded belief (Barlow, 2004). The American Psychological Association Ethical Principles and the Standards for Psychological Testing and Assessment require that clinicians undertake treatment and assessment practices that are founded on scientific evidence (American Educational Research Association, American Psychological Association, & the National Council on Measurement in Education, 2014; American Psychological Association, 2010). By extension, the ethical guidelines also require clinicians to be explicitly cautious when practices sought by a patient, or offered by a clinician, exceed the limits of our scientific knowledge, that is, lack strong scientific support. The methods of evidence-based practice provide some of the most time-efficient techniques to identify practices based on strong evidence and to help identify when assessment or treatment practices exceed the limits of knowledge based on well-designed studies. When supportive evidence from a well-designed study cannot be found, then a clinician is obliged to infer that the assessment or treatment practice does not rest on quality evidence and may be of uncertain value.

CLINICAL EXPERIENCE IS NOT ENOUGH TO GUIDE SCIENTIFIC PRACTICE

Two to three decades ago, it was uncommon to criticize expertise based on authority or clinical experience (Fowler & Matarazzo, 1989; Isaacs & Fitzgerald, 1999; Russell, 2012). Readers familiar with the history of debate in clinical decision-making will appreciate that the discussion of methods underlying evidence-based practice reiterates the historical transition from a reliance on *clinical experience* as the preeminent criterion of professional wisdom (Garb, 2005; Lezak, 1976; Matarazzo, 1990; Walsh, 1985) to, instead, placing greater reliance on more objective knowledge derived from well-designed studies in clinical psychology and clinical neuropsychology (Arkes, 1981; Barlow, 2004; Einhorn, 1986; Fowler & Matarazzo, 1989, Grove & Meehl, 1996; Paul, 2007). The same conclusions regarding the concerns with over-reliance on clinical experience or experiential learning as the arbiter of judgement validity has been widely discussed in the broader human decision-making literature (Brehmer, 1980; Garb, 2005; Shanteau, 1992). For a succinct and humorous analysis of how to ignore the lessons of decision-making research, the reader is directed to David Faust's satirical account of how *not* to be a scientific practitioner (Faust, 1986). One of Faust's many recommendations to ensure that graduate students and young clinicians *do not* become scientific in their thinking is to keep them ignorant of the decision-making literature that highlights the greater fallibility of subjective, intuitive clinical thinking versus the less fallible effects of greater reliance on objective, research-based thinking (Brehmer, 1980; Garb, 2005; Grove & Meehl, 1996).

Sackett's (1995) description of the implementation of evidence-based medicine *at the bedside* outlines many of the changes in clinical thinking that parallel the changes in clinical psychology and clinical neuropsychology regarding the uncertain value of learning by experience. Sackett (1995) argued that traditional approaches to clinical expertise assumed that extensive exposure to patients, together with thorough training in the nature of clinical conditions, was both *necessary* and *sufficient* for valid professional practice. These approaches are readily evident in older, and even some contemporary, textbooks on neuropsychological practice. Instead, Sackett argued that exposure to patients, and their clinical presentations, is necessary for good clinical skills but is also, at times, highly misleading (Faust, 2007; Meehl, 1973). For example, an accurate perspective on *abnormality* (clinical conditions) also requires an accurate and comprehensive understanding of *normality*, including the relevant control statistics.

In the language of psychological criterion–related validity or evidence-based diagnostic validity (see chapters by Bunnage and Riley, this volume), it is not sufficient, for example, to know the diagnostic *sensitivity* of a test (the extent to which the test correctly identifies people with the condition of interest) to know whether the test is a useful diagnostic aid. A clinician must also know the diagnostic *specificity* (the extent to which the test correctly identifies people without the condition of interest (for a detailed description of these diagnostic validity terms, see chapters by Bunnage and Berry, this volume). Having established that a test has useful sensitivity and specificity, a clinician then needs to determine whether the sensitivity and specificity provide useful information across the range of base-rates in the populations to which the test will be applied (Baldessarini, Finklestein, & Arana, 1983; Wood, Garb, & Nezworski, 2007). Perhaps the most common error in the interpretation of valid test scores is to ignore the impact that base-rates have, potentially turning a valid test into a source of misleading information, either at low or high base-rates (Bunnage, this volume; Larrabee, 2011). As noted, contemporary ethical guidelines require that we only use assessment or intervention techniques that have been shown to have useful validity (American Educational Research Association et al., 2014; Kaufman, 1994). Therefore, it is arguably unethical to rely on clinical knowledge gained from experience alone.

Similarly, to identify a new clinical condition, it is not sufficient to provide a detailed clinical case description. It is also necessary to show that the condition is associated with clinical or pathological manifestations that have high sensitivity and specificity in relation to the relevant control population (e.g., Davison & Lazarus, 2007; Devinsky, 2009). Turning to treatment and interventions, the fields of clinical psychology and clinical neuropsychology have accepted for many years that it is not sufficient to show that a treatment is beneficial by only describing anecdotes of single cases that appeared to benefit from the treatment (e.g., Barlow, 2004; Paul, 2007). Instead, to establish that a treatment works, it is necessary to show that the treatment leads to statistically significant and *worthwhile* clinical effects under carefully controlled experimental conditions involving either replicated, randomized controlled trials, replicated observational (cohort) studies, or multiple-baseline, single-case experiments, at a minimum (Barlow, 2004; Paul, 2007; Straus et al., 2011).

Many of the same principles of evidence-based practice were anticipated by earlier accounts of high-quality clinical research in psychology and the logical and information-gathering steps necessary to turn that research into patient-relevant decisions (Meehl, 1973; Paul, 2007). For example, Meehl's (1973) approach to clinical thinking anticipates many of the elements of what we now term "evidence-based practice," well described in his chapter entitled "Why I Do Not Attend Case Conferences" (Meehl, 1973). In that chapter, Meehl highlighted the low standards of scientific thinking evident in some clinical case conferences. Instead, Meehl highlighted the importance of good theory (see Riley and Lee chapters, this volume), careful measurement of theoretically justified clinical constructs (see chapter by Jewsbury and Bowden in this volume), with attention to the reliability properties of relevant test scores and other data used for clinical decision-making (see chapter by Bowden and Finch), and attention to Bayesian inference in diagnostic decisions (see chapters by Berry, Bunnage, and Chelune).

IMPROVING ON THE SCIENTIST-PRACTITIONER MODEL

In line with the recommendations of earlier advocates of high scientific standards (Barlow, 2004; Faust, 1986; Garb, 1988; Meehl, 1973; Paul, 2007; Russell, 2012), evidence-based practice involves three explicit steps not usually evident in descriptions of the widely embraced scientist-practitioner model (for review see Groth-Marnat, 2009). Firstly, evidence-based practice scrutinizes the method quality of published studies to determine the strength of their scientific inference and the risks of bias that may overestimate the importance of the reported findings. Secondly, evidence-based practice encourages re-examination of reported statistical results in any published study to verify the accuracy of reporting and the patient-relevance of statistical findings. Third, evidence-based practice encourages consideration of patient circumstances and careful integration of any important research findings with patient preferences and circumstances (Straus et al., 2011). Methods of evidence-based practice outlined in this volume encourage clinicians to take a rigorous approach to the evaluation of research findings as well as patient circumstances and preferences. Perhaps the most important element of the evidence-based approach is the overt strategy of not taking a study author's interpretation of the importance of study results at face value, but reevaluating reported results for patient relevance (see chapters by Berry, Chelune, Miller, and Schoenberg in this volume).

As noted above, a prominent feature of the evidence-based approach is the reduced emphasis on subjective clinical opinion (Garb, 1998; Straus et al., 2011). This view is not the same as saying the clinical experience has no value. Rather, experiential learning can be informative under certain circumstances, but can also be misleading because many unsuspected biases can influence the way we learn through experience (Brehmer, 1980; Davison & Lazarus, 2007; Einhorn, 1986; Faust, 1986; Garb, 1998). Instead, in a scientifically rigorous profession, insights derived from experience usually need to be subjected to careful scientific scrutiny and verification before assuming that any particular clinical insights are valid (Davison & Lazarus, 2007; Faust, 2012; Garb, 1998). Contemporary students of neuropsychology may not appreciate how dramatic a shift has occurred in the status of clinical experience as a source of knowledge and authority over recent decades.

Haynes, Devereaux, and Guyatt (2002) provide an excellent description of how our understating of expertise has changed. Expertise is no longer thought to be a function of the accumulation of knowledge derived from the scientifically fraught activity of experiential learning. Rather, expertise is now described in terms of the respective practitioner's knowledge of quality evidence derived from well-designed studies, together with an ability to interpret that knowledge in terms of the rules of evidence and patient acceptability (Haynes et al., 2002).

THE PROBLEM OF OVER-RELIANCE ON CLINICAL EXPERIENCE

For many years, neuropsychologists were taught that once a patient was diagnosed with Korsakoff syndrome, then the patient would have the disability associated with the severe amnesia for the rest of his or her life (Butters & Cermak, 1980). Korsakoff syndrome is a severe post-acute phase of Wernicke-Korsakoff syndrome attributable to thiamine deficiency, but most often seen in association with alcohol-use disorders (Bowden, 1990, 2010; Scalzo, Bowden, Ambrose, Whelan, & Cook, 2015). For most of the last century, the prevailing view was that, once acquired, Korsakoff syndrome "usually persisted indefinitely" (*Diagnostic and Statistical Manual of Mental Disorders, Fourth Edition, Text Revision* [DSM-IV-TR]: American Psychiatric Association, 2000, p. 178). No amount of clinical experience in tertiary hospital settings dissuaded clinicians from that view. As a graduate student, this author saw a steady trickle of patients with Korsakoff syndrome with severe amnesia and, on the advice of his teachers, advised these patients and their carers that the condition was permanent. We now know that this view is unnecessarily pessimistic, a product of what the Cohens described as the *clinician's illusion* (Cohen & Cohen, 1984), namely, a view of the clinical characteristics or course of a disorder that is inaccurate, arising from biased sampling of people with the condition. Clinical experience in an academic, tertiary, clinical neuroscience setting was not corrective, and the current author might have spent the rest of his career perpetuating this incorrect view of the chronic course of Wernicke-Korsakoff syndrome and nothing about the repeated exposure to the occasional patient with acute or post-acute symptoms of severe Wernicke-Korsakoff syndrome would have altered that view.

However, this author chose to undertake research on Wernicke-Korsakoff syndrome in a state hospital for long-term care of patients with alcohol use disorders. With a conscientious staff and access to medical records on many clients stretching back several decades, a different view of the chronic course of Wernicke-Korsakoff syndrome became apparent. Medical and nursing staff drew my attention to patients who had been admitted on previous occasions, sometimes years earlier, with "classic" severe, acute-onset Wernicke's encephalopathy followed by a severe, chronic Korsakoff's syndrome who had subsequently recovered to some extent, sometimes apparently showing nearly full or full recovery in cognitive function and resumption of independent living. Perusal of medical files showed that many patients had experienced repeated episodes of WKS with partial or substantial recovery, sometimes with repeated episodes and recovery between the episodes, a view now commonly held (Bowden, 1990; Bowden & Ritter, 2005; Bowden & Scalzo, 2016; Kim et al., 2010; Victor, 1994; Victor, Adams, & Collins, 1971).

The revision in my thinking about Wernicke-Korsakoff syndrome is an illustration of one of the specific *but limited* benefits of descriptive single-case studies or clinical experience (Davison & Lazarus, 2007), namely, that observation of only one patient who showed recovery from severe Korsakoff's amnesia challenged the conventional view that all patients with Korsakoff's amnesia had a permanent amnesia (American Psychiatric Association, 2000, 2013; Kopelman, Thomson, Guerrini, & Marshall, 2009). Armed with clinical observations that appeared to disprove the conventional wisdom about the permanence of Korsakoff syndrome, I then read the literature more thoroughly, only to discover that Korsakoff himself had described the potential for recovery from severe amnesia in his original description (for translation, see Victor & Yakovlev, 1955). Other researchers, who had done long-term-outcome studies on patients admitted to hospital with acute Wernicke-Korsakoff syndrome had shown that many such patients recover to some extent (Victor, 1994; Victor et al., 1971), although we still have a poor understanding of the factors underlying recovery (for reviews, see Bowden, 1990; Bowden & Scalzo, 2016; Svanberg, Withall, Draper, & Bowden, 2015; Victor, 1994). Surprisingly, the view that patients with chronic Wernicke-Korsakoff syndrome will all show a severe, lasting amnesia still persists, although it is now well accepted that the acute Wernicke's phase is extraordinarily variable (Kopelman et al., 2009; Sechi & Serra, 2007).

The illustration of the limited understanding of the variable course and potential recovery from Wernicke-Korsakoff syndrome may not be so exceptional when we rely primarily on knowledge derived from clinical experience.

For example, a similar misunderstanding prevailed for many years regarding the unnecessarily pessimistic view of the chronic course of schizophrenia (see Menezes, Arenovich, & Zipursky, 2006). If we are prone to develop and maintain significant misunderstandings regarding commonly studied, severely disabling conditions, how much more likely is it that we will not fully understand less-common conditions, in the absence of carefully designed studies of the spectrum of severity and course of illness? The principles of evidence-based practice illustrate that we should adopt a scientifically conservative view and assume that, in the absence of relevant, well-designed observational or cohort studies of the course, clinical spectrum, and diagnostic criteria, we should assume that we have an incomplete understanding of that particular disorder. In this volume, Schoenberg's chapter outlines the widely adopted criteria for "best" clinical evidence, and Chelune's chapter illustrates how we can incorporate best-quality evidence into clinical thinking to guide understanding. The same guidelines for best evidence can help us guard against assuming we have a good understanding when our knowledge is based on inadequate or poor-quality studies. Specifically, the methods of critical appraisal allow us to identify high-quality information when it is available, rate the validity of the respective studies, and, hence, rate the validity of our understanding (see chapters by Berry and Miller, this volume).

MISUNDERSTANDING PSYCHOMETRICS

Another essential technical aspect of test score interpretation relates to the understanding of psychometric principles. The dictionary of the International Neuropsychological Society (Loring, 2015) defines *psychometrics* as the "scientific principles underlying clinical and neuropsychological assessment." Although psychometric principles are covered in most graduate courses, many practitioners gain only a relatively superficial appreciation of their importance in the interpretation of test scores. As a consequence, imprecise or frankly indefensible test-score interpretation is sometimes observed in clinical practice and research. Psychometric principles underlie the scientific interpretation of diagnosis or the observation of changes in response to treatment interventions or changing brain function. It is difficult to be a successful evidence-based practitioner if one is using poor assessment tools or does not know how to distinguish good tools from poor (Barlow, 2005). Unfortunately, there is a common view that practitioners are not adequately trained in psychometric principles, and that clinical psychology (including neuropsychology) on one hand, and psychometrics on the other, have diverged as specializations when they should be more closely integrated to better inform clinical practice (Aiken, West, & Millsap, 2008; Cronbach, 1957; Cumming, 2014; Sijtsma, 2009; Soper, Cicchetti, Satz, Light, & Orsini, 1988).

In fact, some unfortunate misunderstandings of psychometrics persist. Rather than psychometrics being seen as the scientific foundation of clinical assessment for diagnosis or evaluation of change, as it should be, it is instead characterized as, for example, an American-style fixed-battery approach to assessment (for diverse views see Macniven, 2016). The diversity of North American approaches to the practice of clinical neuropsychology, including the popularity of flexible approaches, is well described by Russell (2012). In other approaches, psychometrics is described as of lesser importance for true clinical insights that are best derived from a reliance on experience and subjective intuitions, thereby downplaying norms and tests standardization. Any approach that places low emphasis on test norms and test reliability and validity is an illustration of the older understanding of clinical expertise, which elevates the role of subjective judgment and downplays the importance of well-designed research to inform clinical thinking (Isaacs & Fitzgerald, 1999). In this light, a rejection of psychometrics risks throwing the scientific 'baby' out with the psychometric 'bath water' (Meehl, 1973; Wood et al., 2007).

Four chapters in the current volume provide a summary of how psychometric principles of validity and reliability inform theoretical development and assessment precision in clinical neuropsychology. Lee and colleagues describe the ways validity methods have been used to refine models of psychopathology for diagnostic assessment. Riley and colleagues show how assessment of cognitive disorder has been refined using validity methods. Bowden and Finch review the interpretation of reliability and the dramatic impact on precision in clinical assessment associated with use of test scores with lower or unknown reliability. Hinton-Bayre shows how reliable-change criteria can be used to improve precision in the interpretation of clinical change. These four chapters review foundational knowledge in scientific practice of neuropsychology.

PEER REVIEW DOES NOT GUARANTEE QUALITY OF STUDY FINDINGS

Peer review is a basic criterion of credibility in scientific disciplines (Smith, 2006). Yet, it has been recognized for many years that peer review—the process by which most manuscripts are evaluated for eligibility for publication in "peer-reviewed" journals—is a flawed process (Cumming, 2014; Smith, 2006; Straus et al., 2011). Common criticisms of peer review include that the process favors positive (statistically significant) study findings, is subjective and inconsistent, is biased in a variety of ways, and provides inadequate scrutiny of the quality of methodology in studies submitted for publication (Smith, 2006; Straus et al., 2011).

Methods of critical appraisal are specifically designed to overcome some of the limitations of peer-review by providing readers with the skills necessary to identify common methodological flaws and rate the quality of evidence relating to any particular clinical question (Straus et al., 2011). The chapter by Chelune outlines how clinicians can overcome some of the limitations of peer-review by educating themselves in the skills of critical appraisal, skills which build on the EQUATOR network, a framework of quality evidence in health care that has been adopted by a large number of biomedical journals (http://www.equator-network.org/). The chapters by Berry and Miller in this volume give detailed examples of how to undertake critical appraisal of diagnostic validity and treatment studies, respectively.

ORGANIZATION OF THE BOOK

After this introductory chapter, the next three chapters review the validity of evidence for theories of cognitive function and psychopathology relevant to neuropsychological practice. In Chapter 2, Riley and colleagues review the fundamental importance of theoretical refinement in clinical neuropsychology, showing how the validity of tests is always enhanced by a strong theoretical framework. Riley and colleagues show that there is a strong, reciprocal relationship between the quality of our theories of neuropsychological assessment and the validity of our assessment practices. In Chapter 3, Jewsbury and Bowden review current models of cognitive assessment, suggesting that one particular model stands out as a comprehensive schema for describing neuropsychological assessment. These authors provide a provisional taxonomy of neuropsychological tests to guide practice and promote further research. In Chapter 4, Lee and colleagues show that refinements in models of psychopathology provide a strong empirical guide to the assessment of psychopathology across a wide variety of patient populations and clinical settings.

In the subsequent chapters, reviews and applications of the principles of evidence-based practice are explained and illustrated. In Chapter 5, Bowden and Finch outline the criteria for evaluating the reliability of test scores, showing that simple techniques allow clinicians to estimate the precision of their assessments and also to guard against the potentially distracting influences of tests with low reliability, an epistemological trap for the unwary. The specific application of reliability concepts to the detection of change over time is then reviewed by Hinton-Bayre in Chapter 6, showing the variety of techniques that are available to clinicians to improve detection of change related, for example, to therapeutic interventions or changing brain function. Chelune describes, in Chapter 7, the broad framework of evidence-based practice in clinical neuropsychology, showing how clinicians, if they are conversant with the principles, can bring the best evidence to bear on their clinical decisions. Chelune draws together best-evidence techniques that have a long history in clinical psychology and neuropsychology and broader health-care research. In Chapter 8, Bigler describes the current state of evidence supporting the clinical interpretation of neuroimaging studies, delineating imaging techniques that have established clinical validity and those that are under development.

The final chapters in this volume illustrate the clinical application of best-evidence criteria and techniques for evaluation of published studies. Schoenberg describes the EQUATOR network criteria in Chapter 9. These criteria form the basis of study design and reporting standards that have been adopted by a large number of biomedical journals, including an increasing number of neuropsychology journals (e.g., Lee, 2016; Bowden & Loring, 2016). The EQUATOR network criteria highlight the importance of well-designed clinical studies to understanding diagnostic validity and treatment effects. In Chapter 10, Bunnage outlines the primary statistical criteria for demonstrating diagnostic accuracy, criteria that underpin the interpretation of test score utility. The core skills of critical appraisal are demonstrated in Chapters 11 and 12. In the former, Berry and colleagues illustrate the techniques of critical appraisal as applied to a diagnostic test. In the latter, Miller illustrates the application of critical appraisal techniques to the evaluation of an intervention study. Both of these chapters show how clinicians can use quality ratings and rules-of-evidence criteria to decide on the methodological strength and patient-relevance of published findings, helping to overcome some of the limitations of peer review, when necessary. The volume concludes with a summary chapter outlining some the key skills for an evidence-based practitioner of neuropsychology.

REFERENCES

Aiken, L. S., West, S. G., & Millsap, R. E. (2008). Doctoral training in statistics, measurement, and methodology in psychology: Replication and extension of the Aiken, West, Sechrest, and Reno's (1990) survey of PhD programs in North America. *American Psychologist, 63*, 32–50.

American Educational Research Association, American Psychological Association, & National Council on Measurement in Education. (2014). *Standards for Educational and Psychological Testing*. Washington, DC: American Educational Research Association.

American Psychiatric Association. (2000). *Diagnostic and Statistical Manual of Mental Disorders, Fourth Edition, Text Revision*. Washington, DC: Author.

American Psychiatric Association. (2013). *Diagnostic and Statistical Manual of Mental Disorders, Fifth Edition*. Arlington, VA: Author.

American Psychological Association. (2010). *Ethical Principles of Psychologists and Code of Conduct*. Association ethical principles. Available from: http://www.apa.org/ethics/code/. Accessed June 1, 2016.

Arkes, H. R. (1981). Impediments to accurate clinical judgement and possible ways to minimise their impact. *Journal of Consulting and Clinical Psychology, 49*, 323–330.

Barlow, D. H. (2004). Psychological treatments. *American Psychologist, 59*, 869–878.

Barlow, D. H. (2005). What's new about evidence-based assessment? *Psychological Assessment, 17*, 308–311.

Baldessarini, R. J., Finklestein, S., & Arana, G. W. (1983). The predictive power of diagnostic tests and the effect of prevalence of illness. *Archives of General Psychiatry, 40*, 569–573.

Bowden, S. C. (1990). Separating cognitive impairment in neurologically asymptomatic alcoholism from Wernicke-Korsakoff syndrome: Is the neuropsychological distinction justified? *Psychological Bulletin, 107*, 355–366.

Bowden, S. C. (2010). Alcohol related dementia and Wernicke-Korsakoff syndrome. In D. Ames, A. Burns, & J. O'Brien (Eds.), *Dementia* (4th ed., pp. 722–729). London: Edward Arnold.

Bowden, S. C., & Loring, D. W. (2016). Editorial. *Neuropsychology Review, 26*, 107–108.

Bowden, S. C., & Ritter, A. J. (2005). Alcohol-related dementia and the clinical spectrum of Wernicke-Korsakoff syndrome. In A. Burns, J. O'Brien, & D. Ames (Eds.), *Dementia* (3rd ed., pp. 738–744). London: Hodder Arnold.

Bowden, S. C., & Scalzo, S. J. (2016). Alcohol-related dementia and Wernicke-Korsakoff syndrome. In D. Ames, J. O'Brien, & A. Burns. (Eds.), *Dementia* (5th ed., pp. 858–868). Oxford: Taylor & Francis.

Brehmer, B. (1980). In one word: Not from experience. *Acta Psychologica, 45,* 223–241.

Butters, N., & Cermak, L. S. (1980). *Alcoholic Korsakoff's Syndrome: An Information-Processing Approach to Amnesia*. London: Academic Press.

Chelmsford Royal Commission. (1990). *Report of the Royal Commission into Deep Sleep Therapy*. Sydney, Australia: Government Printing Service.

Cohen, P., & Cohen, J. (1984). The clinician's illusion. *Archives of General Psychiatry. 41,* 1178–1182.

Coomarasamy, A., Taylor, R., & Khan, K. (2003). A systematic review of postgraduate teaching in evidence-based medicine and critical appraisal. *Medical Teacher, 25,* 77–81.

Cronbach, L. J. (1957). The two disciplines of scientific psychology. *American Psychologist, 12,* 671–684.

Cumming, G. (2014). The new statistics: Why and how. *Psychological Science, 25,* 7–29.

Davison, G. C., & Lazarus, A. A. (2007). Clinical case studies are important in the science and practice of psychotherapy. In S. Lilienfeld & W. O'Donohue (Eds.), *The Great Ideas of Clinical Science: 17 Principles That Every Mental Health Professional Should Understand* (pp. 149–162). New York: Routledge.

Devinsky, O. (2009). Delusional misidentifications and duplications: Right brain lesions, left brain delusions. *Neurology, 72,* 80–87.

Einhorn, H. J. (1986). Accepting error to make less error. *Journal of Personality Assessment, 50,* 387–395.

Faust, D. (1986). Learning and maintaining rules for decreasing judgment accuracy. *Journal of Personality Assessment, 50,* 585–600.

Faust, D. (2007). Decision research can increase the accuracy of clinical judgement and thereby improve patient care. In S. Lilienfeld & W. O'Donohue (Eds.), *The Great Ideas of Clinical Science: 17 Principles That Every Mental Health Professional Should Understand* (pp. 49–76). New York: Routledge.

Faust, D. (Ed.). (2012). *Coping with Psychiatric and Psychological Testimony* (6th ed.). New York: Oxford University Press.

Fowler, R. D., & Matarazzo, J. (1988). Psychologists and psychiatrists as expert witnesses. *Science, 241,* 1143.

Garb, H. N. (1988). Comment on "The study of clinical judgment: An ecological approach." *Clinical Psychology Review, 8,* 441–444.

Garb, H. N. (1998). *Studying the Clinician: Judgment Research and Psychological Assessment*. Washington, DC: American Psychological Association.

Garb, H. N. (2005). Clinical judgment and decision making. *Annual Review Clinical Psychology, 1,* 67–89.

Gates, N. J., & March, E. G. (2016). A neuropsychologist's guide to undertaking a systematic review for publication: Making the most of PRISMA guidelines. *Neuropsychology Review,* Published online first: May 19, 2016. doi:10.1007/s11065-016-9318-0

Groth-Marnat, G. (2009). *Handbook of Psychological Assessment* (5th ed.). Hoboken, NJ: John Wiley & Sons.

Grove, W. M., & Meehl, P. E. (1996). Comparative efficiency of informal (subjective, impressionistic) and formal (mechanical, algorithmic) prediction procedures: The clinical-statistical controversy. *Psychology, Public Policy, and Law, 2,* 293–323.

Haynes, R. B., Devereaux, P. J., & Guyatt, G. H. (2002). Clinical expertise in the era of evidence-based medicine and patient choice. *Evidence Based Medicine, 7*, 36–38.

Isaacs, D., & Fitzgerald, D. (1999). Seven alternatives to evidence based medicine. *British Medical Journal, 319*, 1618.

Kaufman, A. S. (1994). *Intelligent Testing with the WISC-III*. New York: John Wiley & Sons.

Kim, E., Ku, J., Jung, Y.-C., Lee, H., Kim, S. I., Kim, J.-J., . . . Song, D.-H. (2010). Restoration of mammillothalamic functional connectivity through thiamine replacement therapy in Wernicke's encephalopathy. *Neuroscience Letters, 479*, 257–261.

Kopelman, M. D., Thomson, A. D., Guerrini, I., & Marshall, E. J. (2009). The Korsakoff syndrome: Clinical aspects, psychology and treatment. *Alcohol & Alcoholism, 44*, 148–154.

Larrabee, G. J. (Ed.). (2011). *Forensic Neuropsychology: A Scientific Approach* (2nd ed.). New York: Oxford University Press.

Lee, G. P. (2016). Editorial. *Archives of Clinical Neuropsychology, 31*, 195–196.

Lezak, M. D. (1976). *Neuropsychological Assessment*. New York: Oxford University Press.

Lilienfeld, S. O., Ritschel, L. A., Lynn, S. J., Cautin, R. L., & Latzman, R. D. (2013). Why many clinical psychologists are resistant to evidence-based practice: Root causes and constructive remedies. *Clinical Psychology Review, 33*, 883–900.

Loring, D. W. (2015). *INS Dictionary of Neuropsychology and Clinical Neurosciences*. Oxford, UK: Oxford University Press.

Macniven, J. (Ed.). (2016). Neuropsychological Formulation: A Clinical Casebook. New York: Springer International Publishing.

Matarazzo, J. D. (1990). Psychological assessment versus psychological testing: Validation from Binet to the school, clinic, and courtroom. *American Psychologist, 45*, 999–1017.

Meehl, P. E. (1973). Why I do not attend case conferences. In P. E. Meehl (Ed.), *Psychodiagnosis: Selected Papers* (pp. 225–302). Minneapolis, MN: University of Minnesota Press.

Meehl, P. E. (1997). Credentialed persons, credentialed knowledge. *Clinical Psychology: Science and Practice, 4*, 91–98.

Meehl, P. E., & Rosen, A. (1955). Antecedent probability and the efficiency of psychometric signs, patterns, or cutting scores. *Psychological Bulletin, 52*, 194–216.

Menezes, N. M., Arenovich, T., & Zipursky, R. B. (2006). A systematic review of longitudinal outcome studies of first-episode psychosis. *Psychological Medicine, 36*, 1349–1362.

Paul, G. L. (2007). Psychotherapy outcome can be studied scientifically. In S. Lilienfeld & W. O'Donohue (Eds.), *The Great Ideas of Clinical Science: 17 Principles That Every Mental Health Professional Should Understand* (pp. 119–147). New York: Routledge.

Russell, E. W. (2012). *The Scientific Foundation of Neuropsychological Assessment: With Applications to Forensic Evaluation*. London: Elsevier.

Sackett, D. L. (1995). Applying overviews and meta-analyses at the bedside. *Journal of Clinical Epidemiology, 48*, 61–66.

Scalzo, S. J., Bowden, S. C., Ambrose, M. L., Whelan, G., & Cook, M. J. (2015). Wernicke-Korsakoff syndrome not related to alcohol use: A systematic review. *Journal of Neurology, Neurosurgery, and Psychiatry, 86*, 1362–1368.

Schoenberg, M. R., & Scott, J. G. (Eds.). (2011). *The Little Black Book of Neuropsychology: A Syndrome-Based Approach*. New York: Springer.

Sechi, G., & Serra, A. (2007). Wernicke's encephalopathy: New clinical settings and recent advances in diagnosis and management. *The Lancet. Neurology, 6*, 442–455.

Shanteau, J. (1992). Competence in experts: The role of task characteristics. *Organizational Behavior and Human Decision Processes, 53*, 252–266.

Shlonsky, A., & Gibbs, L. (2004). Will the real evidence-based practice please stand up? Teaching the process of evidence-based practice to the helping professions. *Brief Treatment and Crisis Intervention, 4*, 137–153.

Sijtsma, K. (2009). Reliability beyond theory and into practice. *Psychometrika, 74*, 169–173.

Smith, R. (2006). Peer review: A flawed process at the heart of science and journals. *Journal of the Royal Society of Medicine, 99*, 178–182.

Soper, H. V., Cicchetti, D. V., Satz, P., Light, R., & Orsini, D. L. (1988). Null hypothesis disrespect in neuropsychology: Dangers of alpha and beta errors. *Journal of Clinical and Experimental Neuropsychology, 10*, 255–270.

Straus, S., Richardson, W. S., Glasziou, P., & Haynes, R. B. (2011). *Evidence-Based Medicine: How to Practice and Teach EBM* (4th ed.). Edinburgh, UK: Churchill Livingstone.

Strauss, M. E., & Smith, G. T. (2009). Construct validity: Advances in theory and methodology. *Annual Review of Clinical Psychology, 5*, 1–25.

Svanberg, J., Withall, A., Draper, B., & Bowden, S. (2015). *Alcohol and the Adult Brain*. London: Psychology Press.

Victor, M. (1994). Alcoholic dementia. *The Canadian Journal of Neurological Sciences, 21*, 88–99.

Victor, M., Adams, R. D., & Collins, G. H. (1971). The Wernicke-Korsakoff syndrome: A clinical and pathological study of 245 patients, 82 with post-mortem examinations. *Contemporary Neurology Series, 7*, 1–206.

Victor, M., & Yakovlev, P. I. (1955). S. S. Korsakoff's psychic disorder in conjunction with peripheral neuritis: A translation of Korsakoff's original article with comments on the author and his contribution to clinical medicine. *Neurology, 5*, 394–406.

Walsh, K. W. (1985). *Understanding Brain Damage: A Primer of Neuropsychological Evaluation*. Edinburgh, UK: Churchill Livingstone.

Wood, J. M., Garb, H. N., & Nezworski, M. T. (2007). Psychometrics: Better measurement makes better clinicians. In S. Lilienfeld & W. O'Donohue (Eds.), *The Great Ideas of Clinical Science: 17 Principles That Every Mental Health Professional Should Understand* (pp. 77–92). New York: Routledge.

Wood, J. M., Nezworski, M. T., Lilienfeld, S. O., & Garb, H. N. (2003). *What's Wrong with the Rorschach? Science Confronts the Controversial Inkblot Test*. San Francisco, CA: Jossey-Bass.

2

Theory as Evidence: Criterion Validity in Neuropsychological Testing

ELIZABETH N. RILEY, HANNAH L. COMBS,
HEATHER A. DAVIS, AND GREGORY T. SMITH

In the field of neuropsychology, accurate, clinically useful assessment is crucial for quality treatment and patient care. The importance of quality assessment is great because the stakes are so high and the accuracy with which a patient's cognitive functioning is assessed can have an extraordinary impact on his or her life. For this reason, the field of neuropsychology has strongly emphasized the validity of its assessment tools (Chaytor & Schmitter-Edgecombe, 2003; Franzen, 2000; Long & Kibby, 1995). Certainly, one of the most important considerations for neuropsychologists in choosing assessment tools concerns their criterion validity. Criterion validity is the degree to which variation on a test accurately predicts variation in a criterion of interest, and when an assessment measure displays strong criterion validity, neuropsychologists can draw conclusions from that test with confidence.

Because of the central importance of criterion validity, an important challenge for practitioners is to choose those tests for which there is the most evidence of strong criterion validity. In this chapter, we highlight the importance of well-developed theory to guide clinicians' choices of assessment instruments. We make the following argument: Psychological theories describe networks of relationships among constructs that have been tested and supported empirically. That is, theories are not hypotheses, instead, they are built on hypotheses that have survived empirical tests. Accordingly, when an assessment measure of a neuropsychological construct predicts a form of cognitive functioning as it should, based on an existing theory, the matrix of empirical support for the validity of that predictive relationship includes, not only the successful prediction itself, but also the body of empirical evidence that underlies the theory. One can contrast such a prediction with a criterion validity test conducted in the absence of an underlying, validated theoretical framework. Empirical support for the latter type of predictive relationship rests only on the single prediction itself. It follows that successful, theory-driven criterion validity tests—that is, those with empirical evidence for both criterion validity and the theory underlying the test—are much less likely to represent false positive findings than "stand-alone" predictions. For this reason, we encourage neuropsychologists, when possible, to choose assessment instruments grounded in theory supported by a network of empirical theory tests.

To make this argument, we first consider aspects of the history of validity theory in psychology. We then describe classic psychological assessment examples, contrasting the rich validity basis afforded by established theory with non–theory based, stand-alone prediction of criteria. We next consider different pathways by which theories develop, because of the importance of the different pathways to neuropsychological assessment. We then consider specific examples of neuropsychological assessment tools that vary in the degree to which they are grounded in theory and thus the degree to which one can be confident that they provide valid prediction of criteria. After considering other concerns regarding the use of validated tests, we close with recommendations to practitioners for evaluating the theoretical basis underlying tests.

CRITERION VALIDITY AS PART OF CONSTRUCT VALIDITY

One of the most important developments in the modern history of psychological assessment was the choice, in the middle of the twentieth century, to define *test validity* as *criterion validity.* Tests were considered valid only to the degree that they predicted a criterion of interest. As Anastasi stated in her seminal 1950 paper, "It is only as a measure of a specifically defined criterion that a test can be objectively validated at all . . ." (p. 67). This focus on the prediction of criteria led to enormous advances in the success and utility of psychological assessment. Classic examples include the development of the Minnesota Multiphasic Personality Inventory (MMPI; Butcher, 1995) and the California Personality Inventory (CPI; Megargee, 2008). Those tests were designed to predict specific criteria and generally do so quite well. The MMPI-2 distinguishes between psychiatric inpatients and outpatients and also facilitates treatment planning (Butcher, 1990; Greene, 2006; Nichols & Crowhurst, 2006; Perry et al., 2006). The MMPI-2 has been applied usefully to normal populations (such as in personnel assessment: Butcher, 2001; Derksen et al., 2003), to head-injured populations (Alkemade et al., 2015; Gass, 2002), seizure disorders (King et al., 2002; Whitman et al., 1994) and in correctional facilities (Megargee, 2006). The CPI validly predicts a wide range of psychosocial functioning criteria as well (Gough, 1996).

Over time, defining "validity" as "criterion validity" led to improved prediction and advances in knowledge. As these changes occurred, two limitations in relying solely on criterion validity became apparent. The first is that the criterion validity of a test can only be as good as the criterion that it was designed to predict. Often, when researchers investigate the criterion validity of a new measure, they presume the validity of the criterion, rather than study the validity of the criterion independently. It has become clear that there are many sources of error in criteria. For example, criteria are often based on some form of judgement, such as teacher or parent rating, or classification status using a highly imperfect diagnostic system like the American Psychiatric Association *Diagnostic and Statistical Manual of Mental Disorders* (currently DSM-5: APA, 2013). There are certainly limits to the criteria predicted by neuropsychological tests. This problem will not be the focus of this chapter, although it is of course important to bear in mind.

The second problem is that the criterion validity approach does not facilitate the development of basic theory (Cronbach & Meehl, 1955; Smith, 2005; Strauss & Smith, 2009). When tests are developed for predicting a very specific criterion, and when they are validated only with respect to that predictive task, the validation process is likely to contribute little to theory development. As a result, criterion validity findings tend not to provide a strong foundation for deducing likely relationships among psychological constructs, and hence for the development of generative theory. This limitation led the field of psychology to develop the concept of *construct validity* and to focus on construct validity in test and theory validation (for review, see Strauss & Smith, 2009).

In order to develop and test theories of the relationships among psychological variables, it is necessary to invoke psychological constructs that do not have a single criterion reference point (Cronbach & Meehl, 1955). Constructs such as fluid reasoning, crystallized intelligence, and working memory cannot be directly observed or tied to a single criterion behavior or action, rather, they are inferred entities (Jewsbury et al., 2016; McGrew, 2009). We infer the existence of constructs from data because doing so proves helpful for understanding psychological processes that lead to important individual differences in real-life task performance and in real-life outcomes. We consider it important to study constructs because of their value in understanding, explaining, and predicting human behaviors (Smith, 2005).

An important challenge is how to measure such inferred or hypothetical entities in valid ways. It is not possible to rely on successful prediction of a single criterion, because the inferred meaning of the constructs cannot be operationalized in a single task (Cronbach & Meehl, 1955). Instead, one must show that a measure of a given construct relates to measures of other constructs in systematic ways that are predictable from theory. For inferred constructs, there is no perfect way to show that a measure reflects the construct validly, except to test whether scores on the measure conform to a theory, of which the target construct is a part.

The process of construct validation is complex and may require multiple experiments. Suppose we develop a measure of hypothetical construct A. We can only validate our measure if we have a theoretical argument that, for example, A relates positively to B, is unrelated to C, and relates negatively to D. If we have good reason to propose such a theory, and if we have measures of B, C, and D along with our new measure of A, we can test whether A performed as predicted by the theoretical argument. Imagine that, over time, tests like this one provide repeated support for our hypotheses. As that occurs, we become more confident both that our measure is a valid measure of construct A, and that our theory relating A, B, C, and D has validity. In a very real sense, each test of the validity of our measure of A is simultaneously a test of the theoretical proposition describing relationships among the four constructs. After extensive successful empirical analysis, our evidence supporting the validity of our measure of A comes to rest on a larger, cumulative body of empirical support for the theory of which A is a part.

Then, when it comes to tests of the criterion validity of A with respect to some important neuropsychological function, the criterion validity experiment represent tests of an extension of an existing body of empirical evidence organized as a psychological theory. Because of the matrix of underlying empirical support, positive tests of criterion validity are less likely to reflect false-positive findings. In the contrasting case, in which tests of criterion validity are conducted without such an underlying network of empirical support, there is a greater chance that positive results may not be replicable.

EXAMPLES FROM CLASSIC PSYCHOLOGICAL TESTS

One group of psychological tests that was developed from, and is continually modified in light of, well-supported basic science research is the set of Wechsler intelligence scales. Each new version of the Wechsler Adult Intelligence Scale (WAIS) or Wechsler Intelligence Scale for Children (WISC) involves changes based on findings that have emerged in the basic and applied cognitive literatures on the nature of cognitive functions. The emergence of working memory and processing-speed indices, and now with the WISC-V a fluid-reasoning index, reflects a process in which the assessment of intelligence is grounded in theories of cognitive functioning that have received extensive empirical support (Lichtenberger & Kaufman, 2009; Wechsler, 2008, 2014). As a result, the Wechsler scales have been remarkably successful in predicting both short-term outcomes such as school achievement and long-term outcomes such as educational level and occupational success (Kaufman, 1994; Mayes & Calhoun, 2007; Neisser et al., 1996; Strenze, 2007). There is a large network of theoretically and empirically supported predictions from Wechsler IQ scores, index scores, and even subtests (Nelson, Canivez, & Watkins, 2013). Predictions from the scales appear to be both reproducible and consistent with established theory (Jewsbury et al., 2016; Lichtenberger & Kaufman, 2013; Matarazzo, 1990; McGrew, 2009).

In contrast to the development of the Wechsler scales, items were chosen for inclusion on key scales in the MMPI (Hathaway & McKinley, 1942) solely because they predicted the outcome of interest. The MMPI was developed in the mid-twentieth century, during the heyday of criterion prediction, and for many scales, items were chosen based on criterion validity alone. Over time, researchers drew a distinction between what were referred to as "obvious items" (those whose content mapped closely onto the intended outcome) and what were referred to as "subtle items" (those whose content bore no apparent relationship to the intended outcome: Jackson, 1971; Weed, Ben-Porath, & Butcher, 1990). In general, the content of the obvious items is consistent with emerging theories of psychopathology, but the content of the subtle items tends not to be. Most of the many studies testing the replicability of validity findings using the subtle items have found that those items often do not predict the intended criteria validly and sometimes even predict in the opposite direction (Hollrah, Schottmann, Scott, & Brunetti, 1995; Jackson, 1971; Weed et al., 1990). Although those items were originally chosen based on their criterion validity (using the criterion-keying approach: Hathaway & McKinley, 1942), researchers can no longer be confident that they predict intended criteria accurately. The case of MMPI subtle items is a case in which criterion validity was initially demonstrated in the absence of supporting theory, and the criterion validity findings have generally not proven replicable. The contrasting examples of the Wechsler scales and the MMPI subtle items reflect the body of knowledge in clinical psychology, which indicates the greater success derived from predicting criteria based on measures well supported in theory.

HOW APPLIED PSYCHOLOGICAL THEORIES DEVELOP

We have thus far put a great deal of emphasis on the importance of theoretically driven criterion validity evidence and its relevance to practitioners and assessors in neuropsychology. It thus seems important to consider briefly how theories develop. Scholars who have studied the history of science observe that theory development occurs in many different ways and is often characterized by an iterative process, in which empirical findings lead to modifications in theory over time (Weimer, 1979).

With an understanding of this iterative process in mind, the generation and development of applied psychological theories and assessment measures generally occur in one of two ways. The first involves extension from, or development based on, existing theories in basic psychological science. Often, theories of cognitive functioning lead more or less directly toward theories of cognitive dysfunction. In such cases, the theory of dysfunction, and measures developed to assess it, can be understood as extensions of existing scientific knowledge. Although successful evidence of criterion prediction by tests measured in this context could represent false positive findings or other errors in prediction, such errors are perhaps less likely, because the evidence does rest on existing theoretical and empirical foundations.

The Stroop Test is a classic example of a neuropsychological measure born out of a strong theoretical foundation. As early as 50 years before Stroop introduced his test, Cattell (1886: interestingly, in his doctoral dissertation supervised by Wundt) reported that objects and colors took longer to name out loud than the corresponding words took to read out loud. His theory to explain this phenomenon was that the association between the idea and the name becomes an almost automatic association because of its frequency. In contrast, associating colors with words is required less often, is less automatic, and thus required voluntary and intentional effort (see review by MacLeod, 1991). Cattell's distinction between the automatic and the voluntary has been highly influential in basic psychological science for more than a century (e.g., James, 1890, Posner & Snyder, 1975; Quantz, 1897).

Development and validation of the modern Stroop Test (Stroop, 1935) as a clinical measure thus rests on an impressive basis of theoretical and empirical support. The test has been found to be a relatively robust measure of attention and interference in numerous experimental studies, and psychologists have adopted it for use in the clinical setting. The test has become so popular in clinical settings that several versions and normative datasets have been created. Ironically, the existence of multiple versions creates a separate set of administration and interpretation problems (Mitrushina, 2005). The Stroop Test has proven to be an effective measure of executive disturbance in numerous neurological and psychiatric populations (e.g., schizophrenia, Parkinson's disease, chronic alcoholism, Huntington's disease, attention-deficit hyperactivity disorder [ADHD]: Strauss, Sherman, & Spreen, 2006). Impaired attentional abilities associated with traumatic brain injury, depression, and bipolar disorder all appear to influence Stroop performance (Lezak, Howeison, Bigler, & Tranel, 2012; Strauss et al., 2006). Consistent with these findings, the Stroop has been shown to be sensitive to both focal and diffuse lesions (Demakis, 2004). Overall, the Stroop Test is a well-validated, reliable measure that provides significant information on the cognitive processes underlying various neurological and psychological disorders. As is characteristic of the iterative nature of scientific development, findings from use of the test have led to modifications in the underlying theory (MacLeod, 1991).

Sometimes, researchers attempt to create assessment measures based on theory but the tests do not, after repeated examination, demonstrate good criterion validity. Generally, one of two things happens in the case of these theory-driven tests that ultimately tend not to be useful. First, it is possible that the test being explored was simply not a good measure of the construct of interest. This can lead to important modifications of the measure so that it more accurately assesses the construct of interest and can be potentially useful in the future. The second possibility is that the theory underlying development of the measure is not fully accurate. When the latter is the case, attempts to use a test to predict criteria will provide inconsistent results, characterized by failures to replicate.

An example of this problem is illustrated in the long history of the Rorschach test in clinical psychology. The Rorschach was developed from hypothetical contentions that one's perceptions of stimuli reveal aspects of one's personality (Rorschach, 1964) and that people project aspects of themselves onto ambiguous stimuli (Frank, 1939). This test provides an example of a hypothesis-based test that has produced inconsistent criterion validity results, a test based on a theoretical contention that has since been challenged and deemed largely unsuccessful. One school of thought is that the hypotheses are sound but that the test scoring procedures are flawed. As a consequence, there have been repeated productions of new scoring systems over the years (see Wood, Nezworski, Lilienfeld, & Garb, 2003). To date, each scoring system, including Exner's (1974, 1978) systems, has had limited predictive validity (Hunsley & Bailey, 1999; Wood et al., 2003). The modest degree of support provided by the literature has led to a second interpretation, which is that the hypothesis underlying use of the test lacks validity (Wood et al., 2003).

We believe there are two important lessons neuropsychologists can draw from histories of tests such as the Rorschach. The first is to be aware of the validation history of theories that are the basis for tests one is considering using. Knowing whether underlying theories have sound empirical support or not can provide valuable guidance for the clinician. The second is that it may not be wise to invest considerable effort in trying to alter or modify tests that either lack adequate criterion validity or are not based on a valid, empirically supported theory.

The second manner in which theories develop is through what has been called a "bootstrapping" process. Cronbach and Meehl (1955) described bootstrapping in this context as the iterative process of using the results of tests of partially developed theories to refine and extend the primary theory. Bootstrapping can lead to further refinement and elaboration, allowing for stronger and more precise validation tests. When using the bootstrapping method of theory development in neuropsychology, it is common for researchers to discover, perhaps even accidentally, that some sort of neuropsychological test can accurately identify who has a cognitive deficit based on their inability to perform the test at hand (e.g., Fuster, 2015; Halstead, 1951). Once researchers are able to determine that the test is a reliable indicator of neuropsychological deficit, they can explore what the task actually measures and can begin to formulate a theory about this cognitive deficit based on what they think the test is measuring. In this manner, the discovery and repeated use of a measure to identify neuropsychological deficit can lead to better theories about the cognitive deficits identified by the tests.

The Trail Making Test (TMT) is one of the most well-validated and widely utilized assessments of scanning and visuomotor tracking, divided attention, and cognitive flexibility (Lezak et al., 2012). Despite the strength and utility of the test as it stands today, the test was not originally developed to test brain dysfunction. The TMT is a variation of John E. Partington's Test of Distributed Attribution, which was initially developed in 1938 to evaluate general intellectual ability. Now, however, the Trail Making Test is commonly used as a diagnostic tool in clinical settings. Poor performance is known to be associated with many types of brain impairment. The TMT remains one of the most commonly used neuropsychological tests in both research and clinical practice (Rabin, Barr, & Burton, 2005).

The TMT is an example of a neuropsychological measure that, although it was not originally based on an established theoretical foundation, is able to function well in the context of current psychological theory that emphasizes cognitive flexibility, divided attention, and visuo-motor tracking. The current theory was developed through the utilization of the TMT, a classic example of the bootstrapping approach to theory development. TMT performance is associated with occupational outcome in adulthood after childhood traumatic brain injury

(TBI: Nybo et al., 2004). In addition, TMT parts A and B can predict psychosocial outcome following head injury (Devitt et al., 2006) and are useful for predicting instrumental activities of daily living in older adults (Boyle et al., 2004; Tierney et al., 2001). Tierney et al. (2001) reported that the TMT was significantly related to self-care deficits, use of emergency services, experiencing harm, and loss of property in a study of cognitively impaired people who live alone. At this point in the history of the test, one can say that the TMT has a strong theoretical foundation and an extensive matrix of successful criterion predictions in line with that theory. Inferences made based on the test today are unlikely to be characterized by repeated false positive conclusions.

NEUROPSYCHOLOGICAL TESTS NOT BASED ON THEORY

Although there have been many examples of successful neuropsychological assessments that are grounded in developed theories, there are also assessment measures that are not based on existing theory, have not led to new, generative theory, and that do not consistently demonstrate criterion validity. Nevertheless, these assessments are still used in practice. For example, the Family Pictures Wechsler Memory Scale III (WMS-III) subtest was originally designed to measure "complex, meaningful, visually presented information" (Wechsler, 1997). In this measure, four pictures of individuals in a family are shown to an examinee for ten seconds followed by recall of the persons, a description of what was occurring in the picture, and the locations of the family members (Lezak et al., 2012). However, the test has been heavily criticized because it is instead thought to measure verbal memory as opposed to its intended target, visual memory. The measure has been shown to have a low average stability coefficient ($r \sim .60$; Lichtenberger, Kaufman, & Lai, 2001) and an inadequate floor and ceiling (Flanagan, McGrew, & Ortiz, 2000). Furthermore, Family Pictures does not correlate well with other visual memory measures and it does not effectively discriminate lesion lateralization (Chapin, Busch, Naugle, & Najm, 2009; Dulay, Schefft, Marc, Testa, Fargo, Privitera, & Yeh, 2002). There is good reason to question its accuracy as a measure of visual memory, its use for that purpose could lead to non-optimal prediction of criteria.

RECOMMENDATIONS TO PRACTITIONERS

Theory-Based Assessment

Our first recommendation is the one we have emphasized throughout this chapter: whenever possible, use assessment tools grounded in empirically supported theory. Doing so reduces the chances that one will draw erroneous conclusions from test results. However, we also recognize that neuropsychological tests demonstrating good, theory-driven criterion validity do not exist for every construct that is of clinical interest and importance. There are sometimes serious issues needing assessment and care for which there are no assessment instruments that fit the bill of showing criterion validity based on strong theory. We thus review here some points we believe will be helpful to practitioners who have to make difficult decisions about neuropsychological assessment when no clear guidelines or evidence exist for that specific clinical context.

The Use of Assessment Instruments "Off-Label"

One of the most pressing issues for clinicians in practice is the use of assessment instruments on populations for whom they are not validated. It happens quite frequently that practitioners might use an assessment tool "off-label." Off-label use may occur when clinicians take an assessment instrument that demonstrated strong validity in one population (e.g., aphasia in Alzheimer's disease) and use it to assess the same neuropsychological dysfunction in another population (e.g., aphasia in TBI). Although such a decision seems quite reasonable, it can be problematic. While the use of the test on such a population may ultimately prove to be valuable and informative, one cannot presume that the validity of the instrument extends beyond use in its originally intended population. Simply because a test has been validated in one population does not mean it will produce the same accurate, reliable, and replicable results in the non-validated population. Thus, clinicians should examine closely the evidence for the validity of a measure specifically for the population on which the clinician wants to use it. Indeed, the American Psychological Association *Ethical Principles of Psychologists and Code of Conduct* (2010) specifically states, in Standard 9.02 (b), that "Psychologists use assessment instruments whose validity and reliability have been established for use with members of the population tested. When such validity or reliability has not been established, psychologists describe the strengths and limitations of test results and interpretation."

One neuropsychological measure that has in the past been used "off-label" is the Repeatable Battery for the Assessment of Neuropsychological Status (RBANS; Randolph, Tierney, Mohr, & Chase, 1998). The RBANS was originally developed as a brief test to identify and differentiate dementia severity in elderly individuals (Strauss et al., 2006). The RBANS contains subscales that assess verbal memory, visual memory, visuospatial-construction skills, language, and attention abilities. As the name suggests, the RBANS was designed to facilitate repeat testing and has four versions that examiners can use in order to minimize (but not eliminate) the influence of practice.

Because of the practical usefulness of a repeatable neuropsychological measure, clinicians frequently used the RBANS in non-demented populations (e.g., TBI, stroke, schizophrenia; Gold, Queern, Iannone, & Buchanan, 1999; Larson, Kirschner, Bode, Heinemann, & Goodman, 2005; McKay, Wertheimer, Fichtenberg, & Casey, 2008). This was true even though, at the time, validation data were only available for individuals with dementia (Duff, Patton, Schoenberg, Mold, Scott, & Adams, 2004) and schizophrenia (Wilk, Gold, Humber, Dickerson, Fenton, & Buchanan, 2004), both of which exclude other medical conditions that affect cognitive functioning (e.g., stroke, TBI, Parkinson's disease, etc.).

More recently, the RBANS has been updated to include special group studies for Alzheimer's disease, vascular dementia, HIV dementia, Huntington's disease, Parkinson's disease, depression, schizophrenia, and closed head injury populations (Pearson Clinical, 2016). This change represents an important step in enhancing the criterion-related validity of this measure, the measure can now be used with more confidence in many non-demented populations. Still, clinicians who make decisions to use this (or any other) measure on a population for whom it was not originally created and for which there is not sound validity evidence should closely examine the body of available empirical literature supporting their decision.

Sometimes the "off-label" use of an assessment tool is necessary because there are no assessment instruments available for the problem of interest that have been validated in the population of interest. This is an unfortunately common gap between the state of the research literature and the state of clinical needs. In such a case, off-label assessments must be used with extreme caution and with the knowledge that the use of such instruments is getting ahead of the theory and research on which these assessments were created.

Construct Homogeneity and Heterogeneity

Another crucial issue of consideration for the neuropsychological practitioner is that of construct heterogeneity. "Construct heterogeneity" refers to the idea that many disorders that need to be assessed are multifaceted and complex, such that different individuals will experience different components of a disorder. In practice, the danger of construct heterogeneity occurs when a clinician uses a single test score to represent multiple dimensions (facets) of a construct or disorder. The use of a single score is a problem for two primary reasons (1) one cannot know how specific components of the construct might differentially contribute to the overall score, and (2) the same overall score could represent different combinations of component scores for different individuals (Strauss & Smith, 2009).

A classic example of construct heterogeneity in assessment is the Beck Depression Inventory (BDI; Beck et al., 1996), which is used to provide a single score of depressive symptomatology. This is problematic because depression is a multifaceted collection of very different symptoms, including feelings of high negative affect (such as sadness/worthlessness), low positive affect (anhedonia), sleeping or eating too much or too little, thoughts of suicide, and others. Individuals can obtain the same score on the BDI but actually have very different patterns of symptoms (McGrath, 2005).

In the case of the BDI, the patient answers questions on a scale of 0–3 points based on the severity of that symptom, and the total depressive score is a sum of all the points for all of the questions. A score of 9 points can mean different things for different patients. One patient might get that score due to high negative affect without disturbances in positive affect, sleep, or appetite. Another patient might get the same score due to loss of positive affect in the absence of any significant negative affect or any sleep or appetite problems. Because treatments for high negative affect and low positive affect differ (Chambless & Ollendick, 2001), it is crucial to know the degree to which each of those two constructs contributed to the patient's score. It is far more efficient and accurate to measure negative and positive affect separately, and doing so can provide a clearer picture of the actual clinical experience of the patient. It is important to note, however, that the actual diagnosis of major depressive disorder in the DSM-5 (APA, 2013) is similarly heterogeneous and is based on these varied and conflated constructs. Thus, the construct heterogeneity of the BDI is not merely an assessment problem, and construct heterogeneity in assessment is not merely a neuropsychological problem. The problem of construct heterogeneity extends well into the entire field of clinical psychology and our understanding of health problems as a whole (see also Chapter 4 of this volume).

For the clinician, it is critical to understand exactly what the assessment instrument being used is purported to measure and, related to this, whether the target construct is heterogeneous or homogeneous. A well-validated test that measures a homogenous construct is the Boston Naming Test (BNT: Pedraza, Sachs, Ferman, Rush, & Lucas, 2011). The BNT is a neuropsychological measure that was designed to assess visual naming ability using line drawings of everyday objects (Strauss et al., 2006). Kaplan first introduced the BNT as a test of confrontation naming in 1983 (Kaplan, Goodglass, & Weintraub, 1983). The BNT is sensitive to naming deficits in patients with left-hemisphere cerebrovascular accidents (Kohn & Goodglass, 1985), anoxia (Tweedy & Schulman, 1982), and subcortical disease (Henry & Crawford, 2004, Locascio et al., 2003). Patients with Alzheimer's disease typically exhibit signs of anomia (difficulty with word recall) and show impairment on the BNT (Strauss et al., 2006).

In contrast, there are neuropsychological measures that measure multiple cognitive domains, thus measuring a more heterogeneous construct. For example, the Arithmetic subtest from the WAIS-IV, one of the core subtests of the working memory index, appears to be heterogeneous (Sudarshan et al., 2016). The Wechsler manual describes the Arithmetic test as measuring "mental manipulation, concentration, attention, short- and long-term memory, numerical reasoning ability, and mental alertness" (p. 15). Since the test measures several areas of cognition, it is difficult to pinpoint the exact area of concern when an individual performs poorly (Lezak et al., 2012). Karzmark (2009) noted that, although Wechsler Arithmetic appears to tap into concentration and working memory, it is affected by many other factors and has limited specificity as a concentration measure.

Tests that assess heterogeneous constructs should be used cautiously and interpreted very carefully, preferably at the facet-level or narrow ability level (see Chapter 3 of this volume). Of course, it is likely that, for many patients, there will not be a perfectly constructed and validated test to measure their exact, specific neuropsychological problem. In these cases, where there is a substantial gap between rigorous scientific validity (such as validation evidence only for a heterogeneous measure) and the necessities of clinical practice (such as identifying the precise nature of a deficit), it will be even more important for clinicians to use the tools they do have at their disposal to ensure or preserve whatever level of validity is available to them.

Ecological Validity

Finally, there is the issue of ecological validity in neuropsychological assessment. An important question for clinicians concerns whether variation in test scores maps onto variation in performance of relevant cognitive functions in everyday life. This issue perhaps becomes central when the results of an assessment instrument do not match clinical observation or patient report. When this occurs, the clinician's judgement concerning how much faith to place in the test result should be influenced by the presence or absence of ecological validity evidence for the test. In the absence of good evidence for ecological validity, the clinician might be wise to weigh observation and patient report more heavily. When there is good evidence for ecological validity of a test, the clinician might instead give the test result more weight. There are certainly times when a neuropsychological test will detect some issue that was previously unknown or that the patient did not cite as a concern (for a full review of the importance of ecological validity issues to neuropsychological assessment, see Chaytor & Schmitter-Edgecombe, 2003).

SUMMARY

In the context of good theory, criterion validity evidence is hugely important to the practitioner. It provides a clear foundation for sound, scientifically based clinical decisions. Criterion validity evidence in the absence of theory may well be useful to practitioners, too, but it provides a riskier basis on which to proceed. The recommendations we make to practitioners follow from this logic. Neuropsychological assessments that demonstrate criterion validity and that were created based on an underlying psychological theory of the construct or dysfunction of interest are often more useful for clinicians because of the lower risk of making an error in assessment. Tests that demonstrate criterion validity evidence in the context of underlying theory often produce results that are more reliable, stable, and replicable than tests that are not grounded in a solid theoretical context.

In addition to this core consideration, we recommend the following. Firstly, when clinicians use measures in the absence of established criterion validity for the clinical question or population in which the test is applied, then clinicians should carefully examine the empirical and theoretical justification for doing so. Secondly, clinicians should avoid relying on single scores that represent multiple constructs, because clients with different presentations can achieve the same score. Thirdly, clinicians should be aware of the evidence concerning the ecological validity of their assessment tools and use that evidence as a guide for reconciling discrepancies between test results and observation or patient report. Because the accuracy with which an individual's neuropsychological functioning is assessed can have an extraordinary impact on that person's life, valid and clinically useful assessment is crucial for high-quality patient care.

REFERENCES

Alkemade, N., Bowden, S. C., & Salzman, L. (2015). Scoring correction for MMPI-2 Hs scale in patients experiencing a traumatic brain injury: A test of measurement invariance. *Archives of Clinical Neuropsychology, 30*, 39–48.

American Psychiatric Association. (2013). *Diagnostic and Statistical Manual of Mental Disorders (DSM-5®)*. Washington, DC: American Psychiatric Association.

American Psychological Association. (2010). *Ethical Principles of Psychologists and Code of Conduct*. Retrieved from http://apa.org/ethics/code/index.aspx. Date retrieved: January 19, 2015.

Anastasi, A. (1950). The concept of validity in the interpretation of test scores. *Educational and Psychological Measurement, 10*, 67–78.

Beck, A. T., Steer, R. A., & Brown, G. K. (1996). *Beck Depression Inventory–II*. San Antonio, TX: Psychological Corporation.

Boyle, P. A., Paul, R. H., Moser, D. J., & Cohen, R. A. (2004). Executive impairments predict functional declines in vascular dementia. *The Clinical Neuropsychologist, 18*(1), 75–82.

Butcher, J. N. (1990). *The MMPI-2 in Psychological Treatment*. New York: Oxford University Press.

Butcher, J. N. (1995). *User's Guide for The Minnesota Report: Revised Personnel Report*. Minneapolis, MN: National Computer Systems

Butcher, J. N. (2001). *Minnesota Multiphasic Personality Inventory–2 (MMPI-2) User's Guide for The Minnesota Report: Revised Personnel System* (3rd ed.). Bloomington, MN: Pearson Assessments.

Chambless, D. L., & Ollendick, T. H. (2001). Empirically supported psychological interventions: Controversies and evidence. *Annual Review of Psychology, 52*(1), 685–716.

Chapin, J. S., Busch, R. M., Naugle, R. I., & Najm, I. M. (2009). The Family Pictures subtest of the WMS-III: Relationship to verbal and visual memory following temporal lobectomy for intractable epilepsy. *Journal of Clinical and Experimental Neuropsychology, 31*(4), 498–504.

Chaytor, N., & Schmitter-Edgecombe, M. (2003). The ecological validity of neuropsychological tests: A review of the literature on everyday cognitive skills. *Neuropsychology Review, 13*(4), 181–197.

Cronbach, L. J., & Meehl, P. E. (1955). Construct validity in psychological tests. *Psychological Bulletin, 52*(4), 281–302.

Demakis, G. J. (2004). Frontal lobe damage and tests of executive processing: A meta-analysis of the category test, Stroop test, and trail-making test. *Journal of Clinical and Experimental Neuropsychology, 26*(3), 441–450.

Devitt, R., Colantonio, A., Dawson, D., Teare, G., Ratcliff, G., & Chase, S. (2006). Prediction of long-term occupational performance outcomes for adults after moderate to severe traumatic brain injury. *Disability & Rehabilitation, 28*(9), 547–559.

Duff, K., Patton, D., Schoenberg, M. R., Mold, J., Scott, J. G., & Adams, R. L. (2003). Age- and education-corrected independent normative data for the RBANS in a community dwelling elderly sample. *The Clinical Neuropsychologist, 17*(3), 351–366.

Dulay, M. F., Schefft, B. K., Marc Testa, S., Fargo, J. D., Privitera, M., & Yeh, H. S. (2002). What does the Family Pictures subtest of the Wechsler Memory Scale–III measure? Insight gained from patients evaluated for epilepsy surgery. *The Clinical Neuropsychologist, 16*(4), 452–462.

Exner, J. E. (1974). *The Rorschach: A Comprehensive System.* New York: John Wiley & Sons.

Exner Jr., J. E., & Clark, B. (1978). *The Rorschach* (pp. 147–178). New York: Plenum Press, Springer US.

Flanagan, D. P., McGrew, K. S., & Ortiz, S. O. (2000). *The Wechsler Intelligence Scales and Gf-Gc Theory: A Contemporary Approach to Interpretation.* Needham Heights, MA: Allyn & Bacon.

Frank, L. K. (1939). Projective methods for the study of personality. *The Journal of Psychology, 8*(2), 389–413.

Franzen, M. D. (2000). *Reliability and Validity in Neuropsychological Assessment.* New York: Springer Science & Business Media.

Fuster, J. M. (2015). *The Prefrontal Cortex.* San Diego: Elsevier, Acad. Press.

Gass, C. S. (2002). Personality assessment of neurologically impaired patients. In J. Butcher (Ed.), *Clinical Personality Assessment: Practical Approaches* (2nd ed., pp. 208–244). New York: Oxford University Press.

Gold, J. M., Queern, C., Iannone, V. N., & Buchanan, R. W. (1999). Repeatable Battery for the Assessment of Neuropsychological Status as a screening test in schizophrenia, I: Sensitivity, reliability, and validity. *American Journal of Psychiatry, 156*(12), 1944–1950.

Gough, H. G. (1996). *CPI Manual: Third Edition.* Palo Alto, CA: Consulting Psychologists Press.

Greene, R. L. (2006). Use of the MMPI-2 in outpatient mental health settings. In J. Butcher (Ed.), *MMPI-2: A Practitioner's Guide.* Washington, DC: American Psychological Association.

Halstead, W. G. (1951). Biological intelligence. *Journal of Personality, 20*(1), 118–130.

Hathaway, S. R., & McKinley, J. C. (1942). *The Minnesota Multiphasic Personality Schedule.* Minneapolis, MN, US: University of Minnesota Press.

Henry, J. D., & Crawford, J. R. (2004). Verbal fluency deficits in Parkinson's disease: A meta-analysis. *Journal of the International Neuropsychological Society, 10*(4), 608–622.

Hollrah, J. L., Schlottmann, S., Scott, A. B., & Brunetti, D. G. (1995). Validity of the MMPI subtle items. *Journal of Personality Assessment, 65*, 278–299.

Hunsley, J., & Bailey, J. M. (1999). The clinical utility of the Rorschach: Unfulfilled promises and an uncertain future. *Psychological Assessment, 11*(3), 266–277.

Jackson, D. N. (1971). The dynamics of structured personality tests: 1971. *Psychological Review, 78*(3), 229–248.

James, W. (1890). *Principles of Psychology.* New York: Holt.

Jewsbury, P. A., Bowden, S. C., & Strauss, M. E. (2016). Integrating the switching, inhibition, and updating model of executive function with the Cattell-Horn-Carroll model. *Journal of Experimental Psychology: General, 145*(2), 220–245.

Kaplan, E., Goodglass, H., & Weintraub, S. (1983). *Boston Naming Test (BNT). Manual* (2nd ed.). Philadelphia: Lea and Fabiger.

Karzmark, P. (2009). The effect of cognitive, personality, and background factors on the WAIS-III arithmetic subtest. *Applied Neuropsychology, 16*(1), 49–53.

Kaufman, A. S. (1994). *Intelligent Testing with the WISC-III.* New York: John Wiley & Sons.

King, T. Z., Fennell, E. B., Bauer, R., Crosson, B., Dede, D., Riley, J. L., . . . & Roper, S. N. (2002). MMPI-2 profiles of patients with intractable epilepsy. *Archives of Clinical Neuropsychology, 17*(6), 583–593.

Kohn, S. E., & Goodglass, H. (1985). Picture-naming in aphasia. *Brain and Language, 24*(2), 266–283.

Larson, E. B., Kirschner, K., Bode, R., Heinemann, A., & Goodman, R. (2005). Construct and predictive validity of the Repeatable Battery for the Assessment of Neuropsychological Status in the evaluation of stroke patients. *Journal of Clinical and Experimental Neuropsychology, 27*(1), 16–32.

Lezak, M. D., Howieson, D. B., Bigler, E. D., & Tranel, D. (2012). *Neuropsychological Assessment*. New York: Oxford University Press.

Lichtenberger, E. O., Kaufman, A. S., & Lai, Z. C. (2001). *Essentials of WMS-III Assessment* (Vol. 31). New York: John Wiley & Sons.

Lichtenberger, E. O., & Kaufman, A. S. (2009). *Essentials of WAIS-IV Assessment* (Vol. 50). New York: John Wiley & Sons.

Lichtenberger, E. O., & Kaufman, A. S. (2013). *Essentials of WAIS-IV Assessment* (2nd ed.). New York: John Wiley and Sons.

Locascio, J. J., Corkin, S., & Growdon, J. H. (2003). Relation between clinical characteristics of Parkinson's disease and cognitive decline. *Journal of Clinical and Experimental Neuropsychology, 25*(1), 94–109.

Long, C. J., & Kibby, M. Y. (1995). Ecological validity of neuropsychological tests: A look at neuropsychology's past and the impact that ecological issues may have on its future. *Advances in Medical Psychotherapy, 8*, 59–78.

MacLeod, C. M. (1991). Half a century of research on the Stroop effect: An integrative review. *Psychological Bulletin, 109*(2), 163–203.

Matarazzo, J. D., 1990. Psychological testing versus psychological assessment. *American Psychologist, 45*, 999–1017.

Mayes, S. D., & Calhoun, S. L. (2007). Wechsler Intelligence Scale for Children third and fourth edition predictors of academic achievement in children with attention-deficit/hyperactivity disorder. *School Psychology Quarterly, 22*(2), 234–249.

McGrath, R. E. (2005). Conceptual complexity and construct validity. *Journal of Personality Assessment, 85*, 112–124.

McGrew, K. S. (2009). CHC theory and the human cognitive abilities project: Standing on the shoulders of giants of psychometric intelligence research. *Intelligence, 37*, 1–10.

McKay, C., Wertheimer, J. C., Fichtenberg, N. L., & Casey, J. E. (2008). The Repeatable Battery for the Assessment of Neuropsychological Status (RBANS): Clinical utility in a traumatic brain injury sample. *The Clinical Neuropsychologist, 22*(2), 228–241.

Megargee, E. I. (2006). *Using the MMPI-2 in Criminal Justice and Correctional Settings*. Minneapolis, MN: University of Minnesota Press.

Megargee, E. I. (2008). The California Psychological Inventory. In J. N. Butcher (Ed.), *Oxford Handbook of Personality Assessment* (pp. 323–335). New York: Oxford University Press.

Mitrushina, M. (Ed.). (2005). *Handbook of Normative Data for Neuropsychological Assessment*. New York: Oxford University Press.

Neisser, U., Boodoo, G., Bouchard Jr., T. J., Boykin, A. W., Brody, N., Ceci, S. J., . . . & Urbina, S. (1996). Intelligence: Knowns and unknowns. *American Psychologist, 51*(2), 77–101.

Nelson, J. M., Canivez, G. L., & Watkins, M. W. (2013). Structural and incremental validity of the Wechsler Adult Intelligence Scale–Fourth Edition with a clinical sample. *Psychological Assessment, 25*(2), 618–630.

Nichols, D. S., & Crowhurst, B. (2006). Use of the MMPI-2 in inpatient mental health settings. In *MMPI-2: A Practitioner's Guide* (pp. 195–252). Washington, DC: American Psychological Association.

Nybo, T., Sainio, M., & Muller, K. (2004). Stability of vocational outcome in adulthood after moderate to severe preschool brain injury. *Journal of the International Neuropsychological Society, 10*(5), 719–723.

Pedraza, O., Sachs, B. C., Ferman, T. J., Rush, B. K., & Lucas, J. A. (2011). Difficulty and discrimination parameters of Boston Naming Test items in a consecutive clinical series. *Archives of Clinical Neuropsychology, 26*(5), 434–444.

Perry, J. N., Miller, K. B., & Klump, K. (2006). Treatment planning with the MMPI-2. In J. Butcher (Ed.), *MMPI-2: A Practitioner's Guide* (pp. 143–64). Washington, DC: American Psychological Association.

Posner, M. I., & Snyder, C. R. R. (1975). Facilitation and inhibition in the processing of signals. *Attention and Performance V*, 669–682.

Quantz, J. O. (1897). Problems in the psychology of reading. *Psychological Monographs: General and Applied, 2*(1), 1–51.

Rabin, L. A., Barr, W. B., & Burton, L. A. (2005). Assessment practices of clinical neuropsychologists in the United States and Canada: A survey of INS, NAN, and APA Division 40 members. *Archives of Clinical Neuropsychology, 20*(1), 33–65.

Randolph, C. (2016). The Repeatable Battery for the Assessment of Neuropsychological Status Update (RBANS Update). Retrieved May, 2016, from http://www.pearsonclinical.com/psychology/products/100000726/repeatable-battery-for-the-assessment-of-neuropsychological-status-update-rbans-update.html#tab-details.

Randolph, C., Tierney, M. C., Mohr, E., & Chase, T. N. (1998). The Repeatable Battery for the Assessment of Neuropsychological Status (RBANS): Preliminary clinical validity. *Journal of Clinical and Experimental Neuropsychology, 20*(3), 310–319.

Rorschach, H. E. (1964). Nuclear relaxation in solids by diffusion to paramagnetic impurities. *Physica, 30*(1), 38–48.

Smith, G. T. (2005). On construct validity: Issues of method and measurement. *Psychological Assessment, 17*(4), 396–408.

Strauss, E., Sherman, E. M., & Spreen, O. (2006). *A Compendium of Neuropsychological Tests: Administration, Norms, and Commentary*. New York: Oxford University Press.

Strauss, M. E., & Smith, G. T. (2009). Construct validity: Advances in theory and methodology. *Annual Review of Clinical Psychology, 5*, 1–25.

Strenze, T. (2007). Intelligence and socioeconomic success: A meta-analytic review of longitudinal research. *Intelligence, 35*(5), 401–426.

Stroop, J. R. (1935). Studies of interference in serial verbal reactions. *Journal of Experimental Psychology, 18*(6), 643–662.

Sudarshan, S. J., Bowden, S. C., Saklofske, D. H., & Weiss, L. G. (2016). *Age-Related Invariance of Abilities Measured with the Wechsler Adult Intelligence Scale–IV.* Psychological Assessment, on line ahead of print: http://dx.doi.org/10.1037/pas0000290

Tierney, M. C., Black, S. E., Szalai, J. P., Snow, W. G., Fisher, R. H., Nadon, G., & Chui, H. C. (2001). Recognition memory and verbal fluency differentiate probable Alzheimer disease from subcortical ischemic vascular dementia. *Archives of Neurology, 58*(10), 1654–1659.

Tweedy, J. R., & Schulman, P. D. (1982). Toward a functional classification of naming impairments. *Brain and Language, 15*(2), 193–206.
Wechsler, D. (1997). *Wechsler Memory Scale. Third Edition (WMS).* San Antonio, TX: Pearson.
Wechsler, D. (2008). *Wechsler Adult Intelligence Scale–Fourth Edition (WAIS-IV).* San Antonio, TX: Pearson.
Wechsler, D. (2014). *Wechsler Intelligence Scale for Children–Fifth Edition (WAIS-V).* San Antonio, TX: Pearson.
Weed, N. C., Ben-Porath, Y. S., & Butcher, J. N. (1990). Failure of Wiener and Harmon Minnesota Multiphasic Personality Inventory (MMPI) subtle scales as personality descriptors and as validity indicators. *Psychological Assessment: A Journal of Consulting and Clinical Psychology, 2*(3), 281–285.
Weimer, W. B. (1979). *Notes on the Methodology of Scientific Research.* Hillsdale, NJ: John Wiley & Sons.
Whitman, S., Hermann, B. P., & Gordon, A. C. (1984). Psychopathology in epilepsy: How great is the risk? *Biological Psychiatry, 19*(2), 213–236.
Wilk, C. M., Gold, J. M., Humber, K., Dickerson, F., Fenton, W. S., & Buchanan, R. W. (2004). Brief cognitive assessment in schizophrenia: Normative data for the Repeatable Battery for the Assessment of Neuropsychological Status. *Schizophrenia Research, 70*(2), 175–186.
Wood, J. M., Nezworski, M. T., Lilienfeld, S. O., & Garb, H. N. (2003). *What's Wrong with the Rorschach? Science Confronts the Controversial Inkblot Test.* San Francisco, CA: Jossey-Bass.

3

Construct Validity Has a Critical Role in Evidence-Based Neuropsychological Assessment

PAUL A. JEWSBURY AND STEPHEN C. BOWDEN

Construct validity has a critical role in psychological methodology and in the development of psychological assessments (Cronbach & Meehl, 1955; M. E. Strauss & Smith, 2009). The concept of construct validity was introduced by Meehl and Challman and later elaborated on by others to provide a framework for theoretical development in psychology (American Psychological Association, 1954; Campbell & Fiske, 1959; Cronbach & Meehl, 1955; Loevinger, 1957). Construct validity was proposed as a response to concern for the theoretical progress of psychology and especially the role of theory in psychological science (American Psychological Association, 1954), and supported by an earlier promotion of hypothetical constructs as a legitimate part of a scientific psychology (MacCorquodale & Meehl, 1948). When applied to tests, construct validity has been defined as the scientific inquiry into test score meaning (Messick, 1995). However, to date, there is limited consensus on the construct validity of neuropsychological tests (Dodrill, 1997, 1999; Lezak, Howieson, & Loring, 2004). This chapter will briefly review the models and approaches of the neuropsychological, cognitive, and psychometric literatures, all of which are concerned to model cognitive function. Finally, an integrative approach will be outlined, and some of the relevant literature will be reviewed.

Neuropsychological assessment primarily involves the assessment of cognitive abilities (Lezak et al., 2004), although, in view of the high rates of comorbidity, most neuropsychologists are concerned with evaluating psychopathology and psychosocial function also (Crowe, 1998; see also Chapter 4, this volume). Many neuropsychological models have their historical roots in early localizationist theories (Andrewes, 2001). "Localizationism" is the view that the brain can be partitioned into regions and that each region independently performs a unique and specific function. More recent neuropsychological models have been heavily influenced by Luria's seminal theory of partitioning the brain into three functional units (Luria, 1966, 1973, 1980). Luria's three functional units are (1) the unit for regulating tone and waking and mental states, (2) the unit for receiving, analyzing, and storing information and (3) the unit for programming, regulation, and verification of activity. Luria described neurological substrates for the three functional units (Luria, 1973), and his theory has been used in the interpretation of functional imaging (e.g., Languis & Miller, 1992).

Luria developed his theory based on extensive clinical research of single-cases, such as patients with brain tumors and penetrating injuries (Peña-Casanova, 1989). Luria described his approach as "romantic science" (Luria, 1979), and his approach has been highly influential in defining contemporary neuropsychological assessment, to such an extent that Luria has been described as "the father of modern neuropsychology" (Akhutina, 2003). Luria's third functional unit is of special relevance because it is believed to be responsible for complex cognition and conscious decision-making, or "human intelligence" (Das, 1980). The concept of a system responsible for controlling other systems of the brain was further developed in Baddeley and Hitch's working-memory model (Baddeley & Hitch, 1974). Baddeley and Hitch referred to this system as the "central executive." The central executive controls and allocates resources to two "slave" systems—one specifically responsible for phonological working memory, and one specifically responsible for visuospatial working memory.

Baddeley (1986, 1990) generalized the central-executive concept beyond working memory by equating the central executive to the "supervisory attentional system" hypothesis developed by Norman and Shallice (1986). The supervisory attentional hypothesis proposes that we have routines of automatic behavior that are triggered by environmental stimuli or internal processes, and the supervisory attentional system inhibits and monitors these routines when necessary. The supervisory attentional system is only involved in behavior for some tasks, such as tasks involving planning or impulse inhibition, and complex or novel tasks (Shallice, 1982).

However, the concept of a central executive is scientifically unsatisfactory for several reasons. First, the central executive appears to require all the mental functioning of a human. As such, a model with the central executive "supervising" other mental functions does not simplify the description of cognitive function (Hazy, Frank, & O'Reilly, 2007). Second, the central-executive concept has not produced readily testable hypotheses (Allport, 1993). Third, neurological and functional imaging evidence is inconsistent with the concept of a unitary central executive (Duncan, Johnson, Swales, & Freer, 1997; Parkin, 1998). Not surprisingly, the concept of a central executive has been criticized as offering few helpful insights into how executive functions actually operate, where they are localized in the brain, or how they may be disrupted by brain injury. Inevitably, the central executive is described with little elaboration (Parkin, 1998) and as representing a gap in theory (Hazy et al., 2007).

Some executive theorists have elaborated on the central-executive concept by replacing the unitary central executive with a system of executive sub-processes or *executive functions*. While many different sets of executive functions can be conceived, the most empirically supported and the most popular is described in a confirmatory factor-analytical study by Miyake and colleagues (2000). Miyake and colleagues modeled the executive functions of *switching*, *inhibition*, and *updating*, chosen on the basis of previous research (e.g., Baddeley, 1986; Logan, 1985).

THE ROLE OF SINGLE-CASE STUDIES IN CONSTRUCT VALIDITY

Many executive-system theorists rely on less-formal evaluation of single-cases (e.g., Shallice, 1982). Caramazza (1986) provided a strong defense of single-patient studies, and argued that group studies are invalid for making inferences about the structure of cognition. This argument formalizes the view that group studies in neuropsychology are meaningless because they involve "averaging over" different individuals, who may, for example, have different disease statuses. Some cognitive theorists (e.g., Horn & McArdle, 1992) have discussed the problem of group study averages. For example, group study averages of performance on a cognitive test may be difficult to explain in terms of a cognitive processing theory if not all participants within the group applied the same cognitive strategy on the test. While recognizing this difficulty, these cognitive theorists do not believe it invalidates the approach of group studies to individual assessment.

Caramazza provided the most explicit defense of the view that all predictors of test performance need to be identified and that all variation in test performance is non-random and interpretable so that an exact, non-probabilistic conclusion, independent from any unobserved variable, can be made. This common view can be seen, for example, in some applications of subtest or scatter analysis, where differences between the subtest scores on an intelligence test or another neuropsychological battery are interpreted as indicative of cognitive status. Caramazza's (1986) premise leads to an untenable scientific methodology because his approach assumes that the conditions of brain disease or injury can be fully described with no measurement error. However, ipsative subtest variation, for example, is relatively unreliable (Watkins & Kush, 1994) and prone to high rates of classification errors (Reynolds & Milam, 2012). While the unreliable variance is theoretically determinate, clinical judgement in identifying the cause of the unreliable variance is inaccurate and often wrongly assumes the subtest-difference variance to be reliable (Dawes, Faust, & Meehl, 1989; Reynolds & Milam, 2012). In contrast to approaches aligned with Caramazza's argument, the psychometric approach views measurement of cognition as having random errors that are not indicative of cognitive ability, and that interpretation of any observed assessment needs to accommodate the effects of measurement error (Nunnally & Bernstein, 1994; Strauss & Smith, 2009).

DISSOCIATION METHODS IN CONSTRUCT VALIDITY

The critical tool for identifying the existence of separate mental functions or modules among many neuropsychological theorists is the concept of "double dissociation" (Teuber, 1955; Young, Hilgetag, & Scannell, 2000). In neuropsychology, dissociation is observed when a patient is impaired on one task but not impaired on another task. Double dissociation is observed when there is a dissociation in one patient, and another patient has the opposite pattern of dissociation on the same two tasks (Coltheart, 2001; Crawford, Garthwaite, & Gray, 2003; Ellis & Young, 1996). Double dissociations are seen as evidence that the two tasks measure two separate mental functions, processes, systems, or cognitive modules.

Throughout most of the history of double-dissociation methods, the operational criteria for identifying double dissociations have been vague (for review, see Bates, Appelbaum, Salcedo, Saygin, & Pizzamiglio, 2003; Crawford et al., 2003). The most common approach is to calculate z-scores of patients' performance on tasks in order to calculate the probability of obtaining a z-score of that magnitude or more extreme. If the probability value is below some critical level (e.g., .05) and the patient is poor at the task, the patient is concluded to be deficient in the ability measured by that task. There are many statistical issues that threaten the validity of inferences based on double-dissociation, such as non-normality, small sample sizes, and "double dipping" (Kriegeskorte, Simmons, Bellgowan, & Baker, 2009).

More fundamental is the logical soundness of the dissociation approach in general. Any two tasks by definition cannot involve exactly the same cognitive functioning if they are different tasks. Double-dissociation research, if taken to the extreme, could eventually hypothesize as many mental functions as there are different tasks, leading to endless construct proliferation (Dunn & Kirsner, 2003; van Orden, Pennington, & Stone, 2001).

Another logical concern relates to the common justification for seeking dissociations on the assumption that certain kinds of tests—for example, "psychometric intelligence" tests—are not sensitive to certain types of brain injury (e.g., Ardila, 1999; Lezak et al., 2004; Walsh, 1978). As reviewed above, the original evidence by authors such as Luria (1966) linking what are now termed "executive functions" to the frontal lobes was based on case-study methods that may have included cases with uncertain localization (Andrés, 2003). And patients with lesions confined to the frontal lobes have been found not to have consistent or severe problems, for example, with Luria's problem-solving tests (Canavan, Janota, & Schurr, 1985; Dodrill, 1997; Hécaen & Albert, 1978). In addition, theorists such as Shallice (1988) depended on patients with lesions that extended beyond the frontal lobes to study the function of the frontal lobes (e.g., Burgess & Shallice, 1996a, 1996b; Shallice, 1982).

With contemporary executive tests, studies have sometimes found minimal executive dysfunction when examining patients with strictly focal frontal damage well after surgery (Andrés & Van der Linden, 2001, 2002; Vilkki, Virtanen,

Surma-Aho, & Servo, 1996). Critical reviews of popular executive tests (e.g., Alvarez & Emory, 2006; Andrés, 2003; Mountain & Snow-William, 1993) concluded that, while these tests are usually sensitive to frontal lobe lesions, lesions in other regions can also cause deficits. Early developers of sorting tests, including the forerunners of the Wisconsin Card Sorting Test (WCST; Grant & Berg, 1948), noted the sensitivity of these tests to focal lesions in many brain locations (Goldstein & Scheerer, 1941).

Moreover, as will be shown below, contemporary definitions of executive function have evolved to include concepts overlapping in important ways with definitions derived from contemporary models of cognitive ability, as commonly assessed by intelligence tests. It will be argued later that the concept of executive function has evolved from clinical case-study research and other forms of neuropsychological research to identify many of the same critical cognitive functions that overlap with the critical cognitive functions identified by parallel research in educational, developmental, and broader clinical populations. It may be that there is an opportunity to integrate diverse approaches to cognitive function, an opportunity highlighted when the broad definition of the executive system is considered alongside the contemporary definitions of intelligence. Ironically, rather than disconfirming one or other line of cognitive ability research, the converging lines of evidence lend support to the construct validity evidence obtained from diverse research approaches. Take, for example, one of Lezak's (1995, p. 42) widely cited definitions of executive function "The executive functions consist of those capacities that enable a person to engage successfully in independent, purposive, self-serving behavior." This definition has clear similarities to Wechsler's (1944, p. 3) definition of intelligence "Intelligence is the aggregate or global capacity of the individual to act purposefully, to think rationally and to deal effectively with his (sic) environment." The similarities of the two definitions show that one of the most influential executive function exponents, and one of the most influential intelligence-test developers, sought to measure broadly similar constellations of constructs, and the target constructs may have co-evolved to a similar focus of theoretical and applied research.

A common argument in the neuropsychological literature is that intelligence tests are limited because they fail to assess important cognitive abilities, especially the executive system (e.g., Ardila, 1999). This argument is usually made on the basis of various case-studies of individual frontal lobe–lesioned patients who appear to have dysfunctional executive or other ability and yet normal intelligence scores (e.g., Ackerly & Benton, 1947; Brickner, 1936; Shallice & Burgess, 1991). There are several issues to consider before it is assumed that this line of argument provides definitive evidence for the discriminant validity of executive versus intelligence constructs.

First, the imperfect reliability of test scores in general, and extreme (low) scores, in particular, is often not considered, although the problem of regression to the mean is well recognized in cognitive neuropsychology. In single-case and dissociation studies, test scores and especially less-reliable component or subtest scores are rarely reported with confidence intervals centered on the appropriate score, the predicted true score (Nunnally & Bernstein, 1994). As a consequence, the interpretation of extreme deviation scores often neglects the fact that a patient's true score is expected to be closer to the normal range (see Chapter 5, this volume). Even when the confidence interval is reported, the issue of unreliability is still relevant. In a busy clinic, occurrences of the estimated score falling outside the confidence interval can accrue, on the basis of false-positive findings alone. Just reporting extreme cases is potentially uninformative (Chapman & Chapman, 1983; Strauss, 2001).

Second, case-study methods typically assume, implicitly, that clinical classification of impaired ability to be perfect. The probability of a false positive (FP: see Chapter 10, this volume) diagnosis of impairment on, say, a less reliable test, in the context of an accurate assessment of no impairment by a more reliable intelligence test, will be non-zero. That is, any less reliable test will produce some FPs, and the less reliable the test, the more frequent the FPs (Strauss, 2001). Such cases may accrue and produce a literature of false-positive diagnosed "impaired" single-cases with normal intelligence scores. That is, cases with clinically diagnosed impaired ability but normal intelligence may represent the failure of accurate clinical diagnosis, rather than insensitivity of intelligence tests. Hence, imperfect specificity of clinical diagnosis based on less reliable tests, and imperfect sensitivity of more reliable intelligence tests, are confounded in descriptive case-studies and dissociation studies (Chapman & Chapman, 1983; Strauss, 2001).

Both of these points provide independent reasons for why cases of apparently normal intelligence scores but abnormal clinical diagnoses of cognitive ability will be expected to occur in the absence of a real difference in the assessed abilities and may be published without regard to the underlying problem of FP findings. Therefore, the existence of cases of clinically diagnosed impaired ability with normal intelligence (or any other test) scores does not provide conclusive evidence against psychometric intelligence tests as clinically useful and valid assessment. Alternative techniques are required to resolve this dissociation conundrum more rigorously, including latent-variable analysis of the test scores of interest, as described below.

CONVERGING EVIDENCE ON THE METHODS OF EXECUTIVE FUNCTION AND INTELLIGENCE

The argument that executive tests are fundamentally different from psychometric tests mirrors an earlier distinction proposed by Halstead (1947). Halstead defined the concept of "biological intelligence" as distinct from "psychometric intelligence" due to perceived dissatisfaction with the clinical utility of psychometric intelligence tests such as the Wechsler-Bellevue Intelligence Scale (Wechsler, 1944). Consequently, Halstead and Reitan developed the Halstead-Reitan Neuropsychological Test Battery (Halstead, 1947; Reitan & Wolfson, 1985). However, even if the Halstead-Reitan Neuropsychological Test Battery measures cognitive ability factors not represented by psychometric intelligence tests such as the Wechsler scales, different methodology would not be required for the study of biological intelligence (Larrabee, 2000; Matarazzo, 1990). Rather, established methods of convergent and discriminant validity would provide much informative evidence, again including latent variable or factor analysis, as described in following sections.

The use of factor analysis to investigate convergent and discriminant validity allows for controlled group studies and an account of measurement error as well as *a priori* hypothesis testing of proposed models and plausible alternatives (Strauss & Smith, 2009). The use of factor analysis for executive function research could close the gap between psychometric research of cognitive abilities and neuropsychological research on executive system function. In fact, factor analysis is often used in executive function research, although with limited reference to the enormous body of previous research on cognitive abilities with factor analysis. For example, Miyake and colleagues' (2000) highly cited study of the executive system employs the methodology most commonly used in intelligence research—namely, confirmatory factor analysis—and their study was even conducted with a healthy community population similar to those commonly used in nonclinical psychometric research.

In summary, the single-case and dissociation approach to cognitive models often depends on methodology involving tenuous assumptions and is highly prone to errors of inference, such as confounding measurement error with true discriminant validity in the identification of double-dissociations (for reviews, see Strauss, 2001; van Orden et al., 2001). When stronger methodology is employed, neuropsychology model-building is compatible with the psychometric and intelligence approaches to modelling or cognitive abilities, and there appears to be some important and as yet incompletely explored convergence between current definitions of executive functions and contemporary models of intelligence as multiple-factor cognitive abilities. These questions will be explored in further detail toward the end of this chapter, after brief consideration of other historically important approaches to modelling cognition.

COGNITIVE APPROACHES TO CONSTRUCT VALIDATION

Embretson and Gorin (2001) argue that, in Cronbach and Meehl's (1955) approach to construct validation of psychological assessment, theory plays little role in the design of tests. Instead, theory and meaning are established after the test is developed, based on empirical properties such as correlations of the test with external variables. An alternate approach most prominently advocated by Embretson (1983, 1998, 2007) and Mislevy (2007) is the "construct representation" approach.

The construct representation approach uses the provisional cognitive theory of a construct to guide test-design and item-selection. Based on this theory, a model of the test scores is developed (Embretson, 1984). If the model accurately predicts the test scores, the test has construct validity through the theoretical or construct representation analysis "by design" (Mislevy, 2007).

An example of construct representation described by Embretson (1998) involves the theory of progressive matrices performance developed by Carpenter, Just, and Shell (1990) to successfully model scores on Raven's progressive matrices (Raven, Court, & Raven, 1992). Carpenter and colleagues' theory predicts that matrix problems with a greater number of stimulus relationships require greater working memory capacity. Therefore, modelling matrix problems with varying numbers of relationships can be used to estimate working memory capacity.

Invoking theory to define meaning is also central to mathematical-psychology approaches to modelling cognition, where cognitive task parameters acquire theoretical significance from the accuracy of the model used to predict task behavior (Barchelder, 1998; Townsend & Neufeld, 2010). In contrast to individual differences and clinical assessment research, models in mathematical psychology do not typically involve estimating scores for every individual. Instead, mathematical psychologists tend to focus on modelling the average person or producing idiosyncratic models for a small number of people that are assumed to generalize consistently across members of a population. If parameters for individuals were added into the models, but the same philosophical approach to validity was taken, then the mathematical models would satisfy the requirements of Embretson's (1983) construct representation approach and would be an integration of the mathematical (cognitive) psychology and psychometric approaches. Known as "cognitive psychometrics," researchers have discussed the role that such cognitive-theory–driven mathematical psychology may have in enhancing individual-differences research and assessment (Barchelder, 1998; Townsend & Neufeld, 2010).

Although the construct representation approach may be preferred in terms of empirical rigor and philosophy of science, it does have some limitations. First, it requires, in effect, a cognitive theory as *a priori* given (Bejar, 1993). Second, the construct representation approach requires complex test items that can be decomposed into discrete features that have differential relationships with cognitive constructs, so that these features can be systematically varied and modeled (Daniel & Embretson, 2010; Embretson & Gorin, 2001; Strauss & Smith, 2009). Third, the approach often requires more complex statistical models than the traditional psychometric approach, and these models typically requires stronger assumptions and larger sample sizes (von Davier & Carstensen, 2007). The recommended statistical analysis under the construct representation approach often involves extensions of item-response theory (IRT) and latent class analysis (LCA). While there have been a limited number of applications of IRT to cognitive assessment (Carlozzi, Tulsky, & Kisala, 2011; Mungas & Reed, 2000), in general, IRT and LCA may require relatively large samples due to weaker distributional assumptions. A fourth limitation of the construct representation approach involves its focus on theoretical coherence rather than optimizing psychometric and instrumentalist qualities, meaning that a focus on construct representation may produce tests with good theoretical standing but inferior criterion-related validity and diagnostic utility. However, with computerized adaptive testing

(CAT), construct representation approaches that lend themselves effectively to CAT may eventually become superior in reliability and criterion-related validity (Embretson, 1999).

Like factor analysis, IRT and LCA rests on the assumption of local independence, meaning that the response to any one item in a test is not dependent on responses to other items in the same test, except due to the underlying latent scale, factor, or class (von Davier & Carstensen, 2007). In fact, recent versions of confirmatory factor-analytical software generalize factor analysis to applications that include ordinal-categorical indicators or outcome variables and enable the factor-analysis parameters to be converted into IRT parameters and the generation of familiar IRT tools such as item characteristic curves (ICCs). As such, the distinction between IRT and familiar approaches to confirmatory factor analysis is being bridged (Bandalos, 2008; Millsap & Yun-Tien, 2004).

PSYCHOMETRIC METHODS AND CONSTRUCT VALIDITY

Psychometrics is one of the oldest traditions in research psychology and provides the scientific basis for the interpretation of test scores and assessment results more broadly. Rejection of psychometrics, a view sometimes heard amongst clinicians, involves repudiation of the scientific basis of psychological assessment (Schmidt & Hunter, 1996). Essentially, all factor-analytical work on intelligence stems from Spearman's g theory (Spearman, 1904). Spearman hypothesized that a single factor, g, could fully account for all inter-correlations between cognitive tests, with the standard assumptions of linearity and normality. In contrast to Spearman, Thurstone believed that there were many cognitive abilities, and he proposed the theory of primary mental abilities (Thurstone, 1938; 1947).

Raymond Cattell, a doctoral student of Spearman, expanded Spearman's g into the hierarchical model known as the "Gf-Gc theory." Cattell proposed that general intelligence could be split into "fluid" and "crystallized" intelligence (Cattell, 1941, 1943, 1963). Fluid intelligence, defined as reasoning ability to solve novel problems, was assumed to be largely biological and declined with age in adulthood. In contrast, crystallized intelligence, defined as knowledge-based ability, was assumed to be largely a consequence of education and acculturation, and more resistant to age.

John Horn, a doctoral student of Cattell's, expanded the Gf-Gc theory to include additional abilities such as short-term acquisition and retrieval, long-term storage and retrieval, visual processing, and speed of processing (e.g., Horn, 1965, 1988; Horn & Noll, 1997). These additional abilities were assumed to be as general as Cattell's Gf and Gc abilities.

John Carroll worked relatively independently from Cattell and Horn to produce a monumental survey of cognitive abilities, involving over 460 diverse data sets re-analyzed with exploratory factor analysis (Carroll, 1993). On the basis of these re-analyses, Carroll proposed a hierarchical theory of cognitive abilities. What has become known as the "Cattell-Horn-Carroll (CHC) model" of cognitive abilities will be discussed in more detail in later sections of this chapter.

ALTERNATIVE PSYCHOMETRIC MODELS

Three psychometric cognitive models are popular in contemporary assessment psychology. These are the *multiple-intelligences* theory, the *triarchic theory* of intelligence, and the *CHC model* of cognitive abilities. Although all three theories were influenced by the early psychometric research reviewed above, the CHC model is the natural continuation of the general-research approach that began with Spearman, and is the dominant cognitive-ability theory in psychometrics (McGrew, 2009). In contrast, the multiple-intelligences theory and the triarchic theory of intelligence diverge from pure psychometric methodology by placing more importance on cognitive theory and other forms of evidence. Consequently, constructs in the multiple-intelligences theory and the triarchic theory of intelligence are conceptually broader but also less well defined than the factorial constructs in the psychometric approach of the CHC model.

The multiple-intelligences theory states that intelligence is made up of multiple intelligences, of which there are "probably eight or nine" (Gardner, 2006, p. 503). It is hypothesized that each of these intelligences has an independent information-processing mechanism associated with an independent neural substrate that is specialized by type of information. Each intelligence also has a unique symbol system and separate perceptual and memory resources (Gardner, 1983, 1999, 2006). However, the validity of multiple-intelligences theory has been widely debated, some arguing that support for the theory is not convincing (Allix, 2000; Sternberg, 1994; Sternberg & Grigorenko, 2004; Waterhouse, 2006) and that the theory needs to generate falsifiable hypotheses to be scientifically fruitful (Visser, Ashton, & Vernon, 2006). Gardner has responded that "Multiple-intelligences theory does not lend itself easily to testing through paper-and-pencil assessments or a one-shot experiment" (Gardner & Moran, 2006, p. 230).

Focusing on the aspect of multiple-intelligences theory that is aligned with factor analysis, multiple-intelligences theory seems to be a mix of intelligence and personality factors. Carroll (1993) noted that there are similarities between the Cattell-Horn Gf-Gc model and multiple-intelligences, and suggested that multiple-intelligences may be useful to suggest new possible areas of intelligence (e.g., bodily-kinesthetic) that can be explored with factor analysis (Carroll, pp. 641–642). On the other hand, as a factor model, multiple-intelligences theory makes tenuous claims, in particular, that the intelligences are autonomous and correspond to uncorrelated factors (Messick, 1992).

The triarchic theory of intelligence was championed by Sternberg in several influential publications (e.g., Sternberg, 1985, 2005). The theory comprises three subtheories. The *componential subtheory* addresses the mental mechanisms that underlie intelligent human behavior. The componential subtheory is assumed to describe universal processes and does so in terms of higher-order executive processes (*metacomponents*), specialized lower-order processes that are coordinated by the metacomponents (*performance components*), and finally, learning components (*knowledge acquisition components*). The second subtheory is the *experiential subtheory*, which addresses the effect of experience on intelligence, particularly in terms of how repeated experience with a task can cause that task to change from being novel to being automatized. The third subtheory is the *contextual subtheory*, which proposes that intelligent behavior depends on the sociocultural context and focuses on the relationship between the function of the mental processes and the external world.

The three types of subtheories are thought to lead to three types of abilities. The componential, experiential, and contextual subtheories lead to *analytical*, *creative*, and *practical* abilities, respectively. The creative ability is sometimes split into *automatized* and *novel* (Sternberg, 1991). While Sternberg asserts that the triarchic theory of intelligence incorporates known factorial constructs (Sternberg, 2005), Messick (1992) points out that the tests in the Sternberg Triarchic Abilities Test (Sternberg, 1991) are the same kinds of tests studied outside the context of the triarchic theory of intelligence. Based on previous research on the types of tests in the Sternberg Triarchic Abilities Test (e.g., Guilford & Hoepfner, 1971; Horn, 1986), Messick (1992) argues that the Sternberg Triarchic Abilities Test measures cognitive abilities identified and accommodated in traditional psychometric factorial models of intelligence. Furthermore, Messick (1992) argues that the Sternberg Triarchic Abilities Test only measures a subset of the factors represented in psychometric models. It has also been suggested that the triarchic theory of intelligence is more complex than available evidence (Keating, 1980), and for this reason, Messick (1992, p. 379) describes several aspects of the theory as "nonfactual" or necessarily true (Kline, 1991).

Ultimately, the triarchic theory of intelligence is an ambitious and impressive attempt to integrate a wide range of psychometric and cognitive research under one umbrella, but it relies on metaphors that may not readily facilitate empirical research and does not represent a well-developed scientific theory (Keating, 1980; Messick, 1992; Rabbitt, 1988). Empirically, some key propositions of the triarchic theory of intelligence—for example, that g is not general intelligence but just one type of intelligence (analytical ability), that practical intelligence is distinct from g and as general as g, and that practical intelligence is at least as good an estimator of future success as g—are contradicted by a wide variety of data (Gottfredson, 2003a; see also Sternberg, 2003; and Gottfredson, 2003b).

CONTEMPORARY PSYCHOMETRIC APPROACHES TO CONSTRUCT VALIDATION

The psychometric approach to validity has a long history of progressive refinement and development. Prior to the focus on construct validity in assessment research, the primary method to evaluate the validity or clinical usefulness of a test was criterion-related validation (Kane, 2001). "Criterion-related validity" refers to the effectiveness of a test in predicting a criterion such as a clinical disorder (American Psychological Association, 1966, see also Chapters 2 and 10 of this volume).

The criterion-related validation approach led to the criterion-keying method (Strauss & Smith, 2009), wherein test items were selected based on their predictive validity. An example of a test developed using criterion-keying is the Minnesota Multiphasic Personality Inventory (MMPI; Hathaway & McKinley, 1967). The MMPI was a major advance in personality assessment (Goldberg, 1971; McReynolds, 1975), although the atheoretical development of the MMPI has led some to argue that it became outdated as psychometric thought matured (e.g., Helmes & Reddon, 1993) and has motivated the theoretical refinement of the MMPI in the latest version, namely, the Restructured Form (MMPI-2-RF; see Chapter 4, this volume).

While criterion-related validity has clear importance in the practical application of a test, on its own, it has limited use for facilitating theoretical interpretation of test scores. At best, criterion-related validity provides an indirect contribution to theoretical development (Strauss & Smith, 2009).

"Construct homogeneity" refers to the approach wherein constructs must be unidimensional (Strauss & Smith, 2009). While the definition of unidimensionality depends on the statistical method used, most discussions of unidimensionality appear to implicitly assume a factor-analytical definition of unidimensionality (Nunnally & Bernstein, 1994). That is, a construct is "unidimensional" if it corresponds to a single factor. A "multidimensional construct" is a construct where multiple factors are treated together as a single concept (Law, Wong, & Mobley, 1998).

Of course, the most widely used method for testing unidimensionality, and establishing construct validity in terms of convergent and discriminant validity, is factorial validity (Thompson & Daniel, 1996). "Factorial validity" refers to the use of factor analysis in the evaluation of construct validity, where factors are taken as representations of unidimensional constructs.

Carefully conducted factor analysis is viewed by many psychometricians and researchers as central to the validation of measurement constructs (e.g., Miyake et al., 2000; Nunnally, 1978; Strauss & Smith, 2009). Factor analysis is central to psychological measurement because most, if not all, individual-difference constructs of interest in psychology are hypothesized to be measurable by a number of tests. For example, some constructs of interest in neuropsychology are organizational ability, concentration, and memory capacity (Lezak et al., 2004; Strauss, Sherman, & Spreen, 2006). For a hypothetical construct to be supported, test scores believed to measure the construct should load on the hypothesized factor-construct, and test scores believed not to measure the construct should not load on the same factor-construct. In this way, factor analysis is a primary and powerful tool for evaluating convergent and discriminant validity (Cronbach & Meehl, 1955; Strauss & Smith, 2009).

Unfortunately, in clinical research, factor analysis is often applied in an uncritical way, using software defaults, and without careful consideration of the analytical power and pitfalls of the methods. For example, exploratory factor analysis has long been known as too error prone to produce replicable results across samples or studies without great care in the approach taken (Floyd & Widaman,

1995; Henson & Roberts, 2006; Preacher & MacCallum, 2003; Widaman, 1993). Nevertheless, exploratory factor analysis in general, and principal components analysis in particular, continue to be widely reported in the clinical research literature, giving rise to a proliferation of imprecise and unreplicated models. However, when used in a careful way, factor analysis readily deals with the issues of selecting a parsimonious number of unidimensional constructs. First, factor analysis separates dimensions specific to items (unique variances) from dimensions shared across items (factors), where the factors are expected to be theoretically fruitful and empirically useful. Second, most researchers do not attempt to achieve perfectly fitting factor models (e.g., by not rejecting models with significant chi-square statistics indicating perfect fit), but rather accept models that fit well according to approximate fit indices (Hu & Bentler, 1999; Kline, 2011). Factor analysis guided by approximate fit indices allows for dimensions that are major sources of individual differences to be separated from dimensions specific to each measure as well as dimensions associated with trivial individual-difference variation (Brown, 2006; Kline, 2011).

In summary, the traditional psychometric approach has moved away from defining validity purely in terms of criterion-related validity and towards a greater focus on construct validity. Factor-analytic methodology evolved with early theories of intelligence (Spearman, 1904; Thurstone, 1938, 1947) and remains central to construct validity in personality and assessment psychology (Brown, 2006; Marsh et al., 2010; Strauss & Smith, 2009).

THE CATTELL-HORN-CARROLL MODEL OF COGNITIVE ABILITIES

The CHC model is based on psychometric intelligence and cognitive ability research conducted over much of the last century and pioneered by researchers such as Raymond Cattell, John Horn, Louis Leon Thurstone, and Robert Thorndike (McGrew, 2005). Major impetus for the CHC model was derived from the monumental research project of Carroll (1993) involving over 460 exploratory factor analyses. Due to the similarity of Carroll's model to a model that had developing support in the psychometric literature as a whole (namely, the Cattell-Horn Gf-Gc model), the two models were integrated to become the Cattell-Horn-Carroll model (Daniel, 1997, 2000; McGrew, 1997; Snow, 1998; Sternberg & Kaufman, 1998).

Carroll's (1993) work and the CHC model have been the recipients of much acclaim in the psychometric literature (Burns, 1994; Horn, 1998; Jensen, 2004; McGrew, 2009). For example, the CHC model has been described as a "culmination of over 100 years of psychometric research in human intelligence" (Reynolds, Keith, Flanagan, & Alfonso, 2013). It is the most empirically supported taxonomy of cognitive abilities (Ackerman & Lohman, 2006; Kaufman, 2009; McGrew, 2005; Newton & McGrew, 2010) and has influenced the development of most contemporary intelligence tests (Bowden, 2013; Kaufman, 2009; 2013; Keith & Reynolds, 2010).

The CHC model is a hierarchical model comprising three levels. Stratum III (general) consists solely of a weaker form of Spearman's g. Stratum II (broad) comprises eight to ten abilities comparable to Thurstone's primary mental abilities and Horn's mental abilities. Broad constructs describe familiar aspects of cognition usually derived from factor analysis of cognitive ability batteries (e.g., acquired knowledge, fluid reasoning, short-term memory). The fifth edition of the *Diagnostic and Statistical Manual of Mental Disorders* (DSM-5; American Psychiatric Association, 2013) classification of "cognitive domains" maps closely to the CHC broad (Stratum II) constructs, with the major exception of the conflation of several CHC constructs under the DSM category of Executive Function. CHC broad abilities also correspond closely to many pragmatic classifications of neuropsychological tests (e.g., Zakzanis, Leach, & Kaplan, 1999).

Definitions of the most commonly reported broad CHC abilities are included in Table 3.1 (McGrew, 2009). For example, the fourth edition of the Wechsler Intelligence Scales for adults and children have been described in terms of four or five of the CHC broad abilities defined in Table 3.1 (Weiss, Keith, Zhu, & Chen, 2013a, 2013b), namely, Acquired Knowledge (Gc), Fluid Intelligence (Gf), Visual Processing (Gv), Short-term or Working Memory (Gsm), and Processing Speed (Gs). With the addition of the Wechsler Memory Scale, a Wechsler battery includes further assessment of Gsm and, critically, the addition of long-term memory ability (Glr; for a recent discussion on the interpretation of Glr, see Jewsbury & Bowden, 2016).

Each broad construct has a number of subsidiary Stratum I (narrow) constructs. The narrow constructs are based on the work of Carroll (1993) and are quite specific to the cognitive task (e.g., the ability to recall lists in any order, the ability to rapidly state the name of objects, or the ability to solve a maze). Identifying the narrow construct associated with a test indicates what broad factor the test should be classified under. The narrow abilities allow the CHC model to be defined in great detail and the classification of tests to be undertaken more objectively, but the narrow factors are usually not required to be specified in confirmatory factor analyses of common clinical or educational assessment batteries to achieve good model fit (Keith & Reynolds, 2010). One of the reasons that it is not necessary to define narrow abilities relates to the statistical definition of factors. In general, any well-identified factor should have at least three indicators. But with multiple narrow abilities under each broad factor, the number of tests to statistically identify even a few narrow abilities would require many tests per broad factor, more than could be feasibly administered in any reasonable clinical or educational assessment protocol.

As a consequence, most assessment batteries will typically contain only one or two tests per narrow ability, making it impractical to statistically identify the narrow abilities. Occasional exceptions are observed when multiple versions of a test are administered within one assessment battery, multiple scores are derived from one test as part of a larger battery, or a test is repeated as in the immediate and delayed subtests of the Wechsler Memory Scale (WMS). In the latter case, it is common to observe test-format-specific variance in the

Table 3.1 Description of Selected Cattell-Horn-Carroll Broad Constructs

Construct	Description
Gf	The use of deliberate and controlled mental operations to solve novel problems that cannot be performed automatically. Mental operations often include drawing inferences, concept formation, classification, generating and testing hypotheses, identifying relations, comprehending implications, problem solving, extrapolating, and transforming information. Inductive and deductive reasoning are generally considered the hallmark indicators of Gf. Gf has been linked to cognitive complexity, which can be defined as a greater use of a wide and diverse array of elementary cognitive processes during performance.
Gc	The knowledge of the culture that is incorporated by individuals through a process of acculturation. Gc is typically described as a person's breadth and depth of acquired knowledge of the language, information, and concepts of a specific culture, and/or the application of this knowledge. Gc is primarily a store of verbal or language-based declarative (knowing what) and procedural (knowing how) knowledge acquired through the investment of other abilities during formal and informal educational and general life experiences.
Gsm	The ability to apprehend and maintain awareness of a limited number of elements of information in the immediate situation (events that occurred in the last minute or so). A limited-capacity system that loses information quickly through the decay of memory traces, unless an individual activates other cognitive resources to maintain the information in immediate awareness.
Gv	The ability to generate, store, retrieve, and transform visual images and sensations. Gv abilities are typically measured by tasks (figural or geometric stimuli) that require the perception and transformation of visual shapes, forms, or images and/or tasks that require maintaining spatial orientation with regard to objects that may change or move through space.
Ga	Abilities that depend on sound as input and on the functioning of our hearing apparatus. A key characteristic is the extent to which an individual can cognitively control (i.e., handle the competition between signal and noise) the perception of auditory information. The Ga domain circumscribes a wide range of abilities involved in the interpretation and organization of sounds, such as discriminating patterns in sounds and musical structure (often under background noise and/or distorting conditions) and the ability to analyze, manipulate, comprehend, and synthesize sound elements, groups of sounds, or sound patterns.
Glr*	The ability to store and consolidate new information in long-term memory and later fluently retrieve the stored information (e.g., concepts, ideas, items, names) through association. Memory consolidation and retrieval can be measured in terms of information stored for minutes, hours, weeks, or longer. Some Glr narrow abilities have been prominent in creativity research (e.g., production, ideational fluency, or associative fluency).

(Continued)

Table 3.1 Continued

Construct	Description
Gs	The ability to automatically and fluently perform relatively easy or over-learned elementary cognitive tasks, especially when high mental efficiency (i.e., attention and focused concentration) is required.
Gq	The breadth and depth of a person's acquired store of declarative and procedural quantitative or numerical knowledge. Gq is largely acquired through the investment of other abilities, primarily during formal educational experiences. Gq represents an individual's store of acquired mathematical knowledge, not reasoning with this knowledge.

Adapted from "CHC theory and the human cognitive abilities project: Standing on the shoulders of the giants of psychometric intelligence research" by K. S. McGrew (2009). Table used with permission of the author.
*Recent research suggests that encoding and retrieval memory abilities may be better seen as distinct factors rather than combined as Glr (see Jewsbury & Bowden, 2016; Schneider & McGrew, 2012).

factor analysis of the WMS, for example, between immediate and delayed recall of Logical Memory. But because there are only two indicators (scores) for the "Logical Memory" narrow factor (CHC narrow factor MM under Glr; Schneider & McGrew, 2012), limited information is available to identify a separate factor for Glr-MM, and instead Logical Memory is included in the same factor or broad ability with Verbal Paired Associates (CHC narrow ability MA under Glr). Instead of a separate factor, a correlated uniqueness is included in the model to account for the test-specific or narrow-ability variance with greater parsimony (e.g., Bowden, Cook, Bardenhagen, Shores, & Carstairs, 2004; Bowden, Gregg, et al., 2008; Tulsky & Price, 2003). Notably, both Logical Memory and Verbal Paired Associates may share other narrow abilities, including Free Recall (CHC M6; Schneider & McGrew, 2012), as well as auditory-verbal stimulus content. In sum, because of the practical limitations on modelling narrow abilities, most studies of omnibus or comprehensive batteries will model only the broad abilities, with several tests per broad ability, and will not attempt to model the narrow abilities. Comprehensive description of the CHC model, including definitions of all the narrow factors, are given elsewhere (e.g., McGrew, 2009; Schneider & McGrew, 2012).

Similarly, the general intelligence (Stratum III) factor is often included in confirmatory factor analyses of cognitive ability batteries (e.g., Salthouse, 2005; Weiss et al., 2013a, 2013b). However, requirements for satisfactory statistical definition of a general factor dictate that, unless the top level (general) factor is modeled with more than three subordinate (broad) factors, then the hierarchical model will be either unidentified or statistically equivalent to the factor model that includes only the broad factors, provided the interfactor correlation parameters are freely estimated. The statistical reasons for this challenge in testing hierarchical factor models are beyond the scope of the current chapter but have been discussed in detail elsewhere (Bowden, 2013; Brown, 2006; Kline, 2011; Rindskopf & Rose, 1988).

CURRENT STATUS OF THE CHC MODEL

Earlier research on cognitive factor models focused on analyzing test batteries alone and comparing the results from different studies for conceptual consistency (e.g., Carroll, 1993; Thurstone, 1947). Indeed, the CHC model has been found to be consistent with all major intelligence and some neuropsychological test batteries (Gladsjo, McAdams, Palmer, Moore, Jeste, & Heaton, 2004; Jewsbury et al., 2016a; Keith & Reynolds, 2010; Loring & Larrabee, 2006, 2008; Tuokko, Chou, Bowden, Simard, Ska, & Crossley, 2009). More recent research shows the CHC model satisfies even stricter tests, by analyzing data sets that comprised multiple test batteries to show that the conceptually similar factors from different test batteries are empirically identical (Jewsbury et al., 2016a; Keith & Reynolds, 2010).

Two CHC-related cross-battery studies are especially comprehensive. Woodcock (1990) showed that the Cattell-Horn Gf-Gc model, and by extension the CHC model, were consistent with data sets comprising the Wechsler Intelligence Scale–III with the Kaufman Assessment Battery for Children, the Stanford-Binet IV, the Wechsler Intelligence Scale–III, or the Wechsler Adult Intelligence Scale–Revised. Reynolds and colleagues (2013) used a full information maximum-likelihood approach to missing data to examine the Kaufman Assessment Battery for Children–II (KABC-II) with the Wechsler Intelligence Scale for Children–III, Wechsler Intelligence Scale for Children–IV, Woodcock-Johnson–III and Peabody Individual Achievement Test–revised in a single analysis, where all participants took at least the KABC-II. The results show remarkable consistency of the constructs underlying major test batteries, and the accuracy of the CHC model to correctly specify the factor structure.

MEASUREMENT INVARIANCE—TESTING OF THE PRECISE GENERALITY OF CONSTRUCTS ACROSS POPULATIONS

A formal, statistical test of the generality of theoretical constructs involves the question of whether tests measure the same constructs when administered to different populations. This aspect of generalization is described statistically as *measurement invariance* (American Educational Research Association, American Psychological Association, & National Council on Measurement in Education, 2014; Meredith, 1993; Widaman & Reise, 1997). Measurement invariance applies when the relationship between a set of observed test scores and the underlying latent constructs or factors is identical across populations. In this context, different populations may be, for example, community controls versus people with a particular psychiatric or neurological diagnosis or different populations distinguished by different diagnoses or different populations distinguished by ethnicity or language. Establishing measurement invariance is necessary for assuring the generality of measured constructs across populations.

But establishing measurement invariance has implications beyond establishing the universality of measured constructs, because demonstrating that measurement invariance applies across different populations also means that the broader construct validity framework that comes with the test will also generalize across the respective populations. So establishing measurement invariance permits unambiguous interpretation of convergent and discriminant validity and interpretation of group mean differences (Horn & McArdle, 1992; Meredith & Teresi, 2006; Widaman & Reise, 1997; see also Chapter 2 of this volume). These are the very kinds of validity relationships that underlie the observation of deficit and disability as well as differences in correlations (dissociations) between constructs that have been the focus of interest in clinical neuropsychology for many years. In other words, the observation of measurement invariance confers important and powerful information regarding the generality of constructs, but also the generality of the validity interpretation of the test scores corresponding to those constructs, across different populations. These methodological assumptions underpin most clinical neuropsychological research, although the assumptions of measurement invariance have been evaluated only infrequently, until recently. One reason why measurement invariance has not been extensively investigated, to date, in clinical research is that accessible methods for testing invariance have only become available over the last 15–20 years but are still not well known among applied researchers (Horn & McArdle, 1992; Meredith & Teresi, 2006; Widaman & Reise, 1997).

The methods of measurement have been used, for example, to show that the latent-factor model underlying successive generations of the Wechsler Adult Intelligence Scale is similar in representative community controls and heterogeneous neuroscience and neuropsychiatric samples, including seizure disorders, alcohol-use disorders, psychosis, and heterogeneous adult and child clinical populations (see Jewsbury, Bowden, & Duff, 2016a). Other examples of measurement invariance testing of CHC-consistent factor models have further supported the generality of the CHC model across a range of populations (Jewsbury et al., 2016a).

HOW WELL DOES CHC THEORY DESCRIBE NEUROPSYCHOLOGICAL TESTS?

In an unpublished doctoral thesis, Hoelzle (2008) conducted an analysis of 77 data sets of neuropsychological tests with exploratory principal components analysis and interpreted the components in terms of CHC theory. Although the analysis was impressively extensive in terms of the number of data sets, Hoelzle used exploratory component analysis where confirmatory factor analysis would have provided stronger tests of the latent-variable hypotheses (Widaman, 1993). As well, Hoelzle (2008) included many poorer-quality data sets, which confounded method and test-unique variance into the components, making interpretation of some component analyses difficult. Despite these limitations, Hoelzle obtained overwhelming evidence in support of the compatibility of the CHC theory with neuropsychological assessment practices. Despite Hoelzle's impressive analysis, two important questions remain. The first is whether the CHC model or some other psychometric model is comprehensive and can account for all important cognitive abilities, especially those that are assessed by neuropsychological batteries. The second related question is whether the CHC model needs to be augmented by additional constructs to accommodate executive functions.

More recently, Jewsbury and colleagues reanalyzed published data sets of diverse neuropsychological batteries (Jewsbury, Bowden, & Duff, 2016a; Jewsbury, Bowden, & Strauss, 2016b). The analyses were restricted to 31 data sets that were chosen on *a priori* grounds to provide stronger tests of the comprehensiveness of the CHC theory to account for the underlying latent variables. The analyses included only four data sets in common with Hoelzle's (2008) analysis. Key selection criteria included data sets with multiple test scores to provide more statistically robust tests of each hypothesized construct, test scores that represented commonly used neuropsychological tests, and larger sample sizes.

In every re-analysis, a model of the test scores based on *a priori* CHC definitions (McGrew, 2009; Schneider & McGrew, 2012) provided good-to-excellent fit to the test scores, in each respective data set, without the need for post hoc model re-specification. The CHC-derived model of scores fitted as well as or better than the study authors' own published factor models, whenever the respective authors reported factor models, even though the authors' own models were often derived from post hoc modification to improve fit. Of course, in some studies, the authors' reported models were very similar to a CHC model, although not always recognized or reported as such. In other words, theoretically derived, *a priori* definitions of narrow and broad abilities provided a highly successful, principled description of test scores in multiple, heterogeneous neuropsychological data sets. In no confirmatory factor analysis reanalysis did the modification indices suggest that the CHC model wrongly assigned tests to broad factors (Jewsbury et al., 2016a,b).

A proposed taxonomy of some popular neuropsychological tests, resulting from these theoretically guided re-analyses (Hoelzle, 2008; Jewsbury et al., 2016a,b) in terms of CHC constructs, has been reported by Jewsbury and colleagues (Jewsbury et al., 2016a). This taxonomy provides a provisional set of hypotheses regarding the latent-construct classification of neuropsychological tests, which should guide further taxonomy research and theoretical refinement. Multiple lines of construct validity evidence provide support for the CHC classification as a universal taxonomy of cognitive abilities relevant to diagnostic and educational assessment. Taken together these studies reveal the generality of the CHC model as a theoretical framework for diverse ability batteries and provide direct evidence of the strict statistical equivalence of the CHC constructs measured with diverse test batteries, across diverse populations Finally, the successful *a priori* classification of a very diverse set of neuropsychological tests, a classification requiring no important modification from that based on the principled interpretation of CHC narrow and broad factors is testament to the utility of the CHC model (Hoelzle, 2008; Jewsbury et al., 2016a,b; Keith & Reynolds, 2010; Schneider & McGrew, 2012).

The conclusion from these studies, that conventional psychometric and clinical neuropsychological tests measure the same cognitive constructs is consistent with previous research. Larrabee (2000) reviewed the exploratory factor analyses in outpatient samples of Leonberger, Nicks, Larrabee, and Goldfader (1992) and Larrabee and Curtiss (1992) that showed a common factor structure underlying Wechsler Adult Intelligence Scale–Revised, the Halstead-Reitan Neuropsychological Battery, and various other neuropsychological tests. Larabee (2000) noted that the results were consistent with Carroll's (1993) model of cognitive abilities. The finding that psychometric and clinical tests measure the same constructs has important implications for rationale test-selection in clinical practice, much as the Big-5 model of personality guides the selection of personality and psychopathology tests (see Chapter 4, this volume). Apart from theoretical choices in terms of construct coverage, clinicians should compare tests relevant to the assessment of any particular construct on the basis of how reliable they are (Chapman & Chapman, 1983), and tests with optimal construct measurement and reliability should be first-rank choices in clinical assessment. For executive function, it was found that the factorial representation of putative executive function measures is complex, but little modification to the CHC model was required for the CHC model to account for these measures (Jewsbury et al., 2016a,b). Specifically, the CHC model could both explain datasets used to derive the highly influential model of executive functions of switching, inhibition, and updating (Jewsbury et al., 2016b), as well as accounting for the most common clinical measures of executive function (Jewsbury et al., 2016a) without introduction of additional executive function constructs.

The semantic overlap between various definitions of executive function and CHC constructs, as well as the available empirical evidence, suggest that executive function tests are distributed across a number of CHC constructs, rather than overlapping with a single CHC construct (Jewsbury et al., 2016a,b). This observation has two important implications. First, the available factor-analytic data suggest that there is no unitary executive construct underlying all executive function tests, consistent with arguments by Parkin (1998) based on neurobiological evidence. Second, executive function should not be treated as a separate domain of cognition on the same level as, but separate from, well-defined CHC constructs such as fluid reasoning, working memory, and processing speed. Third, averaging across various executive function tests treated as a single domain of cognition as in the DSM-5 classification (American Psychiatric Association, 2013) leads to conceptually confused and clinically imprecise results. Therefore, it is recommended that executive function not be used as a single domain of cognition in meta-analyses and elsewhere, but recognized as an overlapping set of critical cognitive skills that have been defined in parallel and now can be integrated with the CHC model (Jewsbury et al., 2016a,b). Fourth, the results suggest that equating executive function and Gf (e.g., Blair,

2006; Decker, Hill, & Dean, 2007) does not tell the whole story, as not all executive function tests are Gf tests. While simply equating Gf with executive function would be helpful to integrate the two research traditions of psychometrics and neuropsychology amiably (e.g., Floyd, Bergeron, Hamilton, & Parra, 2010), it may also lead to confusion due to elements of executive function that do not conform to Gf (Jewsbury et al., 2016a,b).

CONCLUSIONS

Carefully developed and replicated factor models have great value in simplifying and standardizing clinical research that is undertaken on the assumption that tests measure general cognitive constructs. As noted above, the notion that every test measures a different, unique clinical phenomenon is still encountered in some clinical thinking but is contradicted by a century of psychometric research on the latent structure of cognitive ability tests (e.g., Carroll, 1993; Nunnally & Bernstein, 1994; Schneider & McGrew, 2012; Vernon, 1950). Ignoring the implications of psychometric construct-validity research risks an unconstrained proliferation of constructs for clinical assessment (Dunn & Kirsner, 1988; 2003; Van Orden et al., 2001), an approach that is incompatible with evidence-based neuropsychological practice. Evidence-based practice requires an accumulation of high-quality criterion-related validity evidence derived from the use of scientifically defensible measures of relevant constructs of cognitive ability. The best way currently available to provide scientifically defensible measures of cognitive ability constructs involves the kinds of converging evidence from multiple lines of research reviewed above, at the center of which is psychometric latent-structure evidence.

Finally, factor models provide a coherent structure to group tests in meta-analyses and clinical case-studies. Typically in neuropsychological meta-analyses, tests are grouped in informal domains, and the properties of tests within each domain are averaged (e.g., Belanger, Curtiss, Demery, Lebowitz, & Vanderploeg, 2005; Irani, Kalkstein, Moberg, & Moberg, 2011; Rohling et al., 2011; Zakzanis et al., 1999). However, unless these domains are supported by theoretically guided factor-analysis (Dodrill, 1997, 1999), averaging across the tests within a domain produces confused results. In fact, many previous classifications of tests conform more or less closely to a CHC classification, sometimes because authors have been mindful of the CHC taxonomy, but most often by force of the cumulative factor-analytic research in neuropsychology that has converged on a similar taxonomy (e.g., American Psychiatric Association, 2013; Rohling et al., 2011; Zakzanis et al., 1999), so the CHC taxonomy should not be seen as radical or unfamiliar, rather as a refinement of long-standing research insights in clinical neuropsychology.

The CHC theory is not a completed theory, but it continues to evolve (Jewsbury & Bowden, 2016; McGrew, 2009). However, accumulating evidence suggests that CHC theory provides an accurate and detailed classification of a wide variety of neuropsychological tests. Perhaps better than any other model of cognitive abilities, CHC theory provides a rationale and comprehensive basis for refining evidence-based neuropsychological assessment.

REFERENCES

Ackerly, S. S., & Benton, A. L. (1947). Report of a case of bilateral frontal lobe defect. *Research Publications: Association for Research in Nervous and Mental Disease, 27*, 479–504.

Ackerman, P. L., & Lohman, D. F. (2006). Individual differences in cognitive function. In P. A. Alexander & P. H. Winne (Eds.), *Handbook of Educational Psychology* (2nd ed., pp. 139–161). Mahwah, NJ: Erlbaum.

Akhutina, T. V. (2003). L. S. Vygotsky and A. R. Luria: Foundations of neuropsychology. *Journal of Russian and East European Psychology, 41*, 159–190.

Allix, N. M. (2000). The theory of multiple intelligences: A case of missing cognitive matter. *Australian Journal of Education, 44*, 272–288.

Allport, A. (1993). Attention and control: Have we been asking the wrong questions? A critical review of twenty-five years. In D. E. Meyer & S. Kornblum (Eds.), *Attention and Performance* (Vol. 14, pp. 183–218). Cambridge, MA: Bradford.

Alvarez, J. A., & Emory, E. (2006). Executive function and the frontal lobes: A meta-analytic review. *Neuropsychology Review, 16*, 17–42.

American Educational Research Association, American Psychological Association, & National Council on Measurement in Education, (2014). *Standards for Educational and Psychological Testing.* Washington, DC: American Educational Research Association.

American Psychiatric Association. (2013). *Diagnostic and Statistical Manual of Mental Disorders, Fifth Edition*. Arlington, VA: APA.

American Psychological Association. (1954). Technical recommendations for psychological tests and diagnostic techniques. *Psychological Bulletin Supplement, 51*, 1–38.

American Psychological Association. (1966). *Standards for Educational and Psychological Tests and Manuals*. Washington, DC: APA.

Andrés, P. (2003). Frontal cortex as the central executive of working memory: Time to revise our view. *Cortex, 39*, 871–895.

Andrés, P., & Van der Linden, M. (2001). Supervisory Attentional System in patients with focal frontal lesions. *Journal of Clinical and Experimental Neuropsychology, 23*, 225–239.

Andrés, P., & Van der Linden, M. (2002). Are central executive functions working in patients with focal frontal lesions? *Neuropsychologia, 40*, 835–845.

Andrewes, D. (2001). *Neuropsychology: From Theory to Practice*. Hove, UK: Psychology Press.

Ardila, A. (1999). A neuropsychological approach to intelligence. *Neuropsychology Review, 9*, 117–136.

Baddeley, A. D. (1986). *Working Memory*. Oxford: Oxford University Press.

Baddeley, A. D. (1990). *Human Memory: Theory and Practice*. Hove, UK: Erlbaum.

Baddeley, A. D., & Hitch, G. J. (1974). Working memory. In G. A. Bower (Ed.), *Psychology of Learning and Motivation* (Vol. 8, pp. 47–90). New York: Academic Press.

Bandalos, D. (2008). Is parceling really necessary? A comparison of results from item parceling and categorical variable methodology. *Structural Equation Modeling, 15*, 211–240.

Barchelder, W. H. (1998). Multinomial processing tree models and psychological assessment. *Psychological Assessment, 10,* 331–344.

Bates, E., Appelbaum, M., Salcedo, J., Saygin, A. P., & Pizzamiglio, L. (2003). Quantifying dissociations in neuropsychological research. *Journal of Clinical and Experimental Neuropsychology, 25,* 1128–1153.

Bejar, I. I. (1993). A generative approach to psychological and educational measurement. In N. Frederiksen, R. J. Mislevy, & I. I. Bejar (Eds.), *Test Theory for a New Generation of Tests* (pp. 323–359). Hillsdale, NJ: Erlbaum.

Belanger, H. G., Curtiss, G., Demery, J. A., Lebowitz, B. K., & Vanderploeg, R. D. (2005). Factors moderating neuropsychological outcomes following mild traumatic brain injury: A meta-analysis. *Journal of International Neuropsychological Society, 11,* 215–227.

Blair, C. (2006). How similar are fluid cognition and general intelligence? A developmental neuroscience perspective on fluid cognition as an aspect of human cognitive ability. *Behavioral and Brain Sciences, 29,* 109–160.

Bowden, S. C. (2013). Theoretical convergence in assessment and cognition. *Journal of Psychoeducational Assessment, 31,* 148–156.

Bowden, S. C., Cook, M. J., Bardenhagen, F. J., Shores, E. A., & Carstairs, J. R. (2004). Measurement invariance of core cognitive abilities in heterogeneous neurological and community samples. *Intelligence, 32,* 363–389.

Bowden, S. C., Gregg, N., Bandalos, D., Davis, M., Coleman, C., Holdnack, J. A., & Weiss, L. G. (2008). Latent mean and covariance differences with measurement equivalence in college students with developmental difficulties versus the Wechsler Adult Intelligence Scale–III/Wechsler Memory Scale–III normative sample. *Educational and Psychological Measurement, 68,* 621–642.

Bowden, S. C., Ritter, A. J., Carstairs, J. R., Shores, E. A., Pead, S., Greeley, J. D., & Clifford, C. C. (2001). Factorial invariance for combined Wechsler Adult Intelligence Scale-Revised and Wechsler Memory Scale-Revised Scores in a sample of clients with alcohol dependency. *The Clinical Neuropsychologist, 15,* 69–80.

Brickner, R. M. (1936). *The Intellectual Functions of the Frontal Lobes: A Study Based upon Observation of a Man After Partial Bilateral Frontal Lobectomy.* New York: Macmillan.

Brown, T. A. (2006). *Confirmatory Factor Analysis for Applied Research: Methodology in the Social Sciences.* New York: The Guilford Press.

Burgess, P. W., & Shallice, T. (1996a). Bizarre responses, rule detection and frontal lobe lesions. *Cortex, 32,* 241–259.

Burgess, P. W., & Shallice, T. (1996b). Response suppression, initiation and strategy use following frontal lobe lesions. *Neuropsychologia, 34,* 263–273.

Burns, R. B. (1994). Surveying the cognitive terrain. *Educational Researcher, 23,* 35–37.

Campbell, D. T., & Fiske, D. W. (1959). Convergent and discriminant validation by the multitrait-multimethod matrix. *Psychological Bulletin, 56,* 81–105.

Canavan, A., Janota, I., & Schurr, P. H. (1985). Luria's frontal lobe syndrome: Psychological and anatomical considerations. *Journal of Neurology, Neurosurgery, and Psychiatry, 48,* 1049–1053.

Carlozzi, N. E., Tulsky, D. S., & Kisala, P. A. (2011). Traumatic brain injury patient-reported outcome measure: Identification of health-related quality-of-life issues relevant to individuals with traumatic brain injury. *Archives of Physical Medicine and Rehabilitation, 92*(10 Suppl), S52–S60.

Caramazza, A. (1986). On drawing inferences about the structure of normal cognitive systems from the analysis of patterns of impaired performance: The case for single-patient studies. *Brain and Cognition, 5*, 41–66.

Carpenter, P. A., Just, M. A., & Shell, P. (1990). What one intelligence test measures: A theoretical account of processing in the Raven's Progressive Matrices Test. *Psychological Review, 97*, 404–431.

Carroll, J. B. (1993). *Human Cognitive Abilities: A Survey of Factor-Analytic Studies.* New York: Cambridge University Press.

Cattell, R. B. (1941). Some theoretical issues in adult intelligence testing. *Psychological Bulletin, 38*, 592.

Cattell, R. B. (1943). The measurement of adult intelligence. *Psychological Bulletin, 3*, 153–193.

Cattell, R. B. (1963). Theory of fluid and crystallized intelligence: A critical experiment. *Journal of Educational Psychology, 54*, 1–22.

Chapman, J. P., & Chapman, L. J. (1983). Reliability and the discrimination of normal and pathological groups. *Journal of Nervous and Mental Disease, 171*, 658–661.

Coltheart, M. (2001). Cognitive neuropsychology and the study of reading. In M. I. Posner & O. S. M. Marin (Eds.), *Attention and Performance XI* (pp. 3–21). Hillsdale, NJ: Erlbaum.

Crowe, S. F. (1998). Neuropsychological Effects of the Psychiatric Disorders. Amsterdam, Harwood Academic Publishers. ISBN 90-5702-377-6.

Crawford, J. R., Garthwaite, P. H., & Gray, C. D. (2003). Wanted: Fully operational definitions of dissociations in single-case studies. *Cortex, 29*, 357–370.

Cronbach, L. J., & Meehl, P. E. (1955). Construct validity in psychological test. *Psychological Bulletin, 52*, 281–302.

Daniel, M. H. (1997). Intelligence testing: Status and trends. *American Psychologist, 52*, 1038.

Daniel, M. H. (2000). Interpretation of intelligence test scores. In R. Sternberg (Ed.), *Handbook of Intelligence* (pp. 477–491). New York: Cambridge University Press.

Daniel, R. C., & Embretson, S. E. (2010). Designing cognitive complexity in mathematical problem-solving items. *Applied Psychological Measurement, 34*, 348–364.

Das, J. P. (1980). Planning: Theoretical considerations and empirical evidence. *Psychological Research, 41*, 141–151.

Dawes, R. M., Faust, D., & Meehl, P. E. (1989). Clinical versus actuarial judgment. *Science, 243*, 1668–1674.

Decker, S. L., Hill, S. K., & Dean, R. S. (2007). Evidence of construct similarity in executive functions and fluid reasoning abilities. *International Journal of Neuroscience, 117*, 735–748.

Dodrill, C. B. (1997). Myths of neuropsychology. *The Clinical Neuropsychologist, 11*, 1–17.

Dodrill, C. B. (1999). Myths of neuropsychology: Further considerations. *The Clinical Neuropsychologist, 13*, 562–572.

Duncan, J., Johnson, R., Swales, M., & Freer, C. (1997). Frontal lobe deficits after head injury: Unity and diversity of function. *Cognitive Neuropsychology, 144*, 713–741.

Dunn, J. C., & Kirsner, K. (1988). Discovering functionally independent mental processes: The principle of reversed association. *Psychological Review, 95*, 91–101.

Dunn, J. C., & Kirsner, K. (2003). What can we infer from double dissociations? *Cortex, 39*, 1–7.

Ellis, A. W., & Young, A. (Eds.). (1996). *Human Cognitive Neuropsychology*. Hove, UK: Erlbaum.

Embretson, S. (1983). Construct validity: Construct representation versus nomothetic span. *Psychological Bulletin, 93*, 179–197.

Embretson, S. (1984). A general latent trait model for response processes. *Psychometrika, 49*, 175–186.

Embretson, S. E. (1998). A cognitive design system approach to generating valid tests: Application to abstract reasoning. *Psychological Method, 3*, 380–396.

Embretson, S. E. (1999). Generating items during testing: Psychometric issues and models. *Psychometrika, 64*, 407–433.

Embretson, S. E. (2007). Construct validity: A universal validity system or just another test evaluation procedure? *Educational Researcher, 36*, 449–455.

Embretson, S., & Gorin, J. (2001). Improving construct validity with cognitive psychology principles. *Journal of Educational Measurement, 38*, 343–368.

Floyd, F. J., & Widaman, K. F. (1995). Factor analysis in the development and refinement of clinical assessment instruments. *Psychological Assessment, 7*, 286–299.

Floyd, R. G., Bergeron, R., Hamilton, G., & Parra, G. R. (2010). How do executive functions fit with the Cattell-Horn-Carroll model? Some evidence from a joint factor analysis of the Delis-Kaplan executive function system and the Woodcock-Johnson III tests of cognitive abilities. *Psychology in the Schools, 47*, 721–738.

Gardner, H. (1983). *Frames of Mind: The Theory of Multiple Intelligences*. New York: Basic Books.

Gardner, H. (1999). *Intelligence Reframed: Multiple Intelligences for the 21st Century*. New York: Basic Books.

Gardner, H. (2006). On failing to grasp the core of MI theory: A response to Visser et al. *Intelligence, 34*, 503–505.

Gardner, H., & Moran, S. (2006). The science of Multiple Intelligences Theory: A response to Lynn Waterhouse. *Educational Psychologist, 41*, 227–232.

Gladsjo, J. A., McAdams, L. A., Palmer, B. W., Moore, D. J., Jeste, D. V., & Heaton, R. K. (2004). A six-factor model of cognition in schizophrenia and related psychotic disorders: Relationships with clinical symptoms and functional capacity. *Schizophrenia Bulletin, 30*, 739–754.

Goldberg, L. R. (1971). A historical survey of personality scales and inventories. In P. McReynolds (Ed.), *Advances in Psychological Assessment*. (Vol. 2, pp. 293–336). Palo Alto, CA: Science and Behavior Books.

Goldstein, K., & Scheerer, M. (1941). Abstract and concrete behavior: An experimental study with special tests. *Psychological Monographs, 53*, i–151.

Gottfredson, L. S. (2003a). Dissecting practical intelligence theory: Its claims and evidence. *Intelligence, 31*, 343–397.

Gottfredson, L. S. (2003b). On Sternberg's "Reply to Gottfredson." *Intelligence, 31*, 415–424.

Grant, D. A., & Berg, E. A. (1948). A behavioral analysis of degree of reinforcement and ease of shifting to a new response in a Weigl-type card-sorting problem. *Journal of Experimental Psychology, 38*, 404–411.

Guilford, J. P., & Hoepfner, R. (1971). *The Analysis of Intelligence*. New York: McGraw-Hill.

Halstead, W. C. (1947). *Brain and Intelligence*. Chicago: University of Chicago Press.

Hathaway, S. R., & McKinley, J. C. (1967). *Minnesota Multiphasic Personality Inventory Manual* (rev. ed.). New York: Psychological Corporation.

Hazy, T. E., Frank, M. J., & O'Reilly, R. (2007). Towards an executive without a homunculus: Computational models of the prefrontal cortex/basal ganglia system. *Philosophical Transactions of the Royal Society B, 362*, 1601–1613.

Hécaen, H., & Albert, M. L. (1978). *Human Neuropsychology*. New York: Wiley.

Helmes, E., & Reddon, J. R. (1993). A perspective on developments in assessing psychopathology: A critical review of the MMPI and MMPI-2. *Psychological Bulletin, 113*, 453–471.

Henson, R. K., & Roberts, J. K. (2006). Use of exploratory factor analysis in published research. Common errors and some comment on improved practice. *Educational and Psychological Measurement, 6*, 393–416.

Hoelzle, J. B. (2008). Neuropsychological Assessment and the Cattell-Horn-Carroll (CHC) Cognitive Abilities Model. Unpublished doctoral dissertation, University of Toledo, Toledo, OH.

Horn, J. L. (1965). Fluid and Crystallized Intelligence: A Factor Analytic and Developmental Study of the Structure Among Primary Mental Abilities. Unpublished doctoral dissertation, University of Illinois, Urbana, IL.

Horn, J. L. (1986). Intellectual ability concepts. In R. J. Sternberg (Ed.), *Advances in the Psychology of Human Intelligence* (Vol. 3, pp. 35–77). Mahwah, NJ: Erlbaum.

Horn, J. L. (1988). Thinking about human abilities. In J. R. Nesselroade (Ed.), *Handbook of Multivariate Psychology* (pp. 645–685). New York: Academic Press.

Horn, J. L. (1998). A basis for research on age differences in cognitive abilities. In J. J. McArdle & R. W. Woodcock (Eds.), *Human Cognitive Abilities in Theory and Practice* (pp. 57–92). Mahwah, NJ: Lawrence Erlbaum.

Horn, J. L., & McArdle, J. J. (1992). A practical and theoretical guide to measurement invariance in aging research. *Experimental Aging Research: An International Journal Devoted to the Scientific Study of the Aging Process, 18*, 117–144.

Horn, J. L., & Noll, J. (1997). Human cognitive capabilities: Gf-Gc theory. In D. P. Flanagan, J. L. Gensaft, & P. L. Harrison (Eds.), *Contemporary Intellectual Assessment: Theories, Tests, and Issues* (pp. 53–91). New York: Guilford.

Hu, L.-T., & Bentler, P. M. (1999). Cutoff criteria for fit indexes in covariance structure analysis: Conventional criteria versus new alternatives. *Structural Equation Modeling, 6*, 1–55.

Irani, F., Kalkstein, S., Moberg, E. A., & Moberg, P. J. (2011). Neuropsychological performance in older patients with schizophrenia: A meta-analysis of cross-sectional and longitudinal studies. *Schizophrenia Bulletin, 37*, 1318–1326.

Jensen, A. R. (2004). Obituary—John Bissell Carroll. *Intelligence, 32*, 1–5.

Jewsbury, P. A., & Bowden, S. C. (2016). Construct validity of Fluency, and implications for the latent structure of the Cattell-Horn-Carroll model of cognition. *Journal of Psychoeducational Assessment*, in press. http://jpa.sagepub.com/content/early/2016/05/11/0734282916648041.abstract

Jewsbury, P. A., Bowden, S. C., & Duff, K. (2016a). The Cattell–Horn–Carroll model of cognition for clinical assessment. *Journal of Psychoeducational Assessment*, in press. http://jpa.sagepub.com/content/early/2016/05/31/0734282916651360.abstract

Jewsbury, P. A., Bowden, S. C., & Strauss, M. E. (2016b). Integrating the switching, inhibition, and updating model of executive function with the Cattell-Horn-Carroll model. *Journal of Experimental Psychology: General, 145*(2), 220–245.

Kane, M. T. (2001). Current concerns in validity theory. *Journal of Educational Measurement, 38*, 319–342.

Kaufman, A. S. (2009). *IQ Testing 101*. New York: Springer.

Kaufman, A. S. (2013). Intelligent testing with Wechsler's Fourth Editions: Perspectives on the Weiss et al. studies and the eight commentaries. *Journal of Psychoeducational Assessment, 31*, 224–234.

Keating, D. P. (1980). Sternberg's sketchy theory: Defining details desired. *Behavioral and Brain Sciences, 3*, 595–596.

Keith, T. Z., & Reynolds, M. R. (2010). Cattell-Horn-Carroll abilities and cognitive tests: What we've learnt from 20 years of research. *Psychology in the Schools, 47*, 635–650.

Kline, P. (1991). Sternberg's components: Non-contingent concepts. *Personality and Individual Differences, 12*, 873–876.

Kline, R. B. (2011). *Principles and Practice of Structural Equation Modeling* (3rd ed.). New York: The Guilford Press.

Kriegeskorte, N., Simmons, W. K., Bellgowan, P. S. F., & Baker, C. I. (2009). Circular analysis in systems neuroscience—the dangers of double dipping. *Nature Neuroscience, 12*, 535–540.

Languis, M. L., & Miller, D. C. (1992). Luria's theory of brain functioning: A model for research in cognitive psychophysiology. *Educational Psychologist, 27*, 493–511.

Larrabee, G. J. (2000). Association between IQ and neuropsychological test performance: Commentary on Tremont, Hoffman, Scott, and Adams (1998). *The Clinical Neuropsychologist, 14*, 139–145.

Larrabee, G. J., & Curtiss, G. (1992). Factor structure of an ability-focused neuropsychological battery (abstract). *Journal of Clinical and Experimental Neuropsychology, 14*, 65.

Law, K. S., Wong, C. S., & Mobley, W. M. (1998). Toward a taxonomy of multidimensional constructs. *Academy of Management Review, 23*, 741–755.

Leonberger, F. T., Nicks, S. D., Larrabee, G. J., & Goldfader, P. R. (1992). Factor structure of the Wechsler Memory Scale–Revised within a comprehensive neuropsychological battery. *Neuropsychology, 6*, 239–249.

Lezak, M. (1995). *Neuropsychological Assessment* (3rd ed.). New York: Oxford University Press.

Lezak, M. D., Howieson, D. B., & Loring, D. W. (2004). *Neuropsychological Assessment* (4th ed.). New York: Oxford.

Loevinger, J. (1957). Objective tests as instruments of psychological theory. *Psychological Reports, 3*, 635–694.

Logan, G. D. (1985). Executive control of thought and action. *Acta Psychologica, 60*, 193–210.

Loring, D. W., & Larrabee, G. J. (2006). Sensitivity of the Halstead and Wechsler test batteries to brain damage: Evidence from Reitan's original validation sample. *The Clinical Neuropsychologist, 20*(2), 221–229. doi:10.1080/13854040590947443

Loring, D. W., & Larrabee, G. J. (2008). "Psychometric intelligence" is not equivalent to "crystallized intelligence," nor is it insensitive to presence of brain damage: A reply to Russell. *The Clinical Neuropsychologist, 22*(3), 524–528. doi:10.1080/13854040701425445

Luria, A. R. (1966). *Higher Cortical Functions in Man*. New York: Basic Books.

Luria, A. R. (1973). *The Working Brain*. Harmondsworth, UK: Penguin.

Luria, A. R. (1979). *The Making of Mind* (M. Cole & S. Cole, Trans.). Cambridge, MA: Harvard University Press.

Luria, A. R. (1980). Neuropsychology in the local diagnosis of brain damage. *International Journal of Clinical Neuropsychology, 2*, 1–7.

MacCorquodale, K., & Meehl, P. E. (1948). On a distinction between hypothetical constructs and intervening variables. *Psychological Review, 55*, 95–107.

Marsh, H. W., Lüdtke, O., Muthén, B., Asparouhov, T., Morin, A. J., Trautwein, U., & Nagengast, B. (2010). A new look at the Big Five factor structure through exploratory structural equation modeling. *Psychological Assessment, 22*, 471–491.

Matarazzo, J. D. (1990). Psychological testing versus psychological assessment. *American Psychologist, 45*, 999–1017.

McGrew, K. S. (1997). Analysis of the major intelligence batteries according to a proposed comprehensive Gf–Gc framework. In D. P. Flanagan, J. L. Genshaft, & P. L. Harrison (Eds.), *Contemporary Intellectual Assessment: Theories, Tests, and Issues* (pp. 151–179). New York: Guilford.

McGrew, K. S. (2005). The Cattell-Horn-Carroll theory of cognitive abilities. In D. P. Flanagan & P. L. Harrison (Eds.), *Contemporary Intellectual Assessment: Theories, Tests, and Issues* (2nd ed., pp. 136–181). New York: Guilford Press.

McGrew, K. S. (2009). CHC theory and the human cognitive abilities project: Standing on the shoulders of giants of psychometric intelligence research. *Intelligence, 37*, 1–10.

McReynolds, P. (1975). Historical antecedents of personality assessment. In P. McReynolds (Ed.), *Advances in Psychological Assessment* (Vol. 3, pp. 477–532). San Francisco: Jossey-Bass.

Meredith, W. (1993). Measurement invariance, factor analysis and factorial invariance. *Psychometrika, 58*, 525–543.

Meredith, W., & Teresi, J. A. (2006). An essay on measurement and factorial invariance. *Medical Care, 44*, S69–S77.

Messick, S. (1992). Multiple intelligences or multilevel intelligence? Selective emphasis on distinctive properties of hierarchy: On Gardner's Frames of Mind and Sternberg's Beyond IQ in the context of theory and research on the structure of human abilities. *Psychological Inquiry, 3*, 365–384.

Messick, S. (1995). Validity of psychological assessment: Validation of inferences from persons' responses and performances as scientific inquiry into score meaning. *American Psychologist, 50*, 741–749.

Millsap, R. E., & Yun-Tein, J. (2004). Assessing factorial invariance in ordered-categorical measures. *Multivariate Behavioral Research, 39*, 479–515.

Mislevy, R. J. (2007). Validity by design. *Educational Researcher, 36*, 463–469.

Miyake, A., Friedman, N. P., Emerson, M. J., Witzki, A. H., Howerter, A., & Wager, T. D. (2000). The unity and diversity of executive functions and their contributions to complex "frontal lobe" tasks: A latent variable analysis. *Cognitive Psychology, 41*, 49–100.

Mountain, M. A., & Snow-William, G. (1993). WCST as a measure of frontal pathology. A review. *Clinical Neuropsychologist, 7*, 108–118.

Mungas, D., & Reed, B. R. (2000). Application of item response theory for development of a global functioning measure of dementia with linear measurement properties. *Statistics in Medicine, 19*, 1631–1644.

Norman, D. A., & Shallice, T. (1986). Attention to action: Willed and automatic control of behavior. In R. J. Davidson, G. E. Schwartz, & D. Shapiro (Eds.), *Consciousness and Self-Regulation: Advances in Research and Theory* (Vol. 4, pp. 1–18). New York: Plenum Press.

Nunnally, J. C. (1978). *Psychometric Theory* (2nd ed.). New York: McGraw-Hill.

Nunnally, J. C., & Bernstein, I. H. (1994). *Psychometric Theory* (3rd ed.). New York: McGraw-Hill.

Parkin, A. J. (1998). The central executive does not exist. *Journal of the International Neuropsychological Society, 4*, 518–522.

Peña-Casanova, J. (1989). A. R. Luria today: Some notes on "Lurianism" and the fundamental bibliography of A. R. Luria. *Journal of Neurolinguistics, 4*, 161–178.

Preacher, K. J., & MacCallum, R. C. (2003). Repairing Tom Swift's electric factor analysis machine. *Understanding Statistics, 2*, 13–43.

Rabbitt, P. (1988). Human intelligence. *The Quarterly Journal of Experimental Psychology Section A, 40*, 167–185.

Raven, J. C., Court, J. H, & Raven, J. (1992). *Manual for Raven's Progressive Matrices and Vocabulary Scale*. San Antonio, TX: Psychological Corporation.

Reitan, R. M., & Wolfson, D. (1985). *The Halstead-Reitan Neuropsychological Test Battery: Theory and Clinical Interpretation*. Tucson, AZ: Neuropsychology Press.

Reynolds, C. R., & Milam, D. A. (2012). Challenging intellectual testing results. In D. Faust (Ed.), *Coping with Psychiatric and Psychological Testimony* (6th ed., pp. 311–334). Oxford, UK: Oxford University Press.

Reynolds, M. R., Keith, T. Z., Flanagan, D. P., & Alfonso, V. C. (2013). A cross-battery, reference variable, confirmatory factor analytic investigation of the CHC taxonomy. *Journal of School Psychology, 51*, 535–555.

Rindskopf, D., & Rose, T. (1988). Some theory and applications for confirmatory second-order factor analysis. *Multivariate Behavioural Research, 23*, 51–67.

Rohling, M. L., Binder, L. M., Demakis, G. J, Larrabee, G. J., Ploetz, D. M., & Langhinrichsen-Rohling, J. (2011). A meta-analysis of neuropsychological outcome after mild traumatic brain injury: Re-analyses and reconsiderations of Binder et al. (1997), Frencham et al. (2005), and Pertab et al. (2009). *The Clinical Neuropsychologist, 25*, 608–623.

Salthouse, T. A. (2005). Relations between cognitive abilities and measures of executive functioning. *Neuropsychology, 4*, 532–545.

Schmidt, F. L., & Hunter, J. E. (1996). Measurement error in psychological research: Lessons from 26 research scenarios. *Psychological Methods, 1*, 199–223.

Schneider, R. J., Hough, L. M., & Dunnette, M. D. (1996). Broadsided by broad traits: How to sink science in five dimensions or less. *Journal of Organizational Behavior, 17*, 639–655.

Schneider, W. J., & McGrew, K. (2012). The Cattell-Horn-Carroll model of intelligence. In D. Flanagan & P. Harrison (Eds.), *Contemporary Intellectual Assessment: Theories, Tests, and Issues* (3rd ed., pp. 99–144). New York: Guilford.

Shallice, T. (1982). Specific impairments of planning. *Philosophical Transactions of the Royal Society of London. Series B, Biological Sciences, 298*, 199–209.

Shallice, T. (1988). *From Neuropsychology to Mental Structure*. New York: Cambridge University Press.

Shallice, T., & Burgess, P. W. (1991). Deficits in strategy application following frontal lobe damage in man. *Brain, 114*, 727–741.

Snow, R. E. (1998). Abilities as aptitudes and achievements in learning situations. In J. J. McArdle & R. W. Woodcock (Eds.), *Human Cognitive Abilities in Theory and Practice* (pp. 93–112). Mahwah, NJ: Erlbaum.

Spearman, C. (1904). "General intelligence," objectively determined and measured. *The American Journal of Psychology, 15*, 201–292.

Sternberg, R. J. (1985). *Beyond IQ: A Triarchic Theory of Human Intelligence.* New York: Cambridge University Press.

Sternberg, R. J. (1994). Commentary: Reforming school reform: Comments on Multiple Intelligences: The theory in practice. *Teachers College Record, 95*, 561–569.

Sternberg, R. J. (2003). Our research program validating the triarchic theory of successful intelligence: Reply to Gottfredson. *Intelligence, 31*, 399–413.

Sternberg, R. J. (2005). The triarchic theory of successful intelligence. In D. P. Flanagan & P. L. Harrison (Eds.), *Contemporary Intellectual Assessment: Theories, Tests, and Issues* (pp. 103–119). New York: Guilford Press.

Sternberg, R. J., Castejón, J. L., Prieto, M. D., Hautamäki, J., & Grigorenko, E. L. (2001). Confirmatory factor analysis of the Sternberg Triarchic Abilities Test in three international samples. *European Journal of Psychological Assessment, 1*, 1–16.

Sternberg, R. J., & Grigorenko, E. L. (2004). Successful intelligence in the classroom. *Theory into Practice, 43*, 274–280.

Sternberg, R. J., & Kaufman, J. C. (1998). Human abilities. *Annual Review of Psychology, 49*, 479–502.

Strauss, E., Sherman, E. M., & Spreen, O. (2006). *A Compendium of Neuropsychological Tests: Administration, Norms, and Commentary* (3rd ed.). New York: Oxford University Press.

Strauss, M. E. (2001). Demonstrating specific cognitive deficits: A psychometric perspective. *Journal of Abnormal Psychology, 110*, 6–14.

Strauss, M. E., & Smith, G. T. (2009). Construct validity. Advances in theory and methodology. *Annual Review of Clinical Psychology, 5*, 1–25.

Teuber, H. L. (1955). Physiological psychology. *Annual Review of Psychology, 6*, 267–296.

Thompson, B., & Daniel, L. G. (1996). Factor analytic evidence for the construct validity of scores: A historical overview and some guidelines. *Educational and Psychological Measurement, 56*, 197–208.

Thurstone, L. L. (1938). *Primary Mental Abilities.* Chicago: University of Chicago Press.

Thurstone, L. L. (1947). *Multiple-Factor Analysis.* Chicago: University of Chicago Press.

Townsend, J. T., & Neufeld, R. W. J. (2010). Introduction to special issue on contributions of mathematical psychology to clinical science and assessment. *Journal of Mathematical Psychology, 54*, 1–4.

Tulsky, D. S., & Price, L. R. (2003). The joint WAIS-III and WMS-III factor structure: Development and cross-validation of a six-factor model of cognitive functioning. *Psychological Assessment, 15*, 149–162.

Tuokko, H. A., Chou, P. H. B., Bowden, S. C., Simard, M., Ska, B., & Crossley, M. (2009). Partial measurement equivalence of French and English versions of the Canadian Study of Health and Aging neuropsychological battery. *Journal of the International Neuropsychological Society, 15*, 416–425.

Van Orden, G. C., Pennington, B. F., & Stone, G. O. (2001). What do double dissociations prove? *Cognitive Science, 25*, 111–172.

Vernon, P. (1950). *The Structure of Human Intellect.* London, UK: Methuen.

Vilkki, J., Virtanen, S., Surma-Aho, O., & Servo, A. (1996). Dual task performance after focal cerebral lesions and closed head injuries. *Neuropsychologia, 34*, 1051–1056.

Visser, B. A., Ashton, M. C., & Vernon, P. A. (2006). G and the measurement of Multiple Intelligences: A response to Gardner. *Intelligence, 34*, 507–510.

von Davier, M., & Carstensen, C. H. (2007). *Multivariate and Mixture Distribution Rasch Models: Extensions and Applications.* New York: Springer.

Walsh, K. W. (1978). *Neuropsychology: A Clinical Approach.* Oxford, UK: Churchill Livingstone.

Waterhouse, L. (2006). Multiple intelligences, the Mozart effect, and emotional intelligence: A critical review. *Educational Psychologist, 41*, 207–225.

Watkins, M. W., & Kush, J. C. (1994). Wechsler subtest analysis: The right way, the wrong way, or no way? *School Psychological Review, 4*, 640–651.

Wechsler, D. (1944). *The Measurement of Adult Intelligence* (3rd ed.). Baltimore: Williams & Wilkins.

Weiss, L. G., Keith, T. Z., Zhu, J., & Chen, H. (2013a). WAIS-IV and clinical validation of the four- and five-factor interpretative approaches. *Journal of Psychoeducational Assessment, 31*, 94–113.

Weiss, L. G., Keith, T. Z., Zhu, J., & Chen, H. (2013b). WISC-IV and clinical validation of the four- and five-factor interpretative approaches. *Journal of Psychoeducational Assessment, 31*, 114–131.

Widaman, K. F. (1993). Common factor analysis versus principal component analysis: Differential bias in representing model parameters? *Multivariate Behavioral Research, 28*, 263–311.

Widaman, K. F., & Reise. S. P. (1997). Exploring the measurement invariance of psychological instruments: Applications in the substance use domain. In K. Bryant & M. Windle (Eds.), *The Science of Prevention: Methodological Advance from Alcohol and Substance Abuse Research* (pp. 281–324). Washington, DC: American Psychological Association.

Woodcock, R. W. (1990). Theoretical foundations of the WJ-R measures of cognitive ability. *Journal of Psychoeducational Assessment, 8*, 231–258.

Young, M. P., Hilgetag, C. C., & Scannell, J. W. (2000). On imputing function to structure from the behavioural effects of brain lesions. *Philosophical Transactions of the Royal Society of London B: Biological Sciences, 355*, 147–161.

Zakzanis, K. K., Leach, L., & Kaplan, E. (1999). *Neuropsychological Differential Diagnosis*. Lisse, Netherlands: Swets & Zeitlinger.

4

Contemporary Psychopathology Assessment: Mapping Major Personality Inventories onto Empirical Models of Psychopathology

TAYLA T. C. LEE, MARTIN SELLBOM,
AND CHRISTOPHER J. HOPWOOD

Having a method of correctly classifying a psychological construct of interest is a cornerstone of effective clinical practice and research. However, existing classification systems for mental disorders, such as those represented in the *Diagnostic and Statistical Manual of Mental Disorders* (DSM) and the *International Classification of Diseases* (ICD), have limitations that prevent clinicians and scientists from achieving correct classification, hampering assessment, intervention, and etiological research efforts. These limitations are primarily related to the polythetic nature of mental disorders represented in current diagnostic systems. Specifically, polythetic definitions result in heterogeneous symptom presentations amongst individuals who purportedly have the same discrete mental disorder, as well as excessive amounts of comorbidity between mental disorders (Brown & Barlow, 2005; Widiger & Clark, 2000; Widiger & Sankis, 2000).

The goal of this chapter is to introduce an alternative, dimensional view of psychopathology that has been emerging in the literature in the last 15–20 years. An overview of how two broadband instruments already available in clinical practice, the *Minnesota Multiphasic Personality Inventory 2–Restructured Form* (MMPI-2-RF: Ben-Porath & Tellegen, 2008/2011; Tellegen & Ben-Porath, 2008/2011) and the *Personality Assessment Inventory* (Morey, 1991/2007), can be used to assess psychopathology within the structural frameworks proposed in this literature is then provided. The chapter ends with implications of using the MMPI-2-RF and Personality Assessment Inventory (PAI) to assess this framework in research and clinical practice, as well as a brief discussion of the limitations of multivariate structural models and directions for future examination.

DIMENSIONAL MODELS OF PSYCHOPATHOLOGY

Large epidemiological studies have demonstrated that comorbidity amongst mental disorders is the rule (not the exception) for most mental disorders (Brady & Sinha, 2005; Grant, Stinson, Dawson, Chou, Dufour, et al., 2004; Grant, Stinson, Dawson, Chou, Ruan, et al., 2004; Kessler et al., 2006; Kessler, Chiu, Demler, & Walters, 2005; Kessler & Wang, 2008; Reiger et al., 1990). These observations led to the development of complex models that attempt to account for associations between numerous discrete disorders at once. In general, the goal of these models is to test whether certain disorders share a portion of their etiologies with one another and whether each individual disorder can be considered a unique manifestation of a broader, underlying predisposition for developing certain types of disorders (Eaton, South, & Krueger, 2010; Krueger & Markon, 2006). These models add to what is understood about comorbidity between disorders, as they can include multiple disorders that are known to be related within the same study. This inclusion allows for links between pairs of disorders to be investigated, while also exploring how the presence of a third disorder (or more) influences that link. These models can also examine whether comorbidity between certain psychiatric disorders result from shared underlying liabilities, non-unique predispositions for developing certain types of disorders, or associations between liabilities (Krueger & Markon, 2006).

MODEL OF INTERNALIZING AND EXTERNALIZING DYSFUNCTION

Several large-scale community studies have provided support for a model of internalizing and externalizing problems that will be referred as the Multivariate Correlated Liabilities Model[1] (MCLM; Kendler, Prescott, Myers, & Neale, 2003; Kramer, Krueger, & Hicks, 2008; Krueger, 1999; Krueger, Capsi, Moffitt, & Silva, 1998; Krueger & Markon, 2006; Krueger, McGue, & Iacono, 2001; Lahey et al., 2008; Slade & Watson, 2006; Vollebergh et al., 2001). A conceptual representation of the MCLM based on the results of these studies is displayed in Figure 4.1. The model has two broad, moderately correlated dimensions, representing predispositions for internalizing and externalizing disorders. These correlated liabilities are displayed in Figure 4.1 as the ovals connected by a double-headed arrow. The externalizing factor is believed to reflect a propensity for excessive disinhibited behaviors. The liability for internalizing dysfunction is hypothesized to reflect a propensity to express distress inwardly.

Individual mental disorders have been linked to each of the liabilities described above (Katz, Cox, Clark, Oleski, & Sacevich, 2011; Kendler et al., 2003; Kramer et al., 2008; Krueger, 1999; Krueger et al., 1998; Krueger & Markon, 2006; Lahey et al., 2008; Slade & Watson, 2006; Vollebergh et al., 2001). These connections between discrete disorders and the different predispositions are displayed in Figure 4.1 as the rectangles connected to the liabilities by a directional arrow, which indicate that the predisposition is believed to be causing the

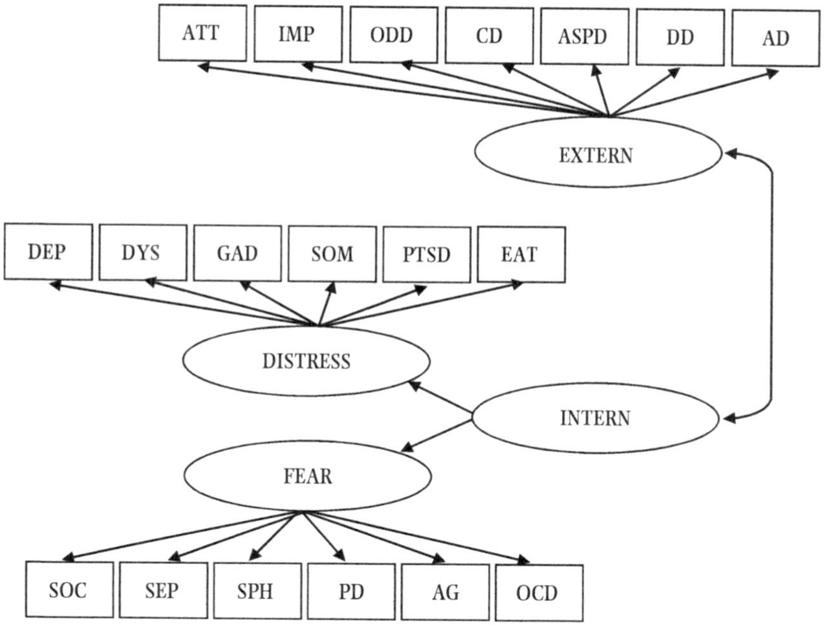

Figure 4.1 The Multivariate Correlated Liabilities Model (MCLM).

EXTERN = Externalizing Liability; ATT = Inattention; IMP = Impulsivity/Hyperactivity; ODD = Oppositional Defiant Disorder; CD = Conduct Disorder; ASPD = Antisocial Personality Disorder; DD = Drug Dependence; AD = Alcohol Dependence; INTERN = Internalizing Liability; DISTRESS = Distress Sub-dimension; DEP = Major Depressive Disorder; DYS = Dysthymic Disorder; GAD = Generalized Anxiety Disorder; SOM = Somatization Disorders; PTSD = Post-Traumatic Stress Disorder; EAT = Bulimia/Binge Eating Disorder; FEAR = Fear Sub-dimension; SOC = Social Phobia; SEP = Separation Anxiety Disorder; SPH = Specific (Simple) Phobias; PD = Panic Disorder; AG = Agoraphobia; OCD = Obsessive-Compulsive Disorder.

manifestation of that distinct type of disorder. Early studies provided evidence to link substance dependence and juvenile/adult antisocial behavior disorders to the externalizing factor. Subsequent studies suggested that antisocial behaviors not meeting criteria for antisocial personality disorder, alcohol and illicit drug abuse, inattention, hyperactivity-impulsivity, and oppositional defiant disorder were also related to the broad, externalizing factor. Disorders including unipolar mood, anxiety, and somatoform disorders have been connected to the broad internalizing factor.

Previous studies that examined the MCLM demonstrated that the internalizing and externalizing factors were moderately to strongly correlated (Krueger, 1999; Krueger et al., 1998; Krueger & Markon, 2006; Slade & Watson, 2006; Vollebergh et al., 2001). The association between the two broad predispositions for dysfunction is displayed in Figure 4.1 as the non-directional arc (double-headed arrow). Subsequent studies in children, adolescents, and adults have suggested that this shared variance likely reflects a genetically driven, higher-order factor describing a generalized predisposition for psychopathology (Caspi et al.,

2013; Lahey et al., 2011, 2012). Broadly, these results strongly indicate that individuals with mental disorders do not always fall into an internalizing or externalizing group. Rather, individuals who are at risk for psychopathology are likely to have some experience of both internalizing and externalizing symptoms.

Additional support has been garnered for the MCLM, as it has been demonstrated to be similar across diverse cultures (Krueger et al., 1998; Krueger, Chentsova-Dutton, Markon, Goldberg, & Ormelet 2003; Krueger et al., 2001; Slade & Watson, 2006; Vollebergh et al., 2001) and across genders (Kramer et al., 2008; Krueger, 1999). There is also an accumulating body of evidence to suggest that this model replicates well across age groups (Kramer et al., 2008; Krueger, 1999; Lahey et al., 2008; Vollebergh et al., 2001). Lastly, predispositions for internalizing and externalizing dysfunction have been demonstrated to be relatively stable over short periods of time (i.e., one year and three years; Krueger et al., 1998; Vollebergh et al., 2001).

Elaborations on the Internalizing Spectrum

In major classification systems, mood and anxiety disorders have typically been organized into two discrete classes of disorders. This conceptualization of mood and anxiety problems is contrary to studies demonstrating that many of these types of difficulties are genetically more similar than they are different (e.g., Kendler et al., 2003) and that all of these disorders are linked in varying degrees to difficulties with negative affect (Watson, 2005). The MCLM resolved this discrepancy by demonstrating that both mood and anxiety disorders could be linked to a latent predisposition for developing internalizing problems. However, "lumping" all mood and anxiety disorders within a single dimension ignored important distinctions between these disorders. Subsequent research demonstrated that the internalizing liability could be bifurcated into two, more distinct predispositions (Krueger, 1999; Krueger & Markon, 2006; Watson, 2005). These sub-factors represent unique manifestations of a broader disposition for internalizing problems and were originally termed "Anxious-Misery" and "Fear." To emphasize the role of distress in the anxious-misery disorders, the Anxious-Misery internalizing sub-factor has been alternatively labeled as "distress" disorders (Watson, 2005). These sub-dimensions are displayed in Figure 4.1 as the two ovals that are connected to the internalizing predisposition by the directional path (one-headed arrow), which indicates that the predisposition for internalizing causes the distinct subtypes of internalizing problems. The Anxious-Misery dimension is hypothesized to represent internalizing problems that have as their primary feature a tendency to experience severe levels of psychological distress. The Fear dimension is hypothesized to represent difficulties whose primary features are related to phobic fearfulness and anxiety sensitivity.

Connections between discrete mood, anxiety, and other disorders and the Distress and Fear subdimensions are displayed in Figure 4.1 as the rectangles connected to the specific liabilities by a directional arrow. Disorders characterized by a generalized dysphoria, including major depression, dysthymic disorder, generalized anxiety disorder, and post-traumatic stress disorder, have been linked to the anxious-misery (distress) subdimension (Cox, Clara, & Enns, 2002; Kendler et al., 2003; Krueger, 1999; Slade & Watson, 2006; Vollebergh, et al., 2001). Disorders not typically conceptualized as mood or anxiety disorders, including somatoform disorder and bulimia/binge eating disorders, have also been tentatively linked to the distress subdimension. Alternatively, disorders with a core feature of fearfulness and phobic anxiety, including social phobia, specific phobia, agoraphobia, panic disorder, and obsessive compulsive disorder, have been linked to the fear subdimension. Notably, in these studies, the association of obsessive compulsive disorder with the Fear subdimension has been less strongly supported than that demonstrated for the other phobia-related disorders.

Elaborations on the Externalizing Spectrum

Previous studies on the MCLM demonstrated support for one higher-order factor underlying disorders of antisocial behavior, impulsivity, and substance dependence (e.g., Krueger et al., 2001). This finding, however, stood in direct contrast to results from behavioral genetics studies indicating that there was substantial unique genetic and environmental variance associated with each externalizing disorder (e.g., Kendler et al., 2003). As such, Krueger and colleagues (Krueger, Markon, Patrick, Benning, & Kramer, 2007) hypothesized that a more comprehensive model of the externalizing liability could be developed if aspects of antisocial behaviors/personality, substance use disorders (SUDs), and disinhibited personality traits were viewed as elements of an externalizing spectrum. Beginning with over 20 constructs describing antisocial, impulsive, and substance-use phenomena drawn from both psychopathology and personality literatures, competing structural models were calculated using data from a large participant sample of college students and correctional inmates. The final, best-fitting model is displayed in Figure 4.2. The model has three uncorrelated factors, Externalizing Problems, Callous-Aggression, and Substance Misuse, which are displayed in Figure 4.2 as the ovals. The model has a bifactor structure, meaning that all measured variables in the model loaded onto the general Externalizing factor, but only specific subsets of the manifest variables loaded on the Callous-Aggression and Substance Misuse factors.

In the elaborated model of externalizing dysfunction, each liability is hypothesized to cause varying observable symptoms and behaviors (Krueger et al., 2007). These are displayed in Figure 4.2 as the rectangles connected to the liabilities by a directional path (one-headed arrow). The broad Externalizing liability was demonstrated to be related to all of the examined behaviors/symptoms, but was most strongly related to measures of irresponsibility and problematic impulsivity. This indicates the core deficits of externalizing problems relate

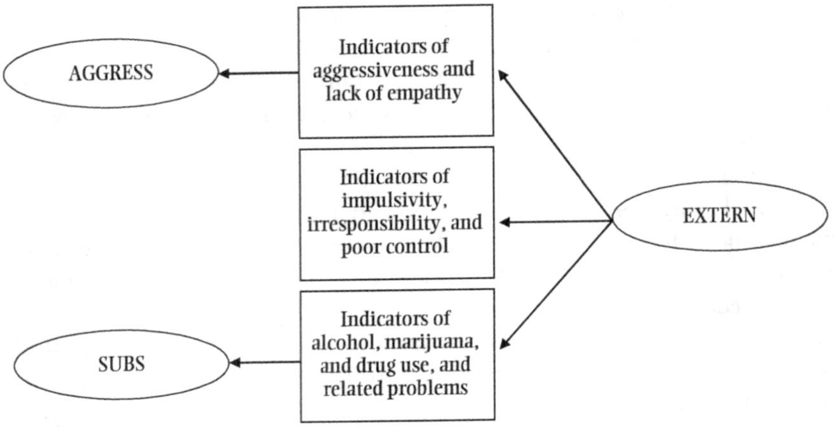

Figure 4.2 Expanded Model of the Adult Externalizing Spectrum.
EXTERN = Externalizing Liability; AGGRESS = Callous-Aggression Dimension; SUBS = Substance Misuse Dimension.

to the inability to approach life in a planful manner. The Callous-Aggression liability was composed of markers of aggressive and unempathetic attitudes. Measures of relational aggression, destructive aggression, and lack of empathy most strongly related to the Callous-Aggression liability. Finally, the third liability, Substance Misuse, was characterized by measures describing the propensity for involvement with substances and substance-related consequences. The Substance Misuse factor was most strongly characterized by measures of marijuana use, marijuana problems, and other illicit drug use.

Theoretically, the emergence of three independent factors suggests that the manifestation of a specific externalizing difficulty is multiply determined (Krueger et al., 2007). More specifically, this model indicates the emergence of an externalizing difficulty can be traced to at least three sources, including the general externalizing propensity, an independent propensity to develop either callous-aggression or substance-related problems, and a highly specific propensity to engage in and experience the measured behavior or symptom. This result represents one of the most important aspects of this study, as the emergence of three independent factors and multiple underlying pathways leading to the same specific outcomes parallels results from genetic studies of the externalizing spectrum, which have demonstrated disorder-specific genetic and environmental risk factors for externalizing disorders (Kendler et al., 2003; Krueger et al., 2002). This result also aligns conceptualization of externalizing disorders characterized by callous-aggression with the extant literature, as this bifactor maps onto features specific to psychopathy (e.g., "meanness," Patrick & Drislane, 2014; or "affective-interpersonal" psychopathy traits; e.g., Hare, 2003) and also resembles what is distinctive about the individual differences antagonism domain found in most omnibus personality models (e.g., DSM-5 Section III; APA, 2013).

EXPANSIONS TO THE MCLM TO INCLUDE LESS FREQUENTLY OCCURRING DIFFICULTIES

Thus far, this discussion of structural models of psychopathology has been limited to disorders that are more prevalent. However, to be useful in research and practice, dimensional models of psychopathology will need to include less frequently occurring and more severe types of mental disorders (e.g., schizophrenia), as well as maladaptive personality patterns. Empirical work that attempts to include these types of difficulties has begun to emerge in the recent literature, though the conclusions that can be drawn from these studies are not as well supported as those just discussed for internalizing and externalizing problems. Nonetheless, there are three relatively robust findings in the emerging literature that warrant inclusion in the current discussion: that of a third independent dimension representing a liability for psychotic disorders, the placement of somatic difficulties in structural models of psychopathology, and the convergence of personality and psychopathology models on similar structures.

A Third Dimension—Psychosis

Earlier studies on the MCLM were primarily conducted in large, community-dwelling samples where the prevalence of psychotic phenomena, such as symptoms of schizophrenia and schizotypal personality disorder, were less common, leaving open to question how these types of difficulties would be best described by structural models of psychopathology. To begin answering this question, Kotov and colleagues (Kotov, Chang, et al., 2011; Kotov, Ruggero, et al., 2011) conducted two large-scale studies using clinical inpatient and outpatient samples in order to determine if these types of symptoms would best be described by existing internalizing and externalizing liability concepts, or if a third, independent factor representing psychotic symptoms would emerge. Results of both studies suggested psychotic symptoms were not well accounted for by a model containing only internalizing and externalizing problems. Rather, results indicated that psychotic symptoms were best conceptualized as manifestations of a third dimension of psychopathology, which they termed "psychosis" (also sometimes referred to as "thought disorders"; Caspi et al., 2014). Subsequent studies in large epidemiological samples from Australia (Wright et al., 2013), New Zealand (Caspi et al., 2014), and the United States (Fleming, Shevlin, Murphy, & Joseph, 2014) have supported the inclusion of a Psychosis liability in the externalizing/internalizing MCLM framework.

The final, best-fitting model in studies that have included a Psychosis liability is displayed in Figure 4.3. The model has three correlated factors—Externalizing, Internalizing, and Psychosis—which are displayed in Figure 4.3 with ovals connected by double-headed arrows. Diverse empirical evidence supports linking to the Psychosis liability such disorders as schizophrenia, schizotypal personality disorder, paranoid personality disorder, and schizoid personality disorder (Caspi et al., 2014; Kotov, Chang, et al., 2011; Kotov, Ruggero, et al., 2011).

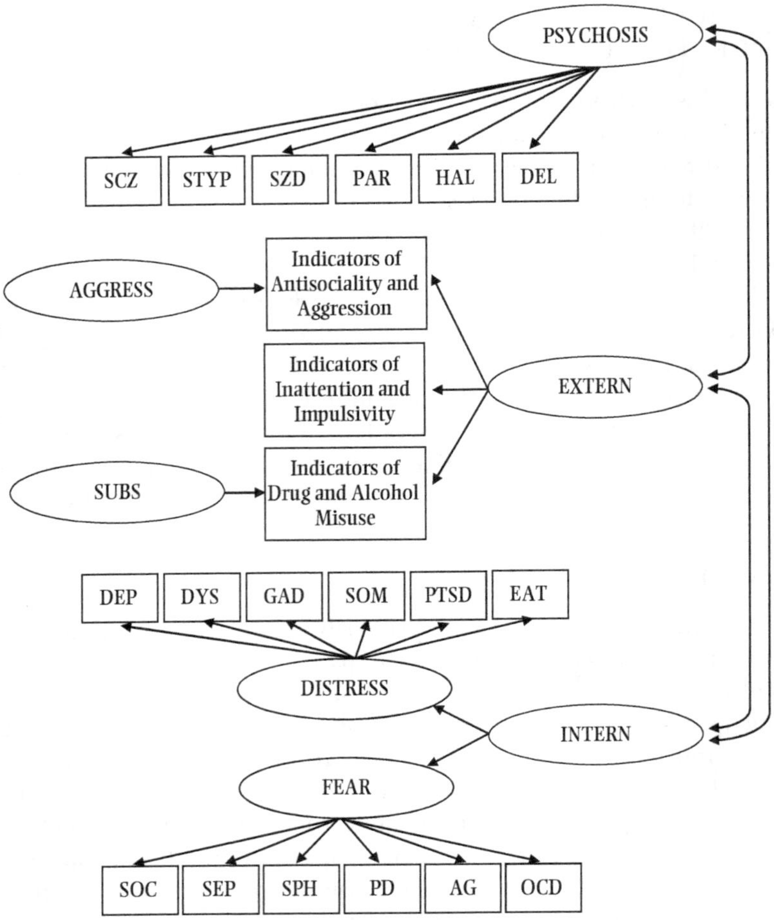

Figure 4.3 The Multivariate Correlated Liabilities Model Incorporating Psychosis Dimension.

PSYCHOSIS = Psychotic Disorders Liability; SCZ = Schizophrenia; STYP = Schizotypal Personality Disorder; SZD = Schizoid Personality Disorder; PAR = Paranoid Personality Disorder; DEL = Delusions regarding thought control and grandiosity; EXTERN = Externalizing Liability; AGGRESS = Callous-Aggression Dimension; SUBS = Substance Misuse Dimension; INTERN = Internalizing Liability; DISTRESS = Distress Sub-dimension; DEP = Major Depressive Disorder; DYS = Dysthymic Disorder; GAD = Generalized Anxiety Disorder; SOM = Somatization Disorders; PTSD = Post-Traumatic Stress Disorder; EAT = Bulimia/Binge Eating Disorder; FEAR = Fear Sub-dimension; SOC = Social Phobia; SEP = Separation Anxiety Disorder; SPH = Specific (Simple) Phobias; PD = Panic Disorder; AG = Agoraphobia; OCD = Obsessive-Compulsive Disorder.

Hallucinations, paranoid delusions, and delusional thoughts regarding controlling others' thinking, believing events have special meaning, and believing one has special powers have also been demonstrated to be best predicted by the predisposition for disordered thinking (Fleming et al., 2014; Wright et al., 2013). All of these symptoms and syndromes are displayed in Figure 4.3 as rectangles. A directional arrow connects the individual syndromes and symptoms with the Psychosis liability, indicating the predisposition for psychosis is hypothesized to cause the discrete disorders.

Somatization—Internalizing or "Other" Dysfunction?

Practitioners in medical, neuropsychological, and forensic disability settings are likely to encounter individuals for whom somatic difficulties dominate the clinical picture. Such manifestations can come in the form of medically unexplained symptoms as well as distress about genuine medical conditions. Therefore, it is important that structural models of psychopathology clearly recognize and account for somatic problems. At this time, somatization is typically not recognized as its own higher-order domain in the psychopathology literature. This is because early studies examining commonly occurring mental difficulties demonstrated somatic problems were related to the Internalizing liability (Krueger et al., 2003). However, accumulating evidence suggests that consideration of whether somatic difficulties would be better described in another way in these models is warranted for two reasons. First, in Krueger and colleagues' (2003) study, the prediction of somatic difficulties by the higher-order internalizing factor was substantially smaller than what it provided for mood and anxiety disorders. Specifically, results indicate that the internalizing factor only accounted for 4% of variance in somatization, which is substantially below conventional standards. Second, Kotov, Ruggero, et al. (2011) demonstrated that somatic difficulties formed a unique liability that was related to, yet distinct from, the liabilities for internalizing, externalizing, and psychotic dysfunctions. Similar results for an independent somatic factor have been suggested in studies examining the structure of broadband instruments, such as the MMPI-2-RF (Anderson et al., 2015; McNulty & Overstreet, 2014). Nonetheless, although these initial findings are promising, additional structural evidence is needed before an independent somatic factor can be formally included in the MCLM.

Moving Further Down in the Hierarchy to Five-Factor Space

Recent elaborations of quantitative personality and psychopathology hierarchies have suggested that the general three-factor structure just reviewed can be further subdivided (e.g., Bagby et al., 2014; Markon, Krueger, & Watson, 2005; Wright et al., 2012). Results from these analyses are consistent with five-factor models in "normative" personality (e.g., Goldberg, 2006) and pathological personality developments (e.g., Harkness & McNulty, 1994; Krueger, Derringer, Markon, Watson, & Skodol, 2012). These models have served as a foundation for the development of the maladaptive personality trait model presented in DSM-5 Section III as an alternative way to operationalize personality psychopathology (e.g., Krueger et al., 2012).

Recent research using Goldberg's (2006) so-called "bass-ackwards" modeling has provided consistent evidence of how the personality-psychopathology hierarchies develop as one systematically descends subsequent levels of abstractions. Several studies have focused on single measures (e.g., Bagby et al., 2014; Kushner, Quilty, Tackett, & Bagby, 2011; Tackett, Quilty, Sellbom, Rector, & Bagby, 2008; Wright et al., 2012), whereas others have examined combinations of measures (e.g., Markon et al., 2005; Wright & Simms, 2014). The results have been strikingly similar, especially at the fifth level of the hierarchy, with factors indicating negative affectivity/neuroticism and detachment/introversion (bifurcation from internalizing); disinhibition/unconscientiousness and antagonism (bifurcation from externalizing), and psychoticism/openness.[2] A visual representation of this structure is provided in Figure 4.4. Moreover, the manifestations of the hierarchy appear slightly different, depending on populations examined. For instance, in patient samples, the big three psychopathology domains reviewed earlier emerge (e.g., Bagby et al., 2014; Chmielewski & Watson, 2007; Kotov, Chang, et al., 2011; Kotov, Ruggero, et al., 2011); whereas, in student or community samples, the negative affectivity/neuroticism, detachment/introversion, and externalizing tend to materialize (e.g., Wright et al.,

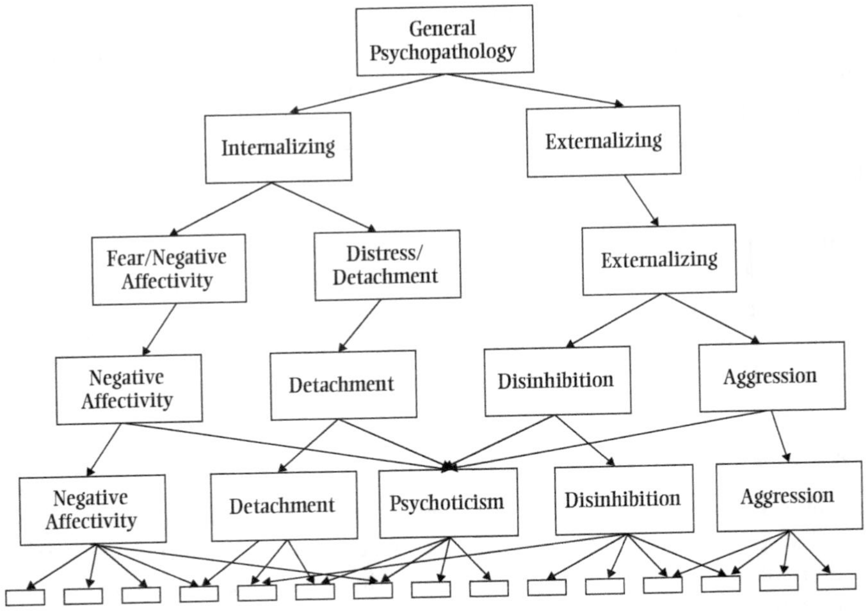

Figure 4.4 Five-Factor Model of Psychopathology/Personality.

Note that the displayed structure is the one that emerges from analyses using community/university samples. In clinical samples, the psychoticism factor emerges higher in the structure (e.g., Bagby et al., 2014). The unidentified boxes at the bottom of the hierarchy represent individual syndromes or items.

2012). These findings make sense, of course, given the construct variations in these different populations. Overall, these hierarchical analyses are important as they demonstrate at least two important things (1) It does not matter which personality model one examines, as they typically map onto each other and represent different levels of analyses within the broader personality hierarchy, and (2) personality and psychopathology variance map onto one another in important ways from an empirical hierarchy perspective.

THE MINNESOTA MULTIPHASIC PERSONALITY INVENTORY–2-RESTRUCTURED FORM

The Minnesota Multiphasic Personality Inventory–2–Restructured Form (MMPI-2-RF; Ben-Porath & Tellegen, 2008) refers to the most recent of the MMPI family of instruments that began with the original MMPI developed in the 1930s and published in 1943 (Hathaway & McKinley, 1943). The MMPI-2-RF is composed of 338 of the original 567 MMPI-2 true/false items, and aggregates onto nine validity and 42 substantive scales. The major aim of this section is to illustrate how the MMPI-2-RF hierarchy of scales maps onto the broader quantitative/empirical structure of psychopathology discussed earlier.

Initial development of the MMPI-2-RF constituted the restructuring of the eight original MMPI clinical scales (Tellegen et al., 2003), which were constructed in the 1930s using an empirical keying method whereby items that differentiated diagnostic groups from healthy controls were included on scales for such disorders. Recognizing the substantial strengths of the clinical scales, which included extensive empirical validation and decades of clinical experience among practitioners, it has been known for some time that the scales themselves were not psychometrically optimal as measures of diagnostic constructs (Tellegen & Ben-Porath, 2008; Tellegen et al., 2003). The primary step in developing these scales was to identify and extract a common general emotional distress dimension (labeled "demoralization") that saturates the clinical scales, elucidate distinct target constructs from each scale, and thereby improve their convergent and discriminant validity. This resulted in a set of nine Restructured Clinical scales (RC scales; Tellegen et al., 2003), including a measure of demoralization and eight other scales assessing key components of the basic Clinical scales (except Scale 5 [Masculinity/Femininity] and 0 [Social Introversion], which do not measure psychopathology constructs), scored on both the MMPI-2 and the MMPI-2-RF.

After the RC scales had been introduced to the MMPI-2, work continued on several other psychometrically efficient scales for a new version of the inventory—the MMPI-2-RF (Ben-Porath & Tellegen, 2008; Tellegen & Ben-Porath, 2008). This version of the MMPI was designed to take advantage of the clinically useful variance of the MMPI-2 item pool in an efficient and psychometrically up-to-date manner. Scales developed for the MMPI-2-RF were intended to assess (a) constructs not directly measured by the RC scales, (b) facets of the broader RC scales, or (c) distinctive core components from the original clinical scales not covered by the RC scales. A set of higher-order scales was also developed to provide a hierarchically organized interpretative framework for the test (Tellegen & Ben-Porath, 2008). Lastly, the MMPI-2-RF contains revised versions of standard MMPI-2 validity scales, as well two new validity scales assessing somatic and cognitive over-reporting.

Higher-Order Structures

Most of the MMPI-2-RF scales are organized in a hierarchical fashion that maps onto the general hierarchical three-factor structure of psychopathology (Kotov, Chang, et al., 2011; Kotov, Ruggero, et al., 2011; Wright et al., 2012). Specifically, the three higher-order (H-O) scales—Emotional-Internalizing Dysfunction (EID), Thought Dysfunction (THD), and Behavioral-Externalizing Dysfunction (BXD)—all map onto the three broad contemporary psychopathology domains. The nine RC scales occupy the middle level of the hierarchy, and the 23 specific problems (SP) scales compose the lowest level with a very narrow, facet-based representation of psychopathology, including specific problems not directly assessed via the broader scales (e.g., suicidal ideation). Extant to the three-level hierarchy, but no less important with respect to empirical psychopathology structures, are the Personality Psychopathology Five (PSY-5; Harkness & McNulty, 1994; see also Harkness, McNulty, Finn, Reynolds, & Shields, 2014) scales that provide a dimensional assessment of maladaptive personality traits from a five-factor perspective akin to that of DSM-5 Section III (APA, 2013).

Although it certainly would be expected that the H-O scales would map onto contemporary psychopathology structures, it is noteworthy that these scales were developed based on factor analysis of the nine RC scales (Tellegen & Ben-Porath, 2008; see also Sellbom, Ben-Porath, & Bagby, 2008b). Tellegen and Ben-Porath (2008) conducted a series of exploratory factor analyses in large outpatient and inpatient samples, and found that three RC scales representing demoralization (RCd), low positive affectivity (RC2), and high negative affectivity (RC7) consistently loaded on an internalizing factor. RC scales reflecting antisocial behavior (RC4), hypomanic activation (RC9), and, to a lesser degree, cynicism (RC3) loaded on an externalizing factor and RC scales indexing persecutory ideation (RC6) and aberrant experiences (RC1) were core markers for a psychoticism factor. Subsequent research has replicated and extended these findings in a variety of samples from North America and Europe. For instance, Hoelzle and Meyer (2008) and Sellbom et al. (2008b) independently reported almost identical findings in large psychiatric samples from the United States and Canada, respectively. Van der Heijden and colleagues (Van der Heijden, Rossi, Van der Veld, Derksen, & Egger, 2013a) replicated Sellbom et al.'s (2008b) findings across five large Dutch clinical and forensic samples, again, finding that the RC scales adhered to a three-factor higher-order structure. Most recently, Anderson et al. (2015) conducted a conjoint exploratory factor analysis using MMPI-2-RF scale sets with the Personality Inventory for DSM-5 (PID-5; Krueger et al., 2012) in a large Canadian psychiatric sample. These authors found that the three higher-order domains could be extracted in analyses using each of the four MMPI-2-RF scale sets in conceptually expected ways. It is noteworthy that, in these latter results using the lower-order scale sets, that a fourth factor representing social detachment, introversion, and low affective arousal consistently emerged. This result is similar to much of the PAI research (reviewed later) on this topic, as well as the five-factor models described earlier (e.g., Wright et al., 2012). Thus, quantitative hierarchical research using the RC scales, which were developed without any particular diagnostic nosology in mind, but rather were grounded in Tellegen's theory of self-reported affect (e.g., Tellegen, 1985; Watson & Tellegen, 1985), strongly suggests the hierarchical organization of the MMPI-2-RF conforms to the same structure as identified in the extant psychopathology epidemiology literature just reviewed.

Domain-Specific Structures

More recent research has emerged to indicate that, within each domain, the SP scales also map onto extant empirically validated structures. Sellbom (2011) demonstrated that the internalizing SP scales conformed to Watson's (2005; see also work by Krueger, 1999; Krueger & Markon, 2006) quantitative hierarchical structure of emotional disorders. Specifically, MMPI-2-RF scales Suicide/Death Ideation (SUI), Helplessness/Hopelessness (HLP), Self-Doubt (SFD), Inefficacy (NFC), and Stress and Worry (STW) loaded on a "distress" factor, whereas Anxiety (AXY), Behavior-Restricting Fears (BRF), and Multiple Specific Fears (MSF) loaded on a "fear" factor in a very large outpatient mental health sample. Sellbom (2010, 2011; see also Sellbom, Marion, et al., 2012) also elaborated on externalizing psychopathology structures in a variety of community, correctional, and forensic samples. By and large, the research has shown that the four externalizing SP scales, including Juvenile Conduct Problems (JCP), Substance Abuse (SUB), Aggression (AGG), and Activation (ACT), load onto a broad externalizing domain, but also can be modeled in accordance with Krueger et al.'s (2007) bifactor structure in which residual subfactors of callous-aggression and substance misuse can be identified. Finally, Sellbom, Titcomb, and Arbisi (2011; see also Titcomb, Sellbom, Cohen, & Arbisi, under review) found that the thought-dysfunction items embedded within RC6 (Ideas of Persecution) and RC8 (Aberrant Experiences) can be modeled according to an overall thought-dysfunction factor, but also isolating a residual, paranoid-ideation subfactor (in a bifactor framework) that corresponds to a neuropsychiatric etiology model that separates paranoid delusions from schizophrenia more broadly (Blackwood, Howard, Bentall, & Murray, 2001).

Research has also established that MMPI-2-RF scale scores map onto the broader five-factor structure of personality and psychopathology (see, e.g., Bagby et al., 2014; Markon et al., 2005; Wright & Simms, 2014; Wright et al., 2012). McNulty and Overstreet (2014) subjected the entire set of MMPI-2-RF scales (corrected for item overlap) to factor analyses in very large outpatient and inpatient mental health samples. They found a six-factor structure, with five of the factors mirroring the aforementioned PSY-5 domains and a sixth factor reflecting somatization. The PSY-5 scales in their own right overlap both conceptually and empirically with the personality trait domains listed in DSM-5 Section III, which provides an alternative model for operationalizing personality disorders (Anderson et al., 2013; see also Anderson et al., 2015). When the PSY-5 domain scales were subjected to a conjoint factor analysis with the DSM-5 Section III personality-trait facets (as operationalized by the PID-5), the five-factor higher-order structure emerged, with the PSY-5 loading on their expected domains (see also Bagby et al., 2014, for analyses with the PSY-5 items). Recent research has further shown that the PSY-5 scales operate similarly to the DSM-5 Section III model in accounting for variance in the formal Section II personality disorders (PD; e.g., Finn, Arbisi, Erbes, Polusny, & Thuras, 2014; Sellbom, Smid, De Saeger, Smit, & Kamphuis, 2014). For instance, Avoidant PD is best predicted by Negative Emotionality/Neuroticism (NEGE-r) and Introversion/Low Positive Emotionality (INTR-r), Antisocial PD by Aggressiveness (AGGR-r) and Disconstraint (DISC-r), Borderline by Negative Emotionality/Neuroticism (NEGE-r) and Disconstraint (DISC-r), Narcissistic by Aggressiveness (AGGR-r), and Schizotypal by Psychoticism (PSYC-r).

CONSTRUCT VALIDITY EVIDENCE FOR THREE-FACTOR MODELS

The three-factor models generally, and the H-O scales specifically, have evinced substantial evidence for construct validity, especially in terms of how they map onto personality trait models and mental health symptomatology. For instance, the MMPI-2-RF Technical Manual presents validity data from a range of medical, mental health, forensic, and nonclinical settings to indicate that these scales are distinctly associated with clinician-rating, interview, record review, and self-report data reflecting psychopathology symptoms of internalizing, externalizing, and thought disorder, with generally very good discriminant validity (Tellegen & Ben-Porath, 2008).

Particularly relevant to contemporary psychopathology models are personality and psychopathology associations, as the differentiation between personality traits and psychopathology symptoms as distinct constructs is becoming less and less tenable (e.g., Hopwood & Sellbom, 2013; Krueger & Markon, 2014). Numerous studies using different personality trait models have revealed a very distinct pattern: EID (or the internalizing factor based on aforementioned factor analyses with RC scales) is primarily associated with trait measures reflecting negative affectivity/neuroticism and introversion/(low) positive emotionality; THD (or the thought disturbance factor) is related to absorption, psychoticism, and peculiarity; and BXD (or the externalizing factor) is generally associated with trait measures of disinhibition, (low) conscientiousness, antagonism/(low) agreeableness, and sensation-seeking (Sellbom et al., 2008b; Tellegen & Ben-Porath, 2008; Van der Heijden, Egger, Rossi, & Derksen, 2012; Van der Heijden, Rossi, Van der Veld, Derksen, & Egger, 2013a, 2013b).

SPECIFIC PSYCHOPATHOLOGY DOMAINS

Internalizing

Research has accumulated to suggest that individual MMPI-2-RF scale scores map onto specific hierarchical models of internalizing psychopathology in ways predicted by theory. In one of the first studies in this regard, Sellbom, Ben-Porath, and Bagby (2008a) examined the utility of Demoralization (RCd), Low Positive Emotions (RC2), and Dysfunctional Negative Emotions (RC7) as markers of an expanded model of temperament in predicting "distress" and "fear" disorders within Watson's (2005) framework for internalizing disorders. They used both clinical and nonclinical samples, and via structural equation modeling, showed that RCd mapped onto the distress disorders, whereas RC7 was preferentially associated with fear disorders. RC2, as expected, differentiated depression (within the distress domain) and social phobia (within the fear domain) from the other disorders. In another study examining PTSD comorbidity, RCd was the best predictor of internalizing/distress psychopathology (Wolf et al., 2008).

Several recent studies have also specifically examined predictors of PTSD within contemporary frameworks. Among the RC scales, RCd seems to consistently be a predictor of global PTSD symptomatology, and in particular, the distress/dysphoria factor associated with this disorder, with RC7 being a meaningful predictor in some as well (Arbisi, Polusny, Erbes, Thuras, & Reddy, 2011; Miller et al., 2010; Sellbom, Lee, Ben-Porath, Arbisi, & Gervais, 2012; Wolf et al., 2008; see also Forbes, Elhai, Miller, & Creamer, 2010). More specifically, among the SP scales, Anxiety (AXY) appears to be the best predictor of PTSD symptoms in various clinical and/or veteran samples (Arbisi et al., 2011; Sellbom, Lee, et al., 2012). Anger Proneness (ANP) is a good predictor of hyperarousal symptoms, and Social Avoidance (SAV) of avoidance symptoms (Sellbom, Lee, et al., 2012; see also Koffel, Polusny, Arbisi, & Erbes, 2012). Finally, Koffel et al. (2012) have begun to identify specific MMPI-2-RF item markers of DSM-5 PTSD symptoms in a large U.S. National Guard sample, but these require further validation before their use can be recommended.

Externalizing

Numerous studies have shown good convergent and discriminant validity of the externalizing RC (RC4 and RC9) and SP (Juvenile Conduct Problems [JCP], Substance Abuse [SUB], Aggression [AGG], and Activation [ACT]) scales that make up the externalizing spectrum. As documented in the Technical Manual and elsewhere, across nonclinical, mental health, and forensic samples, JCP is preferentially associated with crime data and impulsivity. Not surprisingly, SUB is the most potent predictor of alcohol and drug misuse, but it tends to be a good predictor of general externalizing and sensation-seeking as well (Johnson, Sellbom, & Phillips, 2014; Tarescavage, Luna-Jones, & Ben-Porath, 2014; Tellegen & Ben-Porath, 2008). AGG is more specifically associated with behavioral manifestations of both reactive (or angry) and instrumental forms of aggression (Tellegen & Ben-Porath, 2008). ACT is specifically associated with externalizing as reflected in manic or hypomanic episodes (e.g., euphoria, psychological energy, racing thoughts) and is the MMPI-2-RF scale that best differentiates bipolar mood disorder from unipolar mood and psychotic disorders (Sellbom, Bagby, Kushner, Quilty, & Ayearst, 2012; Watson, Quilty, & Bagby, 2011). Finally, the MMPI-2-RF PSY-5 scales AGGR-r and DISC-r, albeit outside of the formal structural hierarchy, provide for dispositional tendencies towards externalizing behavior and, in particular, personality pathology, including antisocial personality disorder, narcissistic personality disorder, and psychopathy as evidenced in a variety of forensic samples (e.g., Sellbom et al., 2014; Wygant & Sellbom, 2012).

In terms of psychopathy (of which the callous-aggression component can be considered a core), Sellbom and colleagues have demonstrated that RC4, RC9, AGGR-r, and DISC-r can predict scores on a variety of psychopathy measures (Phillips, Sellbom, Ben-Porath, & Patrick, 2014; Sellbom, Ben-Porath, Lilienfeld, Patrick, & Graham, 2005; Sellbom, Ben-Porath, & Stafford, 2007; Sellbom, Lee, et al., 2012; Wygant & Sellbom, 2012). Specifically, results indicated that these externalizing scales, in combination with low scores on a variety of internalizing scales (particularly those pertaining to fearfulness), were good predictors of scores on the Psychopathy Checklist: Screening Version (Hart, Cox, & Hare, 1995) and the Psychopathic Personality Inventory (PPI; Lilienfeld & Andrews, 1996) in nonclinical, forensic, and correctional samples.

Thought Dysfunction

Four scales of the MMPI-2-RF are particularly relevant for assessing the psychotic dimension that emerges in structural models of psychopathology, namely the Higher-Order Thought Dysfunction (THD) scale, RC6 (Ideas of Persecution), RC8 (Aberrant Experiences), and the Psychoticism (PSYC-r) scale (Tellegen & Ben-Porath, 2008). Research to date has shown that the two main indicators of specific psychotic symptomatology, RC6 and RC8, are effective in differentiating between paranoid delusional and non-paranoid psychotic presentations. More specifically, in a large inpatient psychiatric sample, Arbisi, Sellbom, and Ben-Porath (2008) and Sellbom et al. (2006) found that RC6 was preferentially associated with a history and active presence of delusions (particularly grandiose and persecutory types), whereas RC8 is a better predictor of hallucinations and non-persecutory delusions. Handel and Archer (2008) replicated these findings in another large inpatient sample. Furthermore, research with the PSY-5 PSYC-r scale has found it to be a good predictor of global thought disturbance and disconnection from reality (Tellegen & Ben-Porath, 2008), as well as Schizotypal Personality Disorder (Sellbom et al., 2014).

Somatization

As discussed earlier, somatization is typically not recognized as its own higher-order domain in the psychopathology literature. However, such measurement is featured on many omnibus personality and psychopathology inventories, including the PAI and MMPI-2-RF, and structural analyses do seem to tentatively support its distinct (from internalizing psychopathology) nature (e.g., Kotov, Ruggero, et al., 2011).

The MMPI-2-RF RC1 (Somatic Complaints) scale is the broadest measure of somatization on the instrument, with five SP scales reflecting preoccupation with general physical debilitation (MLS), gastrointestinal complaints (GIC), head pain complaints (HPC), neurological/conversion symptoms (NUC), and cognitive memory and attention complains (COG). The hierarchical structure of these scales has been supported (Thomas & Locke, 2010). The Technical Manual presents validity evidence that all scales are good predictors of somatic preoccupation with reasonable discriminant validity. Some more specific research has indicated that NUC is a particularly potent predictor of non-epileptic seizures in medical settings (Locke et al., 2010). Gervais, Ben-Porath, and Wygant (2009) have shown that the COG scale is a good predictor of self-report memory complaints in a very large disability sample.

THE PERSONALITY ASSESSMENT INVENTORY

The Personality Assessment Inventory (PAI; Morey, 1991, 2007) is a broadband self-report instrument that is similar to the MMPI-2-RF in many respects. Like the MMPI instruments, the PAI was designed to measure a range of constructs likely to be of interest to practitioners in a variety of personality-assessment settings. Like the MMPI, the PAI includes several validity scales designed to indicate the degree to which an individual's approach to the test affects their responses. Both instruments are interpreted based on large normative samples, including those from the general population and specific samples relevant to the formulation of a particular case (e.g., other pre-employment applicants in a personnel-selection context). Like the MMPI, the PAI is widely used in a host of assessment settings, and a large body of research supports its validity and clinical utility for a range of applications.

However, there are important differences between the PAI and the MMPI-2-RF. Some differences have to do with the format and content of the instruments. For instance, there are specific differences in the scales that are included on each instrument, even though the overall collection is similar in covering personality and psychopathology relatively comprehensively. Also, whereas the MMPI-2-RF items are true/false, the PAI uses a 4-point Likert response scale. Other differences have to do with the approaches taken to developing each test. The most central and unique aspect of the PAI, relative to other instruments, is the use of construct-validation test-development strategies based on the work of Loevinger (1957) and Jackson (1971). Interestingly, the roots of this model of test development go back to the early days of the MMPI, when Meehl and others were using that instrument to transform the approach to test construction and validation in the field (e.g., Cronbach & Meehl, 1955).

A key feature of the construct-validation approach involves establishing content validity by formally articulating the variables that the test is designed to measure, and identifying content that measures those variables as directly as possible. This requires an underlying theory of what is intended to be measured. In the case of the PAI, the "theory" was ultimately practical. The goal was to measure most of the constructs most clinical assessors would be interested in assessing most of the time. A premium was placed on constructs that were used across theoretical orientations and practice settings and that had temporal stability in the clinical assessment lexicon. PAI scales are grouped into four major sections based on the domain of variables they assess. First are validity scales that assess various approaches to test completion. Second are clinical scales that measure psychiatric constructs such as depression, anxiety, alcohol problems, and schizophrenia. Third are treatment-consideration scales designed to measure other features of the person or their environment that may be of clinical interest, including aggression, suicidal ideation, social support, stress, and treatment motivation. Finally, there are two scales that are designed to assess normative interpersonal style. These scales are normative in the sense that they are the only two scales on the PAI for which high scores are not necessarily either good or bad (Morey & Hopwood, 2006). Content validity was broadened via the inclusion of subscales for ten of the 22 PAI full scales. For instance, the depression scale has subscales assessing cognitive (e.g., hopelessness), affective (e.g., subjective sadness), and physiological (e.g., sleep problems) aspects of the construct. Having identified the scales that would be measured, many items were written to directly assess each of these variables, and various empirical procedures were used to trim the measure to its final, 344-item version.

Given their different approaches to test development, it is interesting to note that, like the MMPI-RF, research suggests that the factors that describe the covariance of PAI scales correspond rather well to factor-analytic models of personality and psychopathology (e.g., O'Connor, 2002; Wright et al., 2013). Specifically, several exploratory factor analyses of the PAI scales have consistently suggested three or four factors (Hoelzle & Meyer, 2009; Morey, 2007). When fourth factors sometimes emerge, they often reflect salient features of the sample, such as the substance abuse factor identified by Karlin et al. (2006) in a sample of chronic pain patients for whom opiate abuse is a common issue. Four factors were present in the PAI community and clinical samples. In the community normative sample, the first two factors correspond very closely to internalizing and externalizing dimensions that are commonly found in psychopathology measures. The third factor has to do with antagonistic personality features such as egocentricity, exploitation, and narcissism, which in its more distinct form appears in Krueger et al.'s (2007) externalizing hierarchy ("callous-aggression"). The fourth factor involves social detachment, introversion, and low affective arousal. Interestingly, unlike the MMPI-2-RF analyses (especially with nine RC scales), which tend to yield the three higher-order psychopathology factors, these PAI findings are more akin to what often appears at the "fourth" level in personality/psychopathology structures (e.g., Markon et al., 2005; Tackett et al., 2008; Wright et al., 2012). More specifically, in these structures, "disinhibition" breaks down into specific representations of unconscientiousness and antagonism.

Research also shows that PAI scales are sensitive and specific to direct measures of higher-order factors of personality and psychopathology. For instance, in the initial validation studies, each of the higher-order dimensions of the normal range NEO Personality Inventory (NEO-PI; Costa & McCrae, 1985) was specifically correlated with several PAI scales. Research with instruments whose content focuses on more pathological elements of personality traits, such as the Personality Inventory for DSM-5 (Krueger et al., 2012), shows similar patterns (Hopwood et al., 2013). In the remainder of this section, we provide more specific information about connections between PAI scales and higher-order dimensions of personality and psychopathology.

Internalizing

A general distress factor with strong loadings on PAI scales such as Depression (DEP), Anxiety (ANX), Anxiety-Related Disorders (ARD), Borderline Features (BOR), Suicidal Ideation (SUI), and Stress (STR) is invariably the first factor extracted across studies examining the structure of the PAI scales. As with the MMPI-RF, validity correlations among these scales provide important information about lower-order fear and distress variants of the internalizing dimension. Numerous studies have demonstrated the sensitivity of PAI scales to distress disorders (e.g., major depression) and fear disorders (e.g., panic disorder or phobias), as well as the ability of PAI scales to discriminate between these classes of disorders (e.g., Fantoni-Salvador & Rogers, 1997). Furthermore, Veltri, Williams, and Braxton (2004) found that PAI DEP correlated .55 with MMPI-2-RF RC7 (Dysfunctional Negative Emotions) and .70 with RC2 (Low Positive Emotions), whereas PAI ARD correlated .45 with RC2 and .70 with RC7, suggesting that the PAI and MMPI-2-RF operate similarly in terms of distinguishing fear and distress disorders.

PAI scales are also available for the targeting of specific constructs within this domain. The DEP and ANX scales have the strongest loadings on the internalizing factor. Both of these scales have subscales focused on the affective, cognitive, and physiological aspects of the constructs, which generally tend to be related to the distress aspects of that factor. The one exception is the ANX-Physiological subscale, which, together with the ARD-Phobias subscale, is the most specific to fear symptoms involving panic and phobias among PAI scales. For instance, in the initial validation studies, Morey (1991) showed that ANX-Physiological correlated .62 and ARD-Phobias correlated .60 with the MMPI Wiggins Phobias Content Scale, whereas the average correlation between MMPI Phobias and other PAI ANX and ARD scale correlations was .37.

Several PAI scales can be used to assess other, more specific problems on the internalizing spectrum. For instance, an emerging literature supports the validity of the PAI, and particularly the ARD-Traumatic Stress scale, for assessing post-traumatic symptoms (e.g., Edens & Ruiz, 2005). In addition, the ARD-T scale had a sensitivity of 79% and a specificity of 88% for a PTSD diagnosis based on the Clinician Administered PTSD Scale in a group of women who had been exposed to traumatic events (McDevitt-Murphy, Weathers, Adkins, & Daniels, 2005). The PAI Suicidal Ideation (SUI) scale has been shown to be a valid indicator of suicidal behavior (Hopwood, Baker, & Morey, 2008). The PAI Somatic Complaints (SOM) scale, which typically loads on the internalizing factor of the PAI, focuses on common health concerns, the somatization of psychological symptoms, and the presence of bizarre or unlikely symptoms. The SOM scale has been shown to be sensitive to a variety of health conditions, such as headaches (Brendza, Ashton, Windover, & Stillman, 2005), pain (Karlin et al., 2006), and diabetes (Jacobi, 2002).

Externalizing

The second factor that is typically extracted in factor analyses of the PAI has the strongest loadings on Antisocial Features (ANT), Alcohol Problems (ALC), and Drug Problems (DRG), implying an underlying externalizing dimension. The ANT scale has subscales measuring antisocial behaviors directly, as well subscales that measure psychopathic features including callous egocentricity and sensation-seeking. These scales have demonstrated empirical validity in discriminating disorders from the externalizing spectrum. For instance, Edens, Buffington-Vollum, Colwell, Johnson, and Johnson (2002) reported an area under the curve (AUC) of .70 using the ANT scale to indicate categorical psychopathy diagnoses based on the Psychopathy Checklist–Revised (Hare, 2003), whereas Ruiz, Dickinson, and Pincus (2002) reported an AUC of .84 using the ALC scale to predict interview-based alcohol dependence.

Antagonism

A third factor that is often extracted in factor analyses of the PAI scales has its strongest loadings on Mania (MAN), Dominance (DOM), and Aggression (AGG).[3] Common among these scales is a tendency toward self-importance, controlling behavior, and interpersonal insensitivity, which are collectively similar to the personality construct Antagonism and the liability toward callousness-aggression that emerges in structural psychopathology models. The MAN scale has specific subscales measuring irritability and frustration tolerance, grandiosity and self-esteem, and energy or activity. The Aggression (AGG) scale also generally exhibits strong loadings on the PAI externalizing factors, and has scales sampling behaviors related to an aggressive attitude, verbally aggressive behavior, and physically aggressive behavior. An emerging body of research, mostly in forensic samples, speaks to the validity of AGG to be associated with and predictive of violent and other aggressive behaviors (e.g., Edens & Ruiz, 2005; see also Gardner et al., 2015, for a meta-analysis).

Detachment

In other samples, such as the PAI community normative sample, the fourth factor has its highest loadings on high Nonsupport (NON) and low Warmth (WRM), implying social detachment, disconnection, and introversion, akin to the social-detachment/introversion factor that emerges from structural models of psychopathology and personality discussed earlier. In addition to these scales, numerous PAI scales provide additional information about this aspect of personality and psychopathology. In particular, the Schizophrenia (SCZ) Social Detachment subscale provides a direct assessment of disconnection from the social environment, which is common among psychotic individuals, but is also a common concern among individuals with other forms of psychopathology.

Thought Dysfunction

Although thought disorder is often identified as a major spectrum of psychopathology and is often reflected in one of the major factors explaining covariation in MMPI-2-RF scales, it has not been identified in factor analyses of the PAI full scales. One reason for this finding has to do with participant sampling, insofar as no factor analyses have been based on samples with a high representation of psychotic individuals. A second reason has to do with the proportion of scales on the PAI targeting thought dysfunction. Only two full scales, Schizophrenia (SCZ) and Paranoia (PAR), directly target psychotic content, and several of the subscales of those full scales will tend to relate more strongly to other factors (such as social detachment, as described above). Like other broadband measures with a relatively small number of scales tapping thought dysfunction (e.g., the Schedule for Nonadaptive and Adaptive Personality [SNAP] or Dimensional Assessment of Personality Pathology [DAPP]), the proportion of content on the PAI may not be sufficient to yield a robust thought-dysfunction factor. That being said, the PAI scales have been shown to be empirically effective in distinguishing between individuals with and without psychotic disorders. For example, Klonsky (2004) reported an effect size difference of $d = 1.29$ in distinguishing schizophrenic and non-schizophrenic patients using PAI SCZ.

CONCLUSIONS AND FUTURE DIRECTIONS

In the past several decades, empirical literature has clearly supported a dimensionally based MCLM hierarchy for psychopathology, which defies current thematic organizations represented in diagnostic manuals. These dimensional models are likely to be more useful to neuropsychology and mental health practitioners because research continues to identify and elaborate on neurobiological and psychosocial referents for the liability factors, rather than focus on distinct and fallacious categories of disorder. In this chapter, we have reviewed how two of the most commonly used, omnibus personality inventories in psychological practice, the MMPI-2-RF and PAI, map onto these empirical psychopathology structures. The results are quite impressive for both inventories, and it is important to note that none of these analyses was ever rigged or otherwise set up to confirm the extant structures, rather, exploratory analyses identified them in parallel. Subsequent validity research on both MMPI-2-RF and PAI scale scores clearly indicates that the higher-order structures and the scales that compose them reflect constructs that are located within nomological networks similar to those in the extant literature. Therefore, clinical neuropsychologists and other mental health practitioners who use these inventories in practice can rest assured that their scale scores map onto contemporary and empirically validated models of psychopathology, as well as can be used to generate hypotheses about diagnostic considerations (based on current nosologies) and standing on individual difference personality traits.

Even in light of these sanguine conclusions, there is still much work needed in both empirical investigations of psychopathology structures and the assessment of these structures as we move forward. As would be expected from the methods used to conduct latent-structure analyses, many of our current concepts of the structure of psychopathology, such as that represented in the MCLM, are a result of the types of symptoms and difficulties that were examined, as well as the types of individuals who were included in the studies' samples. We have tried to highlight in this chapter the effects of these methodological issues with our inclusion of three-, four-, and five-factor models of psychopathology. However, our understanding of psychopathology from a dimensional point of view is ever evolving. Future research is needed to reconcile current ambiguities (e.g., an independent somatization factor?) and to further establish a replicable structure that accounts for more of the dysfunctions practitioners encounter in their diverse practices (e.g., impulse-control disorders, eating disorders, paraphilias). Equally important for future work is ensuring that assessment instruments already in use, such as the MMPI-2-RF and the PAI, map onto emerging personality/psychopathology structures. Research of this type allows us to bridge the divide between categorical conceptualizations currently necessary for medical documentation and financial reimbursements and dimensional models that allow large bodies of clinical science research to be more easily applied in routine practice. These efforts will require that both assessment scholars and practitioners move away from the categorical thinking about psychological dysfunctions we have all been trained to use, as well as crystallized beliefs about the distinctions between psychopathology and personality. The previous efforts reviewed in this chapter represent the first steps toward this type of work, both in terms of central liabilities leading to mental difficulties and how our major assessment instruments conform to these structures. However, it should be clear that much additional work is needed, especially concerning mapping existing scales onto more specific liabilities in personality and psychopathology hierarchies.

AUTHOR NOTES

Tayla T. C. Lee is with the Department of Psychological Science, Ball State University, Muncie, Indiana; Martin Sellbom is with the Department of

Psychology, University of Otago, Dunedin, New Zealand; Christopher J. Hopwood is with the Department of Psychology, Michigan State University, East Lansing, Michigan. Lee's work on this chapter was supported by the National Institute on Alcohol Abuse and Alcoholism (T32 AA007462).

Correspondence concerning this chapter should be sent to Assoc. Prof. Martin Sellbom, Department of Psychology, PO Box 56, University of Otago, Dunedin 9054, New Zealand. E-mail: msellbom@psy.otago.ac.nz.

NOTES

1. To our knowledge, the model being described in this chapter has not been given an official name, perhaps because this would not be in the "model in development" spirit that pervades conclusions sections in reports of these studies. For ease of reference, we have given the model a name in this chapter. Although it is a mouthful, we hope the reader will forgive us for choosing "Multivariate Correlated Liabilities Model." We chose this name because the discussed models represent multivariate extensions of the Correlated Liabilities Model (Klein & Riso, 1993; Neale & Kendler, 1995).
2. The latter abstraction is typically psychoticism/thought dysfunction when sufficient indicators of such individual differences are included; however, when predominant measures of the five-factor model are used, openness tends to appear at the fifth level.
3. The nature of the third factor tends to depend on the sample in which the analysis is conducted (see, for example, Morey, 2007; and Hoelzle & Meyer, 2009).

REFERENCES

American Psychiatric Association. (2013). *Diagnostic and Statistical Manual of Mental Disorders, Fifth Edition*. Arlington, VA: APA.

Anderson, J. L., Sellbom, M., Ayearst, L., Quilty, L. C., Chmielewski, M., & Bagby, R. M. (2015). Associations between DSM-5 Section III personality traits and the Minnesota Multiphasic Personality Inventory 2–Restructured Form (MMPI-2-RF) scales in a psychiatric patient sample. *Psychological Assessment, 27*, 801–815.

Anderson, J. L., Sellbom, M., Bagby, R. M., Quilty, L. C., Veltri, C. O. C., Markon, K. E., & Krueger, R. F. (2013). On the convergence between PSY-5 domains and PID-5 domains and facets: Implications for assessment of DSM-5 personality traits. *Assessment, 20*, 286–294.

Arbisi, P. A., Sellbom, M., & Ben-Porath, Y. S. (2008). Empirical correlates of the MMPI-2 Restructured Clinical (RC) scales in an inpatient sample. *Journal of Personality Assessment, 90*, 122–128.

Arbisi, P. A., Polusny, M. A., Erbes, C. R., Thuras, P., & Reddy, M. K. (2011). The Minnesota Multiphasic Personality Inventory–2 Restructured Form in National Guard soldiers screening positive for posttraumatic stress disorder and mild traumatic brain injury. *Psychological Assessment, 23*, 203–214.

Bagby, R. M., Sellbom, M., Ayearst, L. E., Chmielewski, M. S., Anderson, J. L., & Quilty, L. C. (2014). Exploring the hierarchical structure of the MMPI-2-RF Personality Psychopathology Five in psychiatric patient and university student samples. *Journal of Personality Assessment, 96*, 166–172.

Ben-Porath, Y. S., & Tellegen, A. (2008). *MMPI-2-RF (Minnesota Multiphasic Personality Inventory–2 Restructured Form): Manual for Administration, Scoring, and Interpretation*. Minneapolis, MN: University of Minnesota Press.

Blackwood, N. J., Howard, R. J., Bentall, R. P., & Murray, R. M. (2001). Cognitive neuropsychiatric models of persecutory delusions. *American Journal of Psychiatry 158*, 527–539.

Brady, K. T., & Sinha, R. (2005). Co-occurring mental and substance use disorders: The neurobiological effects of chronic stress. *American Journal of Psychiatry, 162*, 1483–1493.

Brendza, D., Ashton, K., Windover, A., & Stillman, M. (2005). Personality Assessment Inventory predictors of therapeutic success or failure in chronic headache patients. *The Journal of Pain, 6*, 81.

Brown, T. A., & Barlow, D. H. (2005). Categorical vs. dimensional classification of mental disorders in DSM-V and beyond. *Journal of Abnormal Psychology, 114*, 551–556.

Caspi, A., Houts, R. M., Belsky, D. W., Goldman-Meilor, S. J., Harrington, H., Israel, S., . . . Moffit, T. E. (2014). The p factor: One general psychopathology factor in the structure of psychiatric disorders? *Clinical Psychological Science, 2*, 119–137.

Chmielewski, M., & Watson, D. (2007, October). *Oddity: The Third Higher Order Factor of Psychopathology.* Poster presented at the 21st Annual Meeting of the Society for Research in Psychopathology, Iowa City, IA.

Costa, P. T. Jr., & McCrae, R. R. (1985). *NEO Personality Inventory Manual.* Odessa, FL: Psychological Assessment Resources.

Cox, B. J., Clara, I. P., & Enns, M. W. (2002). Posttraumatic stress disorder and the structure of common mental disorders. *Depression & Anxiety, 15*(4), 168–171.

Cronbach, L. J, & Meehl, P. E. (1955). Construct validity in psychological tests. *Psychological Bulletin, 52*, 281–302.

Eaton, N. R., South, S. C., & Krueger, R. F. (2010). The meaning of comorbidity among common mental disorders. In T. Millon, R. F. Krueger, & E. Simonson (Eds.), *Contemporary Directions in Psychopathology. Scientific Foundations of the DSM-V and ICD-11* (pp. 223–241). New York: The Guilford Press.

Edens, J. F., Buffington-Vollum, J. K., Colwell, K. W., Johnson, D. W., & Johnson, J. K. (2002). Psychopathy and institutional misbehavior among incarcerated sex offenders: A comparison of the Psychopathy Checklist–Revised and the Personality Assessment Inventory. *International Journal of Forensic Mental Health, 1*, 49–58.

Edens, J. F., & Ruiz, M. A. (2005). *PAI Interpretive Report for Correctional Settings Professional Manual.* Lutz, LF: Psychological Assessment Resources.

Fantoni-Salvador, P., & Rogers, R. (1997). Spanish versions of the MMPI-2 and PAI: An investigation of concurrent validity with Hispanic patients. *Assessment, 4*, 29–39.

Finn, J. A., Arbisi, P. A., Erbes, C. R., Polusny, M. A., & Thuras, P. (2014). The MMPI-2 Restructured Form Personality Psychopathology Five Scales: Bridging DSM-5 Section 2 personality disorders and DSM-5 Section 3 personality trait dimensions. *Journal of Personality Assessment, 96*, 173–184.

Fleming, S., Shevlin, M., Murphy, J., & Joseph, S. (2014). Psychosis within dimensional and categorical models of mental illness. *Psychosis, 6*, 4–15.

Forbes, D., Elhai, J. D., Miller, M. W., & Creamer, M. (2010). Internalizing and externalizing classes in posttraumatic stress disorder: A latent class analysis. *Journal of Traumatic Stress, 23*, 340–349.

Gardner, B. O., Boccaccini, M. T., Bitting, B. S., & Edens, J. F. (2015). Personality Assessment Inventory Scores as predictors of misconduct, recidivism, and violence: A meta-analytic review. *Psychological Assessment, 27*, 534–544.

Gervais, R. O., Ben-Porath, Y. S., & Wygant, D. B. (2009). Empirical correlates and interpretation of the MMPI-2-RF Cognitive Complaints Scale. *The Clinical Neuropsychologist, 23*, 996–1015.

Goldberg, L. R. (2006). Doing it all bass-ackwards: The development of hierarchical factor structures from the top down. *Journal of Research in Personality, 40*, 347–358.

Grant, B. F., Stinson, F. S., Dawson, D. A., Chou, P., Dufour, M. C., Compton, W., . . . Kaplan, K. (2004). Prevalence and co-occurrence of substance use disorders and independent mood and anxiety disorders. *Archives of General Psychiatry, 61*, 807–816.

Grant, B. F., Stinson, F. S., Dawson, D. A., Chou, F. S., Ruan, W. J., & Pickering, R. P. (2004). Co-occurrence of 12-month alcohol and drug use disorders and personality disorders in the United States. *Archives of General Psychiatry, 61*, 361–368.

Handel, R. W., & Archer, R. P. (2008). An investigation of the psychometric properties of the MMPI-2 Restructured Clinical (RC) Scales with mental health inpatients. *Journal of Personality Assessment, 90*, 239–249.

Hare, R. D. (2003). The Hare Psychopathy Checklist–Revised. Toronto: Multi-Health Systems.

Harkness, A. R., & McNulty, J. L. (1994). The Personality Psychopathology Five (PSY-5): Issues from the pages of a diagnostic manual instead of a dictionary. In S. Strack & M. Lorr (Eds.), *Differentiating Normal and Abnormal Personality* (pp. 291–315). New York: Springer.

Harkness, A. R., McNulty, J. L., Finn, J. A., Reynolds, S. M, & Shields, S. M. (2014). The MMPI-2-RF Personality Psychopathology Five (PSY-5) Scales: Development and validity research. *Journal of Personality Assessment, 96*, 140–150.

Hart, S. D., Cox, D. N., & Hare, R. D. (1995). *Manual for the Psychopathy Checklist—Screening Version (PCL-SV)*. Toronto, Ontario: Multi-Health Systems.

Hathaway, S. R., & McKinley, J. C. (1943). *The Minnesota Multiphasic Personality Inventory Manual*. New York: Psychological Corporation.

Hoelzle, J. B., & Meyer, G. J. (2008). The factor structure of the MMPI-2 Restructured Clinical (RC) Scales. *Journal of Personality Assessment, 90*, 443–455.

Hoelzle, J. B., & Meyer, G. J. (2009). The invariant component structure of the Personality Assessment Inventory (PAI) full scales. *Journal of Personality Assessment, 91*, 175–186.

Hopwood, C. J., Baker, K., & Morey, L. C. (2008). Extra-test validity of the Personality Assessment Inventory scales and indicators in an inpatient substance abuse setting. *Journal of Personality Assessment, 90*, 574–577.

Hopwood, C. J., & Sellbom, M. (2013). Implications of DSM-5 personality traits for forensic psychology. *Psychological Injury and Law, 6*, 314–323.

Hopwood, C. J., Wright, A. G. C., Krueger, R. F., Schade, N., Markon, K. E., & Morey, L. C. (2013). DSM-5 pathological personality traits and the Personality Assessment Inventory. *Assessment, 20*, 269–285.

Jackson, D. N. (1971). The dynamics of structured personality tests. *Psychological Review, 78*, 229–248.

Jacobi, S. G. (2002). Effects of Psychological Differentiation on Success with Self-Management of Diabetes. Doctoral dissertation, Columbia University.

Johnson, A. K., Sellbom, M., & Phillips, T. R. (2014). Elucidating the associations between psychopathy, Gray's Reinforcement Sensitivity Theory constructs, and externalizing behavior. *Personality and Individual Differences, 71*, 1–8.

Karlin, B. E., Creech, S. K., Grimes, J. S., Clark, T. S., Meagher, M. W., & Morey, L. C. (2006). The Personality Assessment Inventory with chronic pain patients: Psychometric properties and clinical utility. *Journal of Clinical Psychology, 61*, 1571–1585.

Katz, L. Y., Cox, B. J., Clara, I. P., Oleski, J., & Sacevich, T. (2011). Substance abuse versus dependence and the structure of common mental disorders. *Comprehensive Psychiatry, 52*, 638–643.

Kendler, K. S., Prescott, C. A., Myers, J., & Neale, M. C. (2003). The structure of genetic and environmental risk factors for common psychiatric and substance use disorders in men and women. *Archives of General Psychiatry, 60,* 929–937.

Kessler, R. C., Adler, L., Barkley, R., Biederman, J., Conners, C. K., Demler, O., . . . Zaslavsky, A. M. (2006). The prevalence and correlates of adult ADHD in the United States: Results from the National Comorbidity Survey Replication. *American Journal of Psychiatry, 163,* 716–723.

Kessler, R. C., Chiu, W. T., Demler, O., & Walters, E. E. (2005). Prevalence, severity, and comorbidity of twelve-month DSM-IV disorders in the National Comorbidity Survey Replication (NCS-R). *Archives of General Psychiatry, 62,* 617–627.

Kessler, R. C., & Wang, P. S. (2008). The descriptive epidemiology of commonly occurring mental disorders in the United States. *Annual Review of Public Health, 29,* 115–129.

Klein, D. N., & Riso, L. P. (1993). Psychiatric disorders: Problems of boundaries and comorbidity. In C. G. Costello (Ed.), *Basic Issues in Psychopathology* (pp. 19–66). New York: Guilford Press.

Klonsky, E. D. (2004). Performance of Personality Assessment Inventory and Rorschach indices of schizophrenia in a public psychiatric hospital. *Psychological Services, 1,* 107–110.

Koffel, E., Polusny, M. A., Arbisi, P. A., & Erbes, C. R. (2012). A preliminary investigation of the new and revised symptoms of posttraumatic stress disorder in DSM-5. *Depression and Anxiety, 29,* 731–738.

Kotov, R., Chang, S. W., Fochtmann, L. J., Mojtabai, R., Carlson, G. A., Sedler, M. J., & Bromet, E. J. (2011). Schizophrenia in the internalizing-externalizing framework: A third dimension? *Schizophrenia Bulletin, 37,* 1168–1178.

Kotov, R., Ruggero, C. J., Krueger, R. F., Watson, D., Qilong, Y., & Zimmerman, M. (2011). New dimensions in the quantitative classification of mental illness. *Archives of General Psychiatry, 68,* 1003–1011.

Kramer, M. D., Krueger, R. F., & Hicks, B. M. (2008). The role of internalizing and externalizing liability factors in accounting for gender differences in the prevalence of common psychopathological syndromes. *Psychological Medicine, 38,* 51–62.

Krueger, R. F. (1999). The structure of common mental disorders. *Archives of General Psychiatry, 56,* 921–926.

Krueger, R. F., Capsi, A., Moffitt, T. E., & Silva, P. A. (1998). The structure and stability of common mental disorders (DSM-III-R): A longitudinal-epidemiological study. *Journal of Abnormal Psychology, 107,* 216–227.

Krueger, R. F., Chentsova-Dutton, Y. E., Markon, K. E., Goldberg, D., & Ormel, J. (2003). A cross-cultural study of the structure of comorbidity among common psychopathological syndromes in the general health care setting. *Journal of Abnormal Psychology, 112,* 437–447.

Krueger, R. F., Derringer, J., Markon, K. E., Watson, D., & Skodol, A. E. (2012). Initial construction of a maladaptive personality trait model and inventory for *DSM-5*. *Psychological Medicine, 42,* 1879–1890.

Krueger, R. F., Hicks, B. M., Patrick, C. J., Carlson, S. R., Iacono, W. G., & McGue, M. (2002). Etiologic connections among substance dependence, antisocial behavior, and personality: Modeling the externalizing spectrum. *Journal of Abnormal Psychology, 111,* 411–474.

Krueger, R. F., & Markon, K. E. (2006). Reinterpreting comorbidity: A model-based approach to understanding and classifying psychopathology. *Annual Review of Clinical Psychology, 2,* 111–133.

Krueger, R. F., & Markon, K. E. (2014). The role of the DSM-5 personality trait model in moving toward a quantitative and empirically based approach to classifying personality and psychopathology. *Annual Review of Clinical Psychology, 10,* 477–501.

Krueger, R. F., Markon, K. E., Patrick, C. J., Benning, S. D., & Kramer, M. D. (2007). Linking antisocial behavior, substance use, and personality: An integrative quantitative model of the adult externalizing spectrum. *Journal of Abnormal Psychology, 116,* 645–666.

Krueger, R. F., McGue, M., & Iacono, W. G. (2001). The higher-order structure of common DSM mental disorders: Internalization, externalization, and their connections to personality. *Personality and Individual Differences, 30,* 1245–1259.

Kushner, S. C., Quilty, L. C., Tackett, J. L., & Bagby, R. M. (2011). The hierarchical structure of the dimensional assessment of personality pathology (DAPP–BQ). *Journal of Personality Disorders, 25,* 504–516.

Lahey, B. B., Rathouz, P. J., Van Hulle, C., Urbano, R. C., Krueger, R. F., Applegate, B., Garriock, H. A., . . . Waldman, I. D. (2008). Testing structural models of DSM-IV symptoms of common forms of child and adolescent psychopathology. *Journal of Abnormal Child Psychopathology, 36,* 187–206.

Lahey, B. B., Applegate, B., Hakes, J. K., Zald, D. H., Hariri, A. R., & Rathouz, P. J. (2012). Is there a general factor of prevalent psychopathology during adulthood? *Journal of Abnormal Psychology, 121,* 971–977.

Lahey, B. B., Van Hulle, C. A., Singh, A. L., Waldman, I. D. & Rathouz, P. J. (2011). Higher-order genetic and environmental structure of prevalent forms of child and adolescent psychopathology. *Archives of General Psychiatry, 68,* 181–189.

Lilienfeld, S. O., & Andrews, B. P. (1996). Development and preliminary validation of a self-report measure of psychopathic personality traits in noncriminal population. *Journal of Personality Assessment, 66,* 488–524.

Locke, D. E. C., Kirlin, K. A., Thomas, M. L., Osborne, D., Hurst, D. F., Drazkowsi, J. F., Sirven, J. I., & Noe, K. H. (2010). The Minnesota Multiphasic Personality Inventory Restructured Form in the epilepsy monitoring unit. *Epilepsy and Behavior, 17,* 252–258.

Loevinger, J. (1957). Objective tests as instruments of psychological theory. *Psychological Reports, 3,* 653–694.

Markon, K. E., Krueger, R. F., & Watson, D. (2005). Delineating the structure of normal and abnormal personality: An integrative hierarchical approach. *Journal of Personality and Social Psychology, 88,* 139–157.

McDevitt-Murphy, M. E., Weathers, F. W., Adkins, J. W., & Daniels, J. B. (2005). Use of the Personality Assessment Inventory in the assessment of post-traumatic stress disorder in women. *Journal of Psychopathology and Behavior Assessment, 27,* 57–65.

McNulty, J. L., & Overstreet, S. R. (2014). Viewing the MMPI-2-RF structure through the Personality Psychopathology Five (PSY-5) lens. *Journal of Personality Assessment, 96,* 151–157.

Miller, M. W., Wolf, E. J., Harrington, K. M., Brown, T. A., Kaloupek, D. G., & Keane, T. M. (2010). An evaluation of competing models for the structure of PTSD symptoms using external measures of comorbidity. *Journal of Traumatic Stress, 23,* 631–638.

Morey, L. C. (1991). *Professional Manual for the Personality Assessment Inventory.* Odessa, FL: Psychological Assessment Resources.

Morey, L. C. (2007). *Professional Manual for the Personality Assessment Inventory, Second Edition.* Lutz, FL: Psychological Assessment Resources.

Morey, L. C., & Hopwood, C. J. (200). The Personality Assessment Inventory and the measurement of normal and abnormal personality constructs. In S. Strack (Ed.), *Differentiating Normal and Abnormal Personality* (2nd ed., pp. 451–471). New York: Springer.

Neale, M. C., & Kendler, K. S. (1995). Models of comorbidity for multifactorial disorders. *American Journal of Human Genetics, 57,* 935–953.

O'Connor, B. P. (2002). A quantitative review of the comprehensiveness of the five-factor model in relation to popular personality inventories. *Assessment, 9,* 188–203.

Patrick, C. J., & Drislane, L. E. (2015). Triarchic model of psychopathy: Origins, operationalizations, and observed linkages with personality and general psychopathology. *Journal of Personality, 83,* 627–643.

Phillips, T. R., Sellbom, M., Ben-Porath, Y. S., & Patrick, C. J. (2014). Further development and construct validation of MMPI-2-RF indices of Global Psychopathy, Fearless-Dominance, and Impulsive-Antisociality in a sample of incarcerated women. *Law and Human Behavior, 28,* 34–46.

Reiger, D. A., Farmer, M. E., Rae, D. S., Locke, B. Z., Keith, S. J., Judd, L. L., & Goodwin, F. (1990). Comorbidity of mental disorders with alcohol and other drug abuse. Results from the Epidemiologic Catchment Area (ECA) study. *Journal of the American Medical Association, 264,* 2511–2518.

Ruiz, M. A., Dickinson, K. A., & Pincus, A. L. (2002). Concurrent validity of the Personality Assessment Inventory Alcohol Problems (ALC) scale in a college student sample. *Assessment, 9,* 261–270.

Sellbom, M. (2010, March). *The MMPI-2-RF Externalizing Scales: Hierarchical Structure and Links to Contemporary Models of Psychopathology.* Paper presented at the 2010 Annual Meeting of the American Psychology-Law Society, Vancouver, BC, Canada.

Sellbom, M. (2011, September). *Exploring Psychopathology Structure Empirically Through an Omnibus Clinical Assessment Tool: Reintegrating the MMPI into Contemporary Psychopathology Research.* Paper presented at the 2011 Annual Meeting of the Society for Research on Psychopathology, Boston, MA.

Sellbom, M., Bagby, R. M., Kushner, S., Quilty, L. C., & Ayearst, L. E. (2012). The diagnostic construct validity of MMPI-2 Restructured Form (MMPI-2-RF) scale scores. *Assessment, 19,* 185–195.

Sellbom, M., Ben-Porath, Y. S., & Bagby, R. M. (2008a). On the hierarchical structure of mood and anxiety disorders: Confirmatory evidence and an elaborated model of temperament markers. *Journal of Abnormal Psychology, 117,* 576–590.

Sellbom, M., Ben-Porath, Y. S., & Bagby, R. M. (2008b). Personality and psychopathology: Mapping the MMPI-2 Restructured Clinical (RC) scales onto the five-factor model of personality. *Journal of Personality Disorders, 22,* 291–312.

Sellbom, M., Ben-Porath, Y. S., & Graham, J. R. (2006). Correlates of the MMPI–2 Restructured Clinical (RC) scales in a college counseling setting. *Journal of Personality Assessment, 86,* 88–99.

Sellbom, M., Ben-Porath, Y. S., Lilienfeld, S. O., Patrick, C. J., & Graham, J. R. (2005). Assessing psychopathic personality traits with the MMPI-2. *Journal of Personality Assessment, 85,* 334–343.

Sellbom, M., Ben-Porath, Y. S., & Stafford, K. S. (2007). A comparison of MMPI-2 measures of psychopathic deviance in a forensic setting. *Psychological Assessment, 19,* 430–436.

Sellbom, M., Lee, T. T. C., Ben-Porath, Y. S., Arbisi, P. A., & Gervais, R. O. (2012). Differentiating PTSD symptomatology with the MMPI-2-RF (Restructured Form) in a forensic disability sample. *Psychiatry Research, 197,* 172–179.

Sellbom, M., Marion, B. E., Kastner, R. M., Rock, R. C., Anderson, J. L., Salekin, R. T., & Krueger, R. F. (2012, October). *Externalizing Spectrum of Psychopathology: Associations with DSM-5 Personality Traits and Neurocognitive Tasks*. Paper presented at the 2012 Annual Meeting of the Society for Research on Psychopathology, Ann Arbor, MI.

Sellbom, M., Smid, W., De Saeger, H., Smit, N., & Kamphuis, J. H. (2014). Mapping the Personality Psychopathology Five Domains onto DSM-IV personality disorders in Dutch clinical and forensic samples: Implications for the DSM-5. *Journal of Personality Assessment, 96,* 185–192.

Sellbom, M., Titcomb, C., & Arbisi, P. A. (2011, May). *Clarifying the Hierarchical Structure of Positive Psychotic Symptoms: The MMPI-2-RF as a Road Map*. Paper presented at the 46th Annual Symposium on Recent MMPI-2, MMPI-2-RF, and MMPI-A Research, Minneapolis, MN.

Slade, T., & Watson, D. (2006). The structure of common DSM-IV and ICD-10 mental disorders in the Australian general population. *Psychological Medicine, 35,* 1593–1600.

Tackett, J. L., Quilty, L. C., Sellbom, M., Rector, N. A., & Bagby, R. M. (2008). Additional evidence for a quantitative hierarchical model of the mood and anxiety disorders for DSM-V: The context of personality structure. *Journal of Abnormal Psychology, 117,* 812–825.

Tarescavage, A. M., Luna-Jones, L., & Ben-Porath, Y. S. (2014). Minnesota Multiphasic Personality Inventory–2–Restructured Form (MMPI-2-RF) predictors of violating probation after felonious crimes. *Psychological Assessment, 26,* 1375–1380.

Tellegen, A. (1985). Structures of mood and personality and their relevance to assessing anxiety, with an emphasis on self-report. In A. H. Tuma & J. D. Maser (Eds.), *Anxiety and the Anxiety Disorders* (pp. 681–706). Hillsdale, NJ: Erlbaum.

Tellegen, A., & Ben-Porath, Y. S. (2008). *MMPI-2-RF (Minnesota Multiphasic Personality Inventory–2 Restructured Form): Technical Manual*. Minneapolis, MN: University of Minnesota Press.

Tellegen, A., Ben-Porath, Y. S., McNulty, J. L., Arbisi, P. A., Graham, J. R., & Kaemmer, B. (2003). *MMPI-2 Restructured Clinical (RC) Scales: Development, Validation, and Interpretation*. Minneapolis, MN: University of Minnesota Press.

Thomas, M. L., & Locke, D. E. C. (2010). Psychometric properties of the MMPI-2-RF Somatic Complaints (RC1) scale. *Psychological Assessment, 22,* 492–503.

Titcomb, C., Sellbom, M., Cohen, A., & Arbisi, P. A. (under review). *On the Structure of Positive Psychotic Symptomatology: Can Paranoia Be Modeled as a Separate Liability Factor*? Manuscript submitted for publication.

Van der Heijden, P. T., Egger, J. I. M., Rossi, G., & Derksen, J. J. L. (2012). Integrating psychopathology and personality disorders conceptualized by the MMPI-2-RF and the MCMI-III: A structural validity study. *Journal of Personality Assessment, 94,* 345–347.

Van der Heijden, P. T., Rossi, G. M., Van der Veld, M. M., Derksen, J. J. L., & Egger, J. I. M. (2013a). Personality and psychopathology: Higher order relations between the Five Factor Model of personality and the MMPI-2 Restructured Form. *Journal of Research in Personality, 47,* 572–579.

Van der Heijden, P. T., Rossi, G. M., Van der Veld, M. M., Derksen, J. J. L., & Egger, J. I. M (2013b). Personality and psychopathology: Mapping the MMPI-2-RF on Cloninger's psychobiological model of personality. *Assessment, 20,* 576–584.

Veltri, C. O. C., Williams, J. E., & Braxton, L. (2004, March). MMPI-2 Restructured Clinical scales and the Personality Assessment Inventory in a veteran sample.

Poster presented at the *Annual Meeting of the Society for Personality Assessment*, Chicago, IL.

Vollebergh, W. A. M., Iedema, J., Vijl, R. V., deGraaf, R., Smit, F., & Ormel, J. (2001). The structure and stability of common mental disorders: The NEMESIS study. *Archives of General Psychiatry, 58*, 597–603.

Watson, D. (2005). Rethinking the mood and anxiety disorders: A quantitative hierarchical model for *DSM–V. Journal of Abnormal Psychology, 114*, 522–536.

Watson, C., Quilty, L. C., & Bagby, R. M. (2011). Differentiating bipolar disorder from major depressive disorder using the MMPI-2-RF: A receiver operating characteristics (ROC) analysis. *Journal of Psychopathology and Behavioral Assessment, 33*, 368–374.

Watson, D., & Tellegen, A. (1985). Toward a consensual structure of mood. *Psychological Bulletin, 98*, 219–235.

Widiger, T. A., & Clark, L. A. (2000). Toward DSM-V and the classification of psychopathology. *Psychological Bulletin, 126*, 946–963.

Widiger, T. A., & Sankis, L. M. (2000). Adult psychopathology: Issues and controversies. *Annual Review of Psychology, 51*(1), 377–404.

Wolf, E. J., Miller, M. W., Orazem, R. J., Weierich, M. R., Castillo, D. T., Milford, J., . . . Keane, T. M. (2008). The MMPI-2 Restructured Clinical Scales in the assessment of posttraumatic stress disorder and comorbid disorders. *Psychological Assessment, 20*, 327–340.

Wright, A. G. C., Krueger, R. F., Hobbs, M. J., Markon, K. E., Eaton, N. R., & Slade, T. (2013). The structure of psychopathology: Toward an expanded quantitative empirical model. *Journal of Abnormal Psychology, 122*, 281–294.

Wright, A. G. C., & Simms, L. J. (2014). On the structure of personality disorder traits: Conjoint analyses of the CAT-PD, PID-5, and NEO-PI-3 trait models. *Personality Disorders: Theory, Research, and Treatment, 5*, 43–54.

Wright, A. G. C., Thomas, K. M., Hopwood, C. J., Markon, K. E., Pincus, A. L., & Krueger, R. F. (2012). The hierarchical structure of *DSM–5* pathological personality traits. *Journal of Abnormal Psychology, 121*, 951–957.

Wygant, D. B., & Sellbom, M. (2012). Viewing psychopathy from the perspective of the Personality Psychopathology Five Model: Implications for DSM-5. *Journal of Personality Disorders, 26*, 717–726.

5

When Is a Test Reliable Enough and Why Does It Matter?

STEPHEN C. BOWDEN AND SUE FINCH

It is important to recognize that any obtained score is only one in a probable range of scores whose size is inversely related to the test reliability. (Nunnally & Bernstein, 1994, p. 291)

There has never been any mathematical or substantive rebuttal of the main findings of psychometric theory. (Schmidt & Hunter, 1996, p. 199)

CLINICAL SCENARIO

A 67-year-old male patient is assessed after family physician referral for the evaluation of possible early dementia. In the context of no other significant illness, a family informant provides a history of minor everyday memory failures. Premorbid cognitive ability is judged to be of at least "high average" standing (corresponding to scores of 110 or above on a test of general cognitive ability, with a population mean of 100 and a standard deviation of 15; e.g., Wechsler, 2009) estimated from the patient's educational and occupational attainment. On a well-validated test of anterograde memory function (or long-term retrieval ability: see Chapter 3 in this volume), with the same population mean and standard deviation, the patient scored 115. Assuming a test score reliability of 0.95, a 95% confidence interval (CI) was constructed centered on the predicted true score of 114 (see section below "The Predicted True Score") and using the standard error of estimation (see section "The Family of Standard Errors of Measurement"). The 95% CI ranged from 108–121 (see Table 5.1). This CI includes the estimated premorbid range of ability, namely, above an Index score of 110. Hence the examining clinician concluded there was no objective evidence to infer that anterograde memory function is below that expected on the basis of premorbid estimates, with 95% confidence. The clinician recommends a healthy lifestyle with regular cognitive stimulation and a wait-and-see approach to the diagnosis of early dementia.

Table 5.1 Predicted true scores with 95% confidence intervals (95% CI) for different
of 100 and a standard deviation of 15, illustrated for alternative reliability values
intervals are centered on the predicted true score (**bolded**) and calculated with the
are shown for a range of Intelligence Index scale scores from 55 (z = −3) to 145 (z = +3).

		$r_{xx} = 0.1$, $SE_{est} = 4.5$			$r_{xx} = 0.3$, $SE_{est} = 6.9$			$r_{xx} = 0.5$, $SE_{est} = 7.5$	
Observed score	*z*-score	Lower bound (95%CI)	Predicted True Score	Upper bound (95%CI)	Lower bound (95%CI)	Predicted True Score	Upper bound (95%CI)	Lower bound (95%CI)	Predicted True Score
55	−3	87	**96**	104	73	**87**	100	63	**78**
60	−2.67	87	**96**	105	75	**88**	101	65	**80**
65	−2.33	88	**97**	105	76	**90**	103	68	**83**
70	−2	88	**97**	106	78	**91**	104	70	**85**
75	−1.67	89	**98**	106	79	**93**	106	73	**88**
80	−1.33	89	**98**	107	81	**94**	107	75	**90**
85	−1	90	**99**	107	82	**96**	109	78	**93**
90	−0.67	90	**99**	108	84	**97**	110	80	**95**
95	−0.33	91	**100**	108	85	**99**	112	83	**98**
100	0	91	**100**	109	87	**100**	113	85	**100**
105	0.33	92	**101**	109	88	**102**	115	88	**103**
110	0.67	92	**101**	110	90	**103**	116	90	**105**
115	1	93	**102**	110	91	**105**	118	93	**108**
120	1.33	93	**102**	111	93	**106**	119	95	**110**
125	1.67	94	**103**	111	94	**108**	121	98	**113**
130	2	94	**103**	112	96	**109**	122	100	**115**
135	2.33	95	**104**	112	97	**111**	124	103	**118**
140	2.67	95	**104**	113	99	**112**	125	105	**120**
145	3	96	**105**	113	100	**114**	127	108	**123**

Note: SE_{est} = Standard Error of estimation

OBSERVED TEST SCORES FROM A RANGE OF HYPOTHETICAL TESTS WITH A POPULATION MEAN
AND CORRESPONDING **STANDARD ERRORS OF ESTIMATION** ($SE_{estimation}$) VALUES. THE CONFIDENCE
STANDARD ERROR OF ESTIMATION. THE UPPER AND LOWER LIMITS OF THE CONFIDENCE INTERVALS
PREDICTED TRUE SCORES AND CONFIDENCE LIMITS ARE ROUNDED TO THE NEAREST WHOLE NUMBER

	$r_{xx} = 0.7$, $SE_{est} = 6.9$			$r_{xx} = 0.9$, $SE_{est} = 4.5$			$r_{xx} = 0.95$, $SE_{est} = 3.2$		
Upper bound (95%CI)	Lower bound (95%CI)	Predicted True Score	Upper bound (95%CI)	Lower bound (95%CI)	Predicted True Score	Upper bound (95%CI)	Lower bound (95%CI)	Predicted True Score	Upper bound (95%CI)
92	55	**69**	82	51	**60**	68	51	**57**	64
95	59	**72**	85	55	**64**	73	56	**62**	68
97	62	**76**	89	60	**69**	77	60	**67**	73
100	66	**79**	92	64	**73**	82	65	**72**	78
102	69	**83**	96	69	**78**	86	70	**76**	83
105	73	**86**	99	73	**82**	91	75	**81**	87
107	76	**90**	103	78	**87**	95	79	**86**	92
110	80	**93**	106	82	**91**	100	84	**91**	97
112	83	**97**	110	87	**96**	104	89	**95**	102
115	87	**100**	113	91	**100**	109	94	**100**	106
117	90	**104**	117	96	**105**	113	98	**105**	111
120	94	**107**	120	100	**109**	118	103	**110**	116
122	97	**111**	124	105	**114**	122	108	**114**	121
125	101	**114**	127	109	**118**	127	113	**119**	125
127	104	**118**	131	114	**123**	131	117	**124**	130
130	108	**121**	134	118	**127**	136	122	**129**	135
132	111	**125**	138	123	**132**	140	127	**133**	140
135	115	**128**	141	127	**136**	145	132	**138**	144
137	118	**132**	145	132	**141**	149	136	**143**	149

The patient was seen 18 months later. Self-report no different, family informant reiterating similar symptoms of memory failures, as before, and also increasing social withdrawal. Reassessment with the same test of anterograde memory function resulted in a score of 95. On the basis of test research data, practice effects were judged to be negligible over an 18-month retest interval. To evaluate the consistency of the memory test score at the second assessment with the performance at the first assessment, a 95% prediction interval using the standard error of prediction (see section "Prediction Interval for the True Score Based on the Standard Error of Prediction") was constructed using the 18-month retest reliability estimate of 0.9 available in the test manual. The prediction interval was centered on the predicted true score at Time 1 of 114, and ranged from 101–126 (see Table 5.2). The clinician noted that the Time 2 observed score fell below the lower bound of the prediction interval estimated from the Time 1 assessment, that is, the observed score was outside the range of predicted scores. The clinician concluded that anterograde memory function had most likely deteriorated, with 95% confidence. In this chapter, the methods of interval construction for clinical inference-making will be explained.

THE ROLE OF RELIABILITY IN TEST SCORE INTERPRETATION

Every test score or item of clinical information is less than perfectly reliable. Here, "reliability" is used in the technical sense, where test scores or clinical observations are used to evaluate a patient's current cognitive or broader psychological function. For clinical decision making, reliability is defined as the consistency in the information gathered from tests or other clinical observations. In the hypothetical situation where a test is administered to a person in a stable clinical state on many occasions, and setting aside the issue of practice effects, if the test score is highly reliable, similar scores on the test should be obtained on every occasion. If instead the test score is relatively unreliable, there will be considerable variation in the scores obtained on different occasions. Practice effects add an additional layer of complexity, which will be discussed toward the end of the chapter (see also Chapter 6 of this volume).

As the quote above from Nunnally and Bernstein (1994) describes, the best estimate of a person's score on a test should be accompanied by a measure of the uncertainty of that estimate, captured by a confidence interval (CI). Techniques for estimating CIs for one person's test score will be explained in this chapter. As Schmidt and Hunter (1996) imply, psychometrics—the science of psychological test score interpretation—relies on strong cumulative evidence from statistical theory, providing the scientific foundation for psychological test score interpretation. However, psychometrics is sometimes criticized as though it were incompatible with *pure* clinical judgement. Such a view is, instead, a repudiation of the scientific basis of psychological and neuropsychological assessment (American Educational Research Association, American Psychological Association, & National Council on Measurement in Education, 2014).

In addition, it is a common mistake to assume that consideration of reliability only applies to formal test scores with known reliabilities, and that avoidance of formal tests permits the avoidance of scientific evaluation of reliability and validity. The American Psychological Association Standards on Psychological Testing illustrate that consideration of reliability applies to all information used to evaluate a patient's circumstances, whether that information is derived from formal tests, structured or informal interviews, other professionals, or an informant or collateral source (American Educational Research Association et al., 2014). Every item of clinically relevant information, not just test scores, comes with uncertainty. Scientific psychology allows the quantification of reliability for any test score or any clinical observation and allows incorporation of the effects of the reliability into scientific clinical thinking, whether the reliability is high or low (Nunnally & Bernstein, 1994).

Making explicit the uncertainty in a test score is a core technical skill in psychological assessment. The core techniques involve interval estimation. Most psychology graduates are familiar with the technique of CI estimation for a population mean (Cumming & Finch, 2005; Nunnally & Bernstein, 1994). Here is an important distinction to make. A CI for a population mean, centred on a sample mean, characterizes the uncertainty in the estimate of the mean of a population of individuals. In a clinical setting, with a single individual participating in a clinical assessment, the estimate of interest is an individual true score. In the case of individual assessment, we need to characterize the uncertainty in the estimate of the individual score, using an interval. This uncertainty will be affected by the reliability of the test score.

METHODS FOR ESTIMATING THE RELIABILITY OF TEST SCORES

Detailed description of methods for estimating reliability is beyond the scope of this chapter but is available in a variety of sources (e.g., Anastasi & Urbini, 1997; Brennan, 2006; Nunnally & Bernstein, 1994; Sijtsma, 2009). However, it is important for all clinicians to have an intuitive understanding of what information is conveyed by a reliability coefficient. One of the simplest methods for estimating reliability involves correlating scores on a test administered to the same sample of people on two occasions (Anastasi & Urbini, 1997). If high consistency is sought in a test score, for example, over multiple assessment occasions, then a highly consistent test should show high correlations between pairs of measurements over any two occasions. This concept of reliability as the correlation of a test score obtained on two occasions is often denoted by the symbol r_{xx} to indicate that the reliability coefficient is a correlation of score x, on the two occasions. This property of reliability as test–retest correlation is shown in Figure 5.1 where two tests, one with higher reliability (A) and one with lower reliability (B), were administered to the same sample of clinical participants on two occasions, approximately two years apart. For clarity of illustration, Figure 5.1 shows a small representative sample of 15 participants, drawn from the larger clinical sample. The lines in Figure 5.1 connect the scores for each person on the two occasions.

Table 5.2 PREDICTED TRUE SCORES WITH 95% PREDICTION INTERVALS (95% PI) FOR DIFFERENT
OF 100 AND A STANDARD DEVIATION OF 15, ILLUSTRATED FOR ALTERNATIVE RELIABILITY VALUES
INTERVALS ARE CENTERED ON THE PREDICTED TRUE SCORE (**BOLDED**) AND CALCULATED WITH THE
ARE SHOWN FOR A RANGE OF INTELLIGENCE INDEX SCALE SCORES FROM 55 (Z = −3) TO 145 (Z = +3).

		r_{xx} = .1, SE_{pred} = 14.9			r_{xx} = .3, SE_{pred} = 14.3			r_{xx} = .5, SE_{pred} = 13.0	
Observed score	***z*-score**	**Lower bound (95%PI)**	**Predicted True Score**	**Upper bound (95%PI)**	**Lower bound (95%PI)**	**Predicted True Score**	**Upper bound (95%PI)**	**Lower bound (95%PI)**	**Predicted True Score**
55	−3	66	**96**	125	58	**87**	115	52	**78**
60	−2.67	67	**96**	125	60	**88**	116	55	**80**
65	−2.33	67	**97**	126	61	**90**	118	57	**83**
70	−2	68	**97**	126	63	**91**	119	60	**85**
75	−1.67	68	**98**	127	64	**93**	121	62	**88**
80	−1.33	69	**98**	127	66	**94**	122	65	**90**
85	−1	69	**99**	128	67	**96**	124	67	**93**
90	−0.67	70	**99**	128	69	**97**	125	70	**95**
95	−0.33	70	**100**	129	70	**99**	127	72	**98**
100	0	71	**100**	129	72	**100**	128	75	**100**
105	0.33	71	**101**	130	73	**102**	130	77	**103**
110	0.67	72	**101**	130	75	**103**	131	80	**105**
115	1	72	**102**	131	76	**105**	133	82	**108**
120	1.33	73	**102**	131	78	**106**	134	85	**110**
125	1.67	73	**103**	132	79	**108**	136	87	**113**
130	2	74	**103**	132	81	**109**	137	90	**115**
135	2.33	74	**104**	133	82	**111**	139	92	**118**
140	2.67	75	**104**	133	84	**112**	140	95	**120**
145	3	75	**105**	134	85	**114**	142	97	**123**

Note: SE_{pred} = Standard Error of prediction.

OBSERVED TEST SCORES FROM A RANGE OF HYPOTHETICAL TESTS WITH A POPULATION MEAN
AND CORRESPONDING **STANDARD ERROR OF PREDICTION** ($SE_{prediction}$) VALUES. THE PREDICTION
STANDARD ERROR OF PREDICTION. THE UPPER AND LOWER LIMITS OF THE PREDICTION INTERVALS
PREDICTED TRUE SCORES AND PREDICTION LIMITS ARE ROUNDED TO THE NEAREST WHOLE NUMBER

	r_{xx} = .7, SE_{pred} = 10.7			r_{xx} = .9, SE_{pred} = 6.5			r_{xx} = .95, SE_{pred} = 4.7		
Upper bound (95%PI)	**Lower bound (95%PI)**	**Predicted True Score**	**Upper bound (95%PI)**	**Lower bound (95%PI)**	**Predicted True Score**	**Upper bound (95%PI)**	**Lower bound (95%PI)**	**Predicted True Score**	**Upper bound (95%PI)**
103	48	**69**	89	47	**60**	72	48	**57**	66
105	51	**72**	93	51	**64**	77	53	**62**	71
108	55	**76**	96	56	**69**	81	58	**67**	76
110	58	**79**	100	60	**73**	86	62	**72**	81
113	62	**83**	103	65	**78**	90	67	**76**	85
115	65	**86**	107	69	**82**	95	72	**81**	90
118	69	**90**	110	74	**87**	99	77	**86**	95
120	72	**93**	114	78	**91**	104	81	**91**	100
123	76	**97**	117	83	**96**	108	86	**95**	104
125	79	**100**	121	87	**100**	113	91	**100**	109
128	83	**104**	124	92	**105**	117	96	**105**	114
130	86	**107**	128	96	**109**	122	100	**110**	119
133	90	**111**	131	101	**114**	126	105	**114**	123
135	93	**114**	135	105	**118**	131	110	**119**	128
138	97	**118**	138	110	**123**	135	115	**124**	133
140	100	**121**	142	114	**127**	140	119	**129**	138
143	104	**125**	145	119	**132**	144	124	**133**	142
145	107	**128**	149	123	**136**	149	129	**138**	147
148	111	**132**	152	128	**141**	153	134	**143**	152

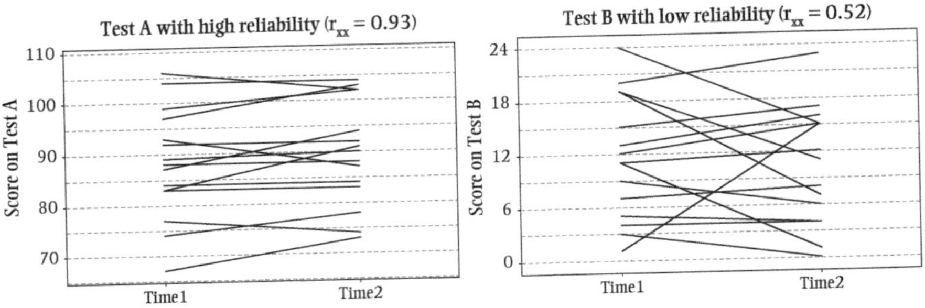

Figure 5.1 Representative sample of 15 people from a homogenous clinical population tested twice, two years apart. Shown are Test A, scores from a test with higher reliability, and Test B, scores from a test with lower reliability.

In the examples shown in Figure 5.1, reliability can be estimated by correlating the scores at Time 1 and Time 2, providing the relationship between the scores is linear. In the left panel (Test A), the Pearson correlation for these data is .93, to two decimal places. The high positive correlation tells us that the ranking of individual scores at Time 2 from highest to lowest is similar to the ranking of scores at Time 1. In other words, a person who scores highly on the test at Time 1 is likely to score highly at Time 2, and a person who obtained a low score at Time 1 is likely to score low at Time 2.

In addition to consistency in relative rank across the two test occasions, the high Pearson correlation tells us that position in relation to the mean is relatively consistent across the two test occasions. A person who scores well above the mean at Time 1 on Test A is likely to score well above the mean at Time 2. Similar consistency in relative position in relation to the means is observed for people who score close to the mean at Time 1, or below the mean at Time 1, respectively.

Thinking of reliability or consistency as a high correlation between scores on a test when administered to the same people on two occasions is a useful way to think about the practical implications of the concept of reliability. Reliability, measured by correlation, tells us about the individual trajectories of each person's score across the two occasions—a high reliability correlation implies consistency in relative rank and relative position in relation to the means. As discussed later in the chapter, it should be noted that reliability measured by correlation characterizes consistency but not absolute agreement. A high correlation between scores on two occasions does not guarantee that the means at Time 1 and Time 2, for example, are the same.

An example of the individual trajectories from the same sample of people, but this time on a test score of lower reliability, is shown in the right panel in Figure 5.1 (Test B). In this figure, the score has a reliability of .52, and many of the individual trajectory lines from Time 1 to Time 2 cross. So, many people's test scores change in relative rank from Time 1 to Time 2 and change in relative position in relation to the sample mean. For example, the person who obtains the highest raw score of 24 at Time 1, scores 14 at Time 2, the same score at Time

2 as two other people, one person who scored 12 at Time 1 and one person who scored 1 on the test at Time 1. In this example, the person who scores highest on the test at Time 1 obtains the same score at Time 2 as a person who obtained the lowest score at Time 1, indicative of the marked lack of consistency in a score with a retest reliability of .52.

A low reliability correlation tells us that, in general, test scores are likely to show little consistency in both absolute and relative scores in relation to other people in the population, from one test occasion to another. Tests are used to generalize about the assessed psychological constructs beyond the immediate assessment occasion. As Figure 5.1 Test B shows, a test with low reliability limits our ability to make precise statements about a person's likely test score and, by inference, the assessed psychological construct, from one occasion to another.

In Figure 5.1, reliability was estimated using a Pearson correlation, so it is important to remember that this assumes a linear relationship between scores, and when calculating the sample correlation, appropriate random sampling from the population of interest. For a detailed discussion of the assumptions underlying use of Pearson correlation, and ways to verify the correct use, see Gravetter and Wallnau (2013).

Sometimes clinicians assert that their clinical expertise or judgement allows them to overcome the limitations of tests, or other clinically relevant information, that display poor reliability. This objection is logically indefensible. Unreliable tests provide poor-quality information, and if interpreted at face-value, they lead to poor-quality clinical inferences (Nunnally & Bernstein, 1994; Schmidt & Hunter, 1996). As will be shown later, unreliable test scores, interpreted at face value, sometimes lead clinicians into logical traps and simple, avoidable errors in clinical judgement. For example, a clinician, who does not interpret test scores or other information in terms of psychometric principles may feel the need to provide a clinical explanation for changes in scores from one occasion to another, when this variability may reflect nothing more than the poor reliability of the test. Similarly, extremely high or low scores derived from unreliable tests may invite specific explanation. Instead, if the observed scores are interpreted in terms of the appropriate psychometric principles (see section "The Predicted True Score") the perceived "extremeness" of one score relative to another may disappear, along with the need to provide ad hoc interpretations (Einhorn, 1986; Faust, 1996; Strauss, 2001; Strauss & Fritsch, 2004).

ALTERNATIVE WAYS TO ESTIMATE RELIABILITY

Another commonly reported method for estimating reliability is an internal consistency coefficient, although this method is now viewed as obsolete (Sijtsma, 2009). Cronbach's alpha is often reported, for example, for interval-scale test items, and an alternative for dichotomous (e.g., True or False) items is the Kuder-Richardson-20 (Anastasi & Urbini, 1997). Internal consistency is the most commonly reported reliability coefficient, perhaps because this method of estimating reliability only requires administration of a test on one occasion, and it appears in many textbooks (Nunnally & Bernstein, 1994; Sijtsma, 2009). An internal consistency coefficient is a measure of the extent to which responses to the items in a single test correlate with each other and is calculated by taking the average of the correlation between the score on each item in a test and the total of all the other items. For a test with 20 items, an internal consistency coefficient is the average of 20 correlations, the correlation between item 1 and the total of items 2–20, the correlation between item 2 and the total of items 1 and 3–20, and so on.

It is important to note that Cronbach's alpha or "coefficient alpha," as it is sometimes termed, is no longer the favored measure of internal consistency, because it may underestimate internal consistency (Cortina, 1993; Sijtsma, 2009). In addition, internal consistency coefficients are often incorrectly used as a measure of the homogeneity or unidimensionality of a test, defined as measurement of a single construct or factor. However, internal consistency is an imprecise and indirect measure of unidimensionality, which is best established through confirmatory factor analysis (Cortina, 1993; Sijtsma, 2009).

Alternative and better measures of internal consistency reliability are available, for example, Guttman's lower bound (λ_3), and interested readers are directed to the relevant references (Brennan, 2006; Cortina, 1993; Sijtsma, 2009). However, the best method for estimating reliability in terms of consistency over time is retest reliability (Nunnally & Bernstein, 1994; Sijtsma, 2009). Clinicians usually wish to make predictions about assessed psychological traits beyond the test situation, especially in terms of future functional status, in coming days, weeks, or years. For this kind of prediction, retest reliability or the special case of long-term retest reliability (sometimes termed "temporal stability"), is most important (Anastasi & Urbini, 1997). Therefore, a clinician should always seek an estimate of reliability most relevant to the clinical question. If the question is about current psychological status around the time of the assessment, then an internal consistency reliability estimate such as Guttman's lower bound may be appropriate (Sijtsma, 2009). If the clinical question is about a patient's capacity to participate in a particular intervention or treatment program over the ensuing weeks, for example, then a retest reliability estimated over a similar period of weeks may be most relevant. If the clinical question relates to functional status over ensuing years, than an estimate of reliability derived from a study of corresponding duration should be used.

Retest reliability may be lower than internal consistency reliability because a retest reliability estimate is susceptible to more sources of unwanted variation (irrelevant, random influences) than an internal consistency reliability estimate (Anastasi & Urbini, 1997). For example, retest reliability may be influenced by fluctuations in the measured psychological trait due to variations in time of day of assessment, day-to-day fluctuations in the patient's psychological well-being, examiner or test-setting influences, or any other extraneous influences that do not affect an internal consistency coefficient obtained from only one test occasion. Similarly, long-term retest reliability estimates may be susceptible to more extraneous influences, or sources of error, than short-term retest reliability estimates.

For a discussion of the cumulative influences of sources of error on reliability estimates as one moves from an internal consistency estimate to a long-term retest reliability, see Anastasi and Urbini (1997). Test authors bear a responsibility to ensure that clinicians have access to the appropriate estimates of reliability corresponding to the ways in which the test is to be used. Conversely, clinicians should be wary if the only estimate of reliability available for a test is in internal consistency coefficient, which may overestimate more clinically relevant retest reliability estimates (Kaufman & Lichtenberger, 2005). As will be shown later, if no estimate of reliability is available for a test, then clinicians should carefully consider whether clinical application of a test is premature.

This discussion reflects the "classical" psychometric approach to the consideration of reliability. Advances in psychometrics have provided more detailed and comprehensive approaches to understanding the reliability of tests scores, which complement and elaborate the classical approach (Brennan, 2006). Generalizability theory provides methods to examine alternative sources of variance that may contribute to reliability in a comprehensive study design (Shavelson & Webb, 1991). For example, generalizability theory enables examination of sources of variance due to items, people, alternative examiners, and multiple assessment occasions in one study. Yet another approach to estimating reliability is available with item-response theory (IRT), which has been widely implemented, for example, in educational testing and adaptive clinical testing (Brennan, 2006; www.nihpromis.org).

In the examples in Figures 5.1, it is assumed there was no practice effect from Time 1 to Time 2. The presence of practice effects (or other sources of bias) in retest scores will reduce the consistency in scores, if consistency is expected in terms of *absolute value* as well as relative rank of tests scores. While some test publishers provide information about expected practice effects, a retest correlation may not provide the best measure of reliability in terms of absolute value or absolute agreement. This problem is illustrated in Figure 5.2, using the same

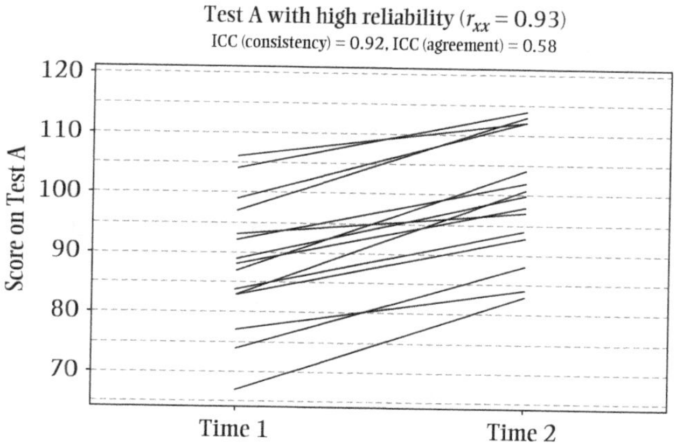

Figure 5.2 Representative sample of 15 people from a homogenous clinical population tested twice, two years apart. These are the same data as in Figure 5.1 Test A, except that a constant of 10 points has been added to the Time 2 score. Values of Pearson reliability and intra-class correlation (ICC) for consistency do not change, but ICC for agreement is lower.

set of scores as were used for Test A in Figure 5.1. However in Figure 5.2, a constant of 10 points has been added to every score at Time 2, to show that the Pearson reliability correlation stays the same at .93. Adding a constant to one set of scores that is used to calculate a correlation does not change the correlation (Gravetter & Wallnau, 2013). In this scenario, the correlation remains high, but the absolute agreement is poor.

In contrast, intra-class correlation coefficients (ICCs) can provide estimates of reliability, depending on whether the focus is on consistency (relative rank and position) or absolute agreement (absolute value). Intra-class correlations are another method for evaluating the reliability of test scores, and, like generalizability theory, they are based on a variance decomposition approach (just as analysis of variance decomposes sources of variance due to explanatory variables and their interactions: Brennan, 2006). Methods for estimating ICCs are available in most statistical software, and ICCs should be used carefully, because misreporting is common. For example, the default ICC reported may include a consistency estimate that assumes the "score" to be interpreted is the sum of scores from every test occasion included in the analysis, which might be two or more occasions. However, if the test is to be interpreted on the basis of a single re-administration, then the simple two-occasion ICC should be reported. The latter may be lower than the multiple test-occasion reliability estimate. In addition, ICCs are available for estimates of consistency, in terms described previously as the correlation between scores on two or more occasions, or as agreement estimates, where the absolute level of scores is also taken into account, and changes due, say, to practice effects, may lower agreement across test occasions. Again, the appropriate estimate should be reported.

In the example in Figure 5.2, the ICC for consistency (assuming persons and test occasions are both random samples of all possible people and test occasions) is equal to .92—high, like the reliability correlation calculated for Test A in Figure 5.1. However, the ICC for absolute agreement is .58, lower than the consistency estimate, because the ICC for agreement estimate takes into account the change in absolute value as well.

As the preceding examples show, different methods for estimating reliability convey different kinds of information. Clinicians need to ensure that they use reliability estimates that are appropriate to the clinical question at hand. Test publishers should ensure that reliability estimates relevant to the intended use of the test are reported in test manuals and that the appropriate interpretation of alternative reliability estimates is communicated effectively to test users.

THE PREDICTED TRUE SCORE

In clinical assessment, knowledge of the reliability of a test score is simply a first step toward scientific test interpretation. The reliability coefficient is of little interest on its own, instead, the reliability of a test score conveys information about the precision of the estimate of the psychological construct or trait that is the target of testing. Explicit consideration of precision involves construction of a CI for the true test score. This concept is analogous to the estimation of a CI for a population mean (Cumming & Finch, 2005). In the same vein, a CI around a person's test score allows estimation of the precision of the estimate of the true score. Calculating CIs also facilitates testing hypotheses using observed scores, as illustrated in the clinical scenario at the beginning of this chapter.

In the familiar research scenario of calculating a CI for a population mean, the center for the CI is the observed sample mean. However, a CI for an individual true test score is centered, not on the observed test score, but on a value known as the predicted true score (PTS: Nunnally & Bernstein, 1994). The PTS takes into account the statistical trend for an observed score obtained on any one occasion to shift toward the population mean if observed on another occasion. The more extreme the deviation of the observed score from the population mean, above or below, the more the adjustment of the observed score toward the population mean. Formally, the PTS takes into account the statistical phenomenon known as "regression to the mean." This regression toward the mean is an important property of test scores that is well known, for example, in single-case studies and in personnel selection (Barlow, Nock, & Hersen, 2009; Crawford & Garthwaite, 2007; Hausknecht, Halpert, Di Paolo, & Moriarty Gerrard, 2007). A well-known source of artifactual "recovery" in single-case studies and in cohort studies without a control group arises from selection of patients on the basis of extremely low scores at pre-test. Improvement at post-test may be a function of an intervention but may also be due to regression to the mean. Selection on the basis of predicted true scores at pre-test, not observed scores, reduces the risk of this misinterpretation (Hausknecht et al., 2007). Calculation of the PTS is shown as Formula 5.1 (see Dudek, 1979; Nunnally & Bernstein, 1994):

$$\text{Formula 5.1: } PTS = xr_{xx} + \mu(1 - r_{xx})$$

where x is the observed score,
μ is the population mean for the test, and
r_{xx} is the reliability of the test score.

Worked example of PTS:

If the observed score, $x = 70$,
$r_{xx} = 0.5$,
and μ is 100, then

$$PTS = 70 \times 0.5 + 100 \times (1 - 0.5) = 35 + 50 = 85$$

Several examples of observed scores and PTS for alternative reliability values are shown in Table 5.3, on an Intelligence Index scale with a mean of 100. Whether the observed score is above or below the population mean, the PTS is always *closer* to the population mean, and the relative difference between the observed score and the PTS in relation to the population mean is directly proportional to the reliability coefficient for the score. Note that the calculation of the PTS does *not* require knowledge of the population standard deviation. As can be seen in Table 5.3, the PTS for an observed score of 70 is much closer to the population

Table 5.3 Values of the Predicted True Score (PTS) for Alternative Observed Scores on an Intelligence Index Scale with a Population Mean, μ, of 100. Values of the PTS are Shown for Three Different Reliability Values, Representing Different Tests. (Note that the Standard Deviation of Test Scores Does Not Enter into Calculation of the PTS.)

	Predicted true scores for alternative reliability values r_{xx}		
Observed score	0.5	0.7	0.9
70	85	79	73
80	90	86	82
90	95	93	91
100	100	100	100
110	105	107	109
120	110	114	118
130	115	121	127

mean if the test score reliability is 0.5 (PTS = 85) than if the test score reliability is 0.9 (PTS = 73). So, to reiterate, the PTS provides the appropriate center for the CI for an individual true test score. Note that as a consequence of centering on the PTS, the CI is *not* symmetrical around the observed score, but instead is symmetrical around the respective PTS (Nunnally & Bernstein, 1994). It can be seen from Table 5.3 that the PTS has an important property. If a test has high reliability, the PTS will be weighted towards the observed score. If, however, the test has low reliability, the PTS will be weighted toward the population mean.

TRUE SCORE CONFIDENCE INTERVALS

In research with samples, interval estimation for a population mean involves calculation of a *standard error*, the estimate of the standard deviation of a sampling distribution (Gravetter & Wallnau, 2013; Nunnally & Bernstein, 1994). For CI estimation for one person's true test score, the underlying sampling distribution is somewhat abstract. It can be thought of as the distribution of scores arising from testing that person a large number of times, with parallel or alternate forms of the test, under the assumption of no change in that person's psychological state and no practice effects. This distribution is centered at the individual's PTS—the quantity we wish to estimate. In psychometric theory, the standard deviation of this distribution is referred to as the "standard error of measurement." As will be seen later, there is, in fact, a family of three standard errors of measurement, defined in different ways, and correct test-score interpretation relies on use of the appropriate standard error in the particular application. Interval estimation is one of the core techniques in psychological assessment, conferring greater scientific accuracy on the interpretation of cognitive and other psychological traits, a skill that psychologists can uniquely contribute to the evaluation of behavior in clinical care.

Consider two hypothetical scenarios contrasting the extremes of reliability. First, suppose that a test score is perfectly reliable, that is, $r_{xx} = 1.0$. If the test were administered to one person on many occasions, what would happen to the test score? The score would not change, because the test is perfectly reliable or consistent—the score obtained on the every other occasion will be the same as that obtained on the first occasion. The implication is that it is possible to predict perfectly the score on any occasion from the score at Time 1.

In the second scenario, assume instead that the test score has zero reliability, that is, $r_{xx} = 0$. The score at Time 1 provides no information about the likely score at Time 2, so it is not possible to predict the Time 2 score from the Time 1 score at all. Indeed, the score obtained on the second occasion could fall anywhere in the range of the population scores on the test. The scores, and by inference the assessed psychological construct, may be very different from one test occasion to the next in a way that is unpredictable. Of course, clinical reality always lies between these two hypothetical extremes. So the CI calculated using the appropriate standard error of measurement conveys information about the precision of the estimated true score.

THE FAMILY OF STANDARD ERRORS OF MEASUREMENT

In this section, we describe three standard errors (standard deviations) of the sampling distribution of an individual test score. There is a variety of abbreviations for these measures, so any psychologist should be careful to ensure they know which standard error is being described in test manuals, texts, or journal articles. The three members of the family of standard errors of measurement are defined as follows:

$SE_{measurement}$	the *standard error of measurement*, as it is most commonly defined
$SE_{estimation}$	the *standard error of estimation*
$SE_{prediction}$	the *standard error of prediction*

The *standard error of measurement*, $SE_{measurement}$, is calculated as shown in Formula 5.2:

$$\text{Formula 5.2: } SE_{measurement} = \sigma\sqrt{1 - r_{xx}}$$

where σ is the population standard deviation on the test score, and r_{xx} is the reliability of the test score.

The value of the standard error of measurement is a function of the reliability of the test, r_{xx} and the population standard deviation σ of the test score. Note that this standard deviation refers to the standard deviation of the population scores on the test. Formula 5.2 shows that as the reliability of the test r_{xx} increases towards 1, then the standard error of measurement decreases toward zero. In other words, as the reliability of a test score increases, the variation in the scores for any given individual decreases. Conversely, when the reliability of the test is zero, then the $SE_{measurement}$ is equal to the value of the standard deviation of the

Table 5.4 VALUE OF THE STANDARD ERROR OF MEASUREMENT ($SE_{measurement}$) FOR SELECTED VALUES OF RELIABILITY (r_{xx}) FOR A TEST WITH A POPULATION STANDARD DEVIATION OF 15

r_{xx}	$SE_{measurement}$
0.0	15.0
0.2	13.4
0.4	11.6
0.6	9.5
0.8	6.7
1.0	0.0

test in the population. This latter circumstance implies that when the reliability is zero, the variability in the scores of any one individual is the same as the variability among individuals in the population. Table 5.4 shows values for the standard error of measurement for selected values of the reliability coefficient between 0 and 1 for a test with a standard deviation of 15. As can be seen, when the reliability of the test score is 0.2, then the $SE_{measurement}$ is 13.4, almost as large as the population standard deviation of 15. Even when the reliability is 0.8, the value of $SE_{measurement}$ is 6.7, almost half the magnitude of the population standard deviation.

Another way to illustrate the effects of the reliability coefficient on the size of the standard error of measurement is shown by the function relating the reliability coefficient to the standard error of measurement, where the latter is expressed as a proportion of the population standard deviation. The curve generated by this function is shown in the left panel in Figure 5.3 where the x-axis represents the reliability of the test and the y-axis represents the standard error of measurement ($SE_{measurement}$) as a proportion of the population standard deviation on the test. As can be seen in Figure 5.3, as the reliability increases toward a value of 1.0 (to the right on the x-axis), the value of the standard error of measurement as a proportion of the population standard deviation decreases toward zero (toward the lowest point of the y-axis). In contrast, as the reliability coefficient tends toward zero, the standard error of measurement as a proportion of the population standard deviation tends toward 1.0. For example, it can be seen in Figure 5.3 that if the reliability coefficient is 0.8 (on the x-axis), then the standard error of measurement as a proportion of the population standard deviation on the test is 0.45 (on the y-axis), approximately. If the population standard deviation were 15, then the standard error of measurement for that test would be $15 \times 0.45 = 6.7$. This is the same value as in the example calculation in Table 5.4.

Note also the shape of the curve for the $SE_{measurement}$ in Figure 5.3. The $SE_{measurement}$ does not become a small proportion of the population standard deviation until the reliability coefficient is close to one. The shape of this function is the reason why psychometricians suggest that the reliability coefficient for a test score used for individual assessment should be high, preferably in excess of 0.9 (Nunnally &

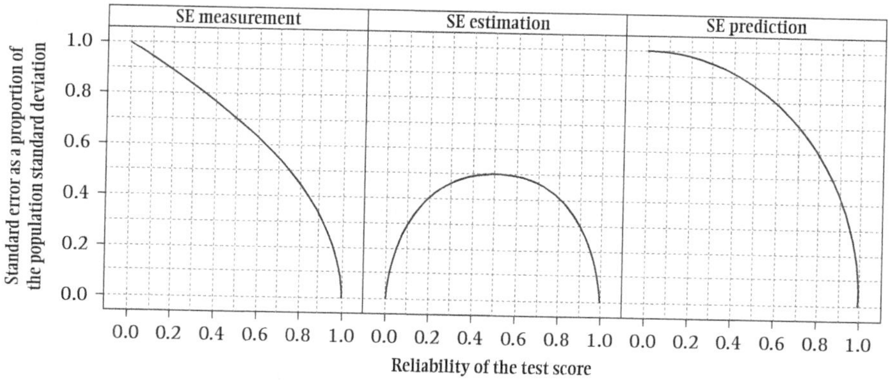

Figure 5.3 The family of standard errors (SE) of measurement. The relationship is shown between the reliability of the test (x-axis) and each of the three standard errors, respectively, as a proportion of the population standard deviation (y-axis).

Bernstein, 1994). With lower reliabilities, the value of the standard error of measurement is large and too close to the value of population standard deviation, so the precision in the estimation of a person's true score on the test is inexact.

Most textbooks on psychological assessment describe only the $SE_{measurement}$, as we have defined it here, without indicating that there is a family of standard errors for individual testing, and the best choice of standard error depends on the clinical assessment question (Dudek, 1979). While choice of standard error makes little difference if the reliability coefficient for a test is very high, choice of standard error has a big impact with lower reliabilities, in the range of reliabilities reported for many published tests (see Franzen, 2000). The $SE_{measurement}$ (Formula 5.2) described previously, and reported in many textbooks on assessment, is, technically, the standard deviation of the distribution of observed scores estimated from a fixed (known) true score (Nunnally & Bernstein, 1994). There are two alternative standard errors that are most useful in clinical assessment and are described in the next sections. The advantage of these alternatives is that they make better use of the relationship between the observed score and the true score.

THE STANDARD ERROR OF ESTIMATION

The first of these alternative standard errors is the standard error of estimation ($SE_{estimation}$). Formula 5.3 shows the calculation for the standard error of estimation, a formula that appears to be related to the formula for the standard error of measurement described previously. However, in terms of statistical theory, the standard error of estimation is quite different from the standard error of measurement. The standard error of estimation arises from a regression framework, describing the error involved in estimating the true score from an observed score (Nunnally & Bernstein, 1994). Using the PTS allows us to describe how the true score is estimated from the observed score. Combined with the formula for the standard error of estimation, we can estimate the average true score from an observed score and provide a CI around this estimate.

$$\text{Formula 5.3: } SE_{estimation} = \sigma\sqrt{r_{xx}\left(1 - r_{xx}\right)}$$

where σ is the population standard deviation on the test score, and r_{xx} is the reliability of the test score.

The function relating the reliability of the test to the standard error of estimation as a proportion of the population standard deviation is shown in the centre panel in Figure 5.3. Immediately, the reader will notice that this function has a peculiar property, namely, that the standard error of estimation is smaller, as a proportion of the population standard deviation, for both higher and lower reliabilities. We can understand this apparent paradox by noting that the standard error of estimation reflects the error in estimating the true score. When the reliability of the test is low, the estimate of the true score (PTS) will be heavily weighted towards the population mean and there will be relatively less error involved than if the estimate was weighted towards the observed score.

In what context should we use the standard error of estimation? Consider a clinician who is undertaking a single assessment of a given patient and is wishing to test a hypothesis about that patient's true score. A CI for the true score is best calculated with the standard error of estimation (Dudek, 1979; Nunnally & Bernstein, 1994). This kind of assessment situation will arise when a clinician wishes to consider the patient's true score in relation to a known criterion such as the second percentile in the case of a possible diagnosis of learning difficulty (intellectual disability), or in relation to a cutting score for identification of suboptimal effort on a performance validity test, to cite just two examples.

CONFIDENCE INTERVAL FOR THE TRUE SCORE BASED ON ASSESSMENT ON ONE OCCASION

Calculation of a CI using the standard error of estimation follows principles for calculating CIs for sample parameters, based on a normal distribution. A worked example using Formula 5.3 is shown in Table 5.5. The choice of the confidence coefficient, be it 95% or 99% for example, should be made *a priori*. It may appear that this choice is arbitrary, but consistency in professional practice should be based on a consistent standard of confidence. Across disciplines the most commonly used standard level of confidence is 95%. Choice of any alternative confidence coefficient should be made thoughtfully. Most neuropsychological assessments involve administration of a large number of tests and interpretation of an even larger number of test scores. Therefore, confidence levels that reduce the false-positive rate of inferred difference or abnormality (e.g., 95% or 99% CIs) are preferable to lower confidence levels under most circumstances (e.g., 68% or 90%). If a 95% confidence level is chosen, then expect 95% of CIs calculated to include the true score when testing over a large number of occasions (e.g., 95 out of 100,

Table 5.5 Calculation of a confidence interval for a true score using the predicted true score and the standard error of estimation.

A 95% confidence interval for the true score, allowing comparison to clinical or other criteria, is provided by the formula –

$$PTS \pm 1.96 \times SE_{estimation}$$

More generally,

$$PTS \pm z \times SE_{estimation}$$

where z is the value from the standard Normal distribution (z-score) corresponding to the desired confidence level, for a x% confidence level, z is the cutoff for total symmetrical tail areas of (100-x)%.

Worked example:

For an intelligence test score with a population mean of 100, standard deviation of 15, and reliability of 0.8, a patient obtains a score of 46. The clinician wishes to determine whether this patient's true score falls below the commonly used criterion for learning difficulty or intellectual disability of 70.

From Formula 5.1 in this chapter, the predicted true score for this patient on this occasion is 57.

From Formula 5.3
$$\begin{aligned} SE_{estimation} &= 15\sqrt{r_{xx}\left(1 - r_{xx}\right)} \\ &= 15\sqrt{.8\ (1 - .8\ )} \\ &= 6 \end{aligned}$$

So a 95% confidence interval for this score is:
= 57 ± 1.96 x 6
= 57 ± 12, rounding to the nearest whole number.

So the 95% confidence interval for the true score ranges from 45 (the lower limit) to 69 (the upper limit). This confidence interval does not include the value of 70. So the plausible values for the patient's true score described by the confidence interval are consistent with the inference that the true score falls below 70.

---

950 of 1000). Choice of a 68% CI (PTS ± 1 x standard error, approximately), for example, is generally not to be recommended as only two-thirds of such intervals will, in the long run include the true score. Such intervals are potentially misleadingly narrow.

A set of worked examples of 95% CIs constructed using the standard error of estimation for a range of Intelligence Index scores from 55–145 is shown in Table 5.1 and rounded to whole numbers. Again, these examples are based on a population mean of 100 and standard deviation of 15. Each column in the body of Table 5.1 shows 95% CIs for selected reliability values for different hypothetical test scores. As can be seen in the first row of Table 5.1, if the reliability of the test is 0.1, the 95% CI for the true score when the observed score is 55 covers a range of 17 Index points, centered on a PTS of 96. The limits of the CI are 87 and

104. Notably, in this instance of extremely low test reliability, the observed score is not included in the 95% CI. This should not be surprising since, if the reliability is very poor, the PTS will be heavily weighted towards the population mean. If instead the reliability of the test score is 0.5, then the CI based on the same observed score of 55 covers a range of over 29 Index points, bounds from 63–92 and centered on a PTS of 78. Finally, if the reliability of the test score is .95, then the CI based on an observed score of 55 covers a range of 13 Index points, centered on a PTS of 57 (see Table 5.1). The varying CI widths reflect varying levels of precision in the estimate of the true score.

PREDICTION INTERVAL FOR THE TRUE SCORE BASED ON THE STANDARD ERROR OF PREDICTION

In a standard linear regression framework, an interval can be described where a future observed score is likely to fall. This is a special form of a CI referred to as a "prediction interval." In many clinical contexts, finding a prediction interval for a future observed score on a test can be useful. This prediction interval is calculated using the standard error of prediction ($SE_{prediction}$; see Formula 5.4), *not* the standard error of estimation. And the prediction interval is also centered at the PTS observed at Time 1.

As the formula suggests, the standard error of prediction will be greater than the standard error of estimation (unless the reliability is zero). This makes sense because there will be greater uncertainty in predicting an observed score on a test score than in predicting the average true score.

Consider a common clinical scenario involving evaluation of test scores across two assessment occasions. On the basis of an observed score at Time 1, a (95%) prediction interval describing a plausible range for future observed scores is calculated. The prediction interval is centered on the PTS at Time 1 and uses the standard error of prediction. The clinician may ask if an observation made in the future, at Time 2, is consistent with the prediction interval estimated from Time 1. If the observed score at Time 2 falls within the prediction interval based on the Time 1 score, the clinician has evidence that the performance is consistent over the two occassions. If instead the score observed at Time 2 falls outside the 95% prediction interval, the clinician has evidence that the new score is not consistent with that predicted on the basis of the Time 1 score. The clinician might then draw the inference that there has been a change in the score over time.

$$\text{Formula 5.4: } SE_{prediction} = \sigma\sqrt{1-(r_{xx} \times r_{xx})}$$

where σ is the population standard deviation on the test score, and r_{xx} is the reliability of the test score.

Of course, there may be some practice effect between Times 1 and 2, particularly over shorter retest intervals, and so it would be reasonable to deduct the practice effect from the Time 2 score. An alternative is to take the closely related reliable-change approach outlined in Chapter 6 of this volume. Appropriate information for calculation of practice effects should be available from the test manual or other research with the test. If the magnitude of the practice effect is not clear, then sensitivity analyses may need to be conducted, contrasting the impacts of different practice effects. All of these calculations need to be handled with care and reported in a clearly communicated way so that colleagues will understand the basis of the interpretation. The same patient may be tested on a third or subsequent occasion, and in that case, the same logic can be applied, for example, to evaluate the consistency of the observed score at Time 3 compared with the prediction interval based on performance at Time 1.

A set of worked examples of 95% prediction intervals constructed using the standard error of prediction for a range of Intelligence Index scores from 55–145 is shown in Table 5.2. Each column in the body of Table 5.2 shows prediction intervals for selected reliability values for different hypothetical test scores (all with the same population mean of 100 and standard deviation of 15). As can be seen in the second-to-last row of Table 5.2, the 95% prediction interval based on an observed score of 140, from a test with a reliability of 0.1, is centered on a PTS of 104 and covers a range of 58 Index points, from 75–133. If instead the reliability of the test score is 0.9, then the prediction interval for the same observed score of 140 is centered on a PTS of 136 and covers a range of 26 Index points from 123–149 (see Table 5.2).

RELEVANCE OF TEST SCORE RELIABILITY FOR EVIDENCE-BASED PRACTICE

As has been shown, every estimate arising from an observed test score comes with a CI (or prediction interval), and the interval quantifies the uncertainty in the estimate of the true score for that patient. As shown in Chapters 10 through 12 of this volume, classification decisions—for example, for a diagnosis or for eligibility for an intervention—usually require the use of cut-scores or numerical decision rules based on test results. Similarly, risk-reduction analysis for a successful treatment requires classification of treatment outcomes as successful or not. Categorical classifications come with CIs also. Remember that in this chapter, *test result* is a term used broadly to include any information relevant to a clinical decision. So, for example, classification criteria for DSM-V involve a combination of clinical item-ratings to reach a threshold for diagnosis. The rating scale "score" comes with a CI also, although the CI is usually not considered in explicit terms (Wittchen, Höfler, Gloster, Craske, & Beesdo, 2011).

It follows that whenever a test score or rating scale is used to assess clinically relevant behavior and to estimate a true score, the interpretation of that estimate should include consideration of the upper and lower limits of the respective CI, not just the point estimate. Clinical confidence in the use of any test or behavior-rating will be greatly enhanced if the interpretation of the test score for classification works well for the likely range of true scores, quantified by the upper and lower bounds of that particular CI, not just for the point-estimate.

These issues can be illustrated with information in Table 5.1. Suppose the assessment question is to identify a person with a learning difficulty or intellectual disability, which usually requires an intelligence scale score less than 70. Suppose, for this example, an observed score of 60 is obtained on a test with a reliability of 0.5. It can be seen from the second row of Table 5.1 that the lower and upper limits of the 95% CI are 65 and 95, respectively, centered on a PTS of 80. While the clinician may note that the CI is consistent with a true score below 70, she can also note that the CI is consistent with many true scores much higher than 70. The width of the CI highlights the relatively poor precision here.

In contrast, suppose the reliability of the test was .95, again with an observed score of 60. It can be seen in the second row of Table 5.1 that the lower and upper bounds of the 95% CI are 56 and 68, respectively, centered on a PTS of 62. In this case, the clinician should infer, with 95% confidence, that the patient's true score was clearly below the criterion score of 70. The relatively narrow CI supports this interpretation.

Obviously, as is illustrated in these examples, test scores with lower reliability will be associated with CIs that may be inconveniently wide. Then classification decisions combining cut-points and the respective upper and lower limits of the CI are likely to show that clinical interpretation of the test score has low precision.

THE IMPACT OF TEST RELIABILITY ON THE INTERPRETATION OF TEST VALIDITY

Correlations between test scores are often interpreted as evidence of the extent to which the tests measure the same psychological constructs. Interpretation of correlations between test scores in fact underlies an old approach to theoretical enquiry in neuropsychology, namely, dissociation methods. Dissociations can be investigated through examination of correlations or via inspections of elements of bivariate scatter plots (Bates, Appelbaum, Salcedo, Saygin, & Pizzamiglio, 2003; Chapman & Chapman, 1983; Crawford, Garthwaite, & Gray, 2003; Dunn & Kirsner, 2003). However, the value of "dissociations" in theory-building in neuropsychology is controversial and interpretation of dissociations is often ambiguous or uncertain (see the special issue of the journal *Cortex, Issue 1* in 2003; also, van Orden, Pennington, & Stone, 2001, and Chapter 3 of this volume).

However, interpretation of correlations as evidence of theoretical similarity or dissimilarity is best done under the general framework of convergent and discriminant validity. The convergent and discriminant validity framework was originally devised to aid theoretical refinement in psychology in general (Strauss & Smith, 2009). Convergent validity is observed when tests theorized to measure the same or similar constructs correlate more highly. Discriminant validity is observed when tests thought to measure different constructs correlate less strongly. Note that distinctions between high and low correlations for convergent and discriminant validity interpretation may be relative and do not rely on any fixed or arbitrary definition of what is a high or low correlation.

For example, the positive manifold of correlations between cognitive abilities (Spearman, 1904) shows that all cognitive ability tests are expected to correlate positively.

Interpretation of correlations between tests, at face value, for the purpose of inferring convergent and discriminant validity relationships is often problematic. As a consequence, current methodological approaches recommend careful use of confirmatory factor analysis to evaluate theoretical predictions regarding correlations (Strauss & Smith, 2009). Instead, when clinicians seek to interpret correlations between observed test scores, they need to be aware of a logical risk in the interpretation of correlations for theoretical purposes. The limitation is that a low correlation between two tests may indicate that the two tests measure different constructs, or the tests may measure the same construct but in an unreliable way.

In other words, the explanation for an observed correlation between two test scores may be ambiguous. One reason for this ambiguity lies in the fact that, if a test does not correlate highly on repeat assessments—one of the definitions of reliability described previously—then the test will not correlate highly with other tests of the same construct, on average. This effect of unreliable measurement in lowering observed correlations is well-recognized by psychometricians and usually described as the "attenuating" effect of low reliability (Schmidt & Hunter, 1996). In other words, it is naïve to interpret a low correlation as evidence of discriminant validity (theoretical divergence) without considering the attenuating effect of reliability. In these circumstances, tests that converge but have unreliable scores may be wrongly interpreted as showing evidence of discriminant validity. Many discussions of the dissociation approach appear to overlook the attenuating effect of unreliable measurement, instead seeming to suggest that correlations between test scores can, in effect, be interpreted at face value for theoretical meaning (see special issue of the journal *Cortex* in 2003; also Chapman, & Chapman, 1983). Such an incautious approach, potentially, will lead to endless construct proliferation (Chapman & Chapman, 1983; van Orden et al., 2001).

The major safeguard against mistakenly interpreting convergent validity in the context of unreliable measurement as evidence of discriminant validity is to "disattenuate" validity correlations before theoretical interpretation. Schmidt and Hunter (1996) provide a detailed account of the adjustment of observed correlations by reducing the attenuating effects of unreliability. These authors also describe numerous research scenarios where researchers may misinterpret correlations on their face value, without taking into account the attenuating effects of unreliable measurement. Since construct fidelity underpins accurate assessment practices, careful interpretation of convergent and discriminant validity evidence is a cornerstone of evidence-based practice in psychology (see Chapters 2–4 of this volume). Clinicians and researchers need to guard against unnecessary construct-proliferation because the greater the number of constructs that need to be assessed, the more time and greater practical challenges will be involved in reliable estimation of those multiple constructs.

CONCLUSIONS—THE MANY IMPLICATIONS OF TEST RELIABILITY

The reliability of test scores has profound implications for precision in measurement and accuracy of clinical decisions. Within a coherent and systematic theoretical framework, clinicians need to strive to use the most reliable test scores available. Since most clinicians are consumers rather than developers of published tests, then a heavy onus rests on test publishers to provide the necessary reliability information to guide clinical interpretation and to provide tests that optimize the accuracy of assessments. Unfortunately, many tests are sold to clinicians when those tests do not meet adequate standards of precision. As a consequence, the quality of clinical decision making is compromised. In these circumstances, clinicians need to be critical consumers of test products and be wary of using tests with unknown or inadequate reliability.

Understanding the principles of interval estimation empowers clinicians to become test-consumers working in an informed way, within the limitations of our science. Neglect or avoidance of the concepts of interval estimation risks exposing clinicians to uncontrolled distractions from the unrecognized impact of measurement error in assessment.

REFERENCES

American Educational Research Association, American Psychological Association, & National Council on Measurement in Education. (2014). *Standards for Educational and Psychological Testing*. Washington, DC: American Educational Research Association.

Anastasi, A., & Urbini, S. (1997). *Psychological Testing* (7th ed.). Upper Saddle River, NJ: Prentice Hall.

Barlow, D. H., Nock, M. K., & Hersen, M. (2009). *Single Case Experimental Designs: Strategies for Studying Behavior Change* (3rd ed.). Boston, MA: Pearson.

Bates, E., Appelbaum, M., Salcedo, J., Saygin, A. P., & Pizzamiglio, L. (2003). Quantifying dissociations in neuropsychological research. *Journal of Clinical and Experimental Neuropsychology, 25,* 1128–1153.

Brennan, R. L. (Ed.). (2006). *Educational Measurement* (4th ed.). Westport, CT: Praeger Publishers.

Chapman, J. P., & Chapman, L. J. (1983). Reliability and the discrimination of normal and pathological groups. *Journal of Nervous and Mental Disease, 171,* 658–661.

Cortina, J. M. (1993). What is coefficient alpha? An examination of theory and applications. *Journal of Applied Psychology, 78,* 98–104.

Crawford, J. R., & Garthwaite, P. H. (2007). Using regression equations built from summary data in the neuropsychological assessment of the individual case. *Neuropsychology, 21,* 611–620.

Crawford, J. R., Garthwaite, P. H., & Gray, C. D. (2003). Wanted: Fully operational definitions of dissociations in single-case studies. *Cortex, 29,* 357–370.

Cumming, G., & Finch, S. (2005). Inference by eye: Confidence intervals and how to read pictures of data. *American Psychologist, 60,* 170–180.

Dudek, F. J. (1979). The continuing misinterpretation of the standard error of measurement. *Psychological Bulletin, 86,* 335–337.

Dunn, J. C., & Kirsner, K. (2003). What can we infer from double dissociations? *Cortex, 39,* 1–7.

Einhorn, H. J. (1986). Accepting error to make less error. *Journal of Personality Assessment, 50,* 387–395.

Faust, D. (1996). Learning and maintaining rules for decreasing judgment accuracy. *Journal of Personality Assessment, 50,* 585–600.

Franzen, M. (2000). *Reliability and Validity in Neuropsychological Assessment* (2nd ed.). New York: Kluwer Academic/Plenum Publishers.

Gravetter, F. J., & Wallnau, L. B. (2013). *Statistics for the Behavioral Sciences* (9th ed.). Belmont, CA: Wadsworth, Cengage Learning.

Hausknecht, J. P., Halpert, J. A., Di Paolo, N. T., & Moriarty Gerrard, M. O. (2007). Retesting in selection: A meta-analysis of coaching and practice effects for tests of cognitive ability. *Journal of Applied Psychology, 92,* 373–385.

Kaufman, A. S., & Lichtenberger, E. O. (2005). *Assessing Adolescent and Adult Intelligence*. Hoboken, NJ: John Wiley & Sons.

Nunnally, J. C., & Bernstein, I. H. (1994). *Psychometric Theory* (3rd ed.). New York: McGraw-Hill.

Shavelson, R. J., & Webb, N. M. (1991). *Generalizability Theory*. Newbury Park, CA: Sage Publications.

Schmidt, F. L., & Hunter, J. E. (1996). Measurement error in psychological research: Lessons from 26 research scenarios. *Psychological Methods, 1,* 199–223.

Sijtsma, K. (2009). On the use, the misuse, and the very limited usefulness of Cronbach's alpha. *Psychometrika. 74,* 107–120.

Spearman, C. (1904). "General intelligence," objectively determined and measured. *The American Journal of Psychology, 15,* 201–292.

Strauss, M. E. (2001). Demonstrating specific cognitive deficits: A psychometric perspective. *Journal of Abnormal Psychology, 110,* 6–14.

Strauss, M. E., & Fritsch, T. (2004). Factor structure of the CERAD neuropsychological battery. *Journal of the International Neuropsychological Society, 10,* 559–565.

Strauss, M. E., & Smith, G. T. (2009). Construct validity: Advances in theory and methodology. *Annual Review of Clinical Psychology, 5,* 1–25.

Van Orden, G. C., Pennington, B. F., & Stone, G. O. (2001). What do double dissociations prove? *Cognitive Science, 25,* 111–172.

Wechsler, D. (2009). *Wechsler Memory Scale—Fourth Edition*. San Antonio, TX: Pearson.

Wittchen, H. U., Höfler, M., Gloster, A. T., Craske, M. G., & Beesdo, K. (2011). Options and dilemmas of dimensional measures for DSM-5: Which types of measures fare best in predicting course and outcome. In D. Regier, W. Narrow, E. Kuhl, & D. Kupfer (Eds.), *The Conceptual Evolution of DSM-5* (pp. 119–146). Washington, DC: American Psychiatric Publishing.

6

Best Practice Approaches for Evaluating Significant Change for Individuals

ANTON D. HINTON-BAYRE AND KARLEIGH J. KWAPIL

In the age of evidence-based practice, psychologists increasingly value the establishment of consensus statements and guidelines to facilitate the appropriate selection and delivery of effective treatment interventions. Randomized control trials (RCTs) are considered the best practice methodology for evaluating the effectiveness of therapeutic interventions in most situations. Longitudinal observational studies, including prospective cohort and case-control designs, are also important for the assessment of the natural history of disease states, related risk factors, and where RCTs are not appropriate. In such situations, statistically significant change is evaluated at the level of the group, whereby a null hypothesis (that there is no relationship between variables) is either accepted or rejected. "Change" in the clinical group or individual is considered relative to any difference observed in the control or comparison group and is usually indexed as a significance level or effect size. Consensus guidelines such as those provided within the Consolidated Standards of Reporting Trials statement (CONSORT; Schulz, Altman, & Moher, 2010) and Strengthening the Reporting of Observational Studies in Epidemiology (STROBE; von Elm, Egger, Altman, Pocock, Gotzsche, & Vandenbroucke, 2007) provide clear parameters for minimum reporting standards in communicating methodology and results. Implementation of such guidelines will ultimately provide for greater ease of interpretation, critique, meta-analysis, and replication of findings.

In clinical settings, it is more often the case that an examiner wishes to monitor a change in particular test scores for an individual over time. For example, the examiner might want to assess improvement in neuropsychological test performance following an insult to the brain. Traditional mean- or group-based analyses of statistical significance are important for making conclusions about treatment effects or associations, but they have limited application in clinical situations when information regarding change is desired at an individual level. In biological and medical science, an outcome for an individual is often coded dichotomously as being either present or absent, such as a disease. In the psychological sciences, dependent variables or outcomes are frequently assessed on a continuous scale. Furthermore, the distribution of what is considered "normal" often overlaps with the range of scores derived from a group whose scores are considered "abnormal." Reliable change indices (RCIs) were first popularized over 20 years ago (Jacobson & Truax, 1991) and offer a statistical solution for evaluating "significant change" at the individual level. RCIs allow clinicians or researchers to make conclusions about a client's performance level over time or to determine the effects of an intervening event. Like group-based analyses, RCIs evaluate statistical significance for individual change or a difference score to determine whether the observed change exceeds any confounding influence of systematic error (e.g., practice effects), as well as random error (e.g., measurement error). RCIs can be conceptualized loosely as repeated measures *t*-tests for the individual. Early applications of RCI models in clinical research included baseline and subsequent retesting following epilepsy surgery, coronary artery bypass grafting, and sports-related concussion (Martin, Sawrie, Gilliam, et al., 2002; Kneebone, Andrew, Baker, & Knight, 1998; Hinton-Bayre, Geffen, Geffen, McFarland, & Friis, 1999). As clinical applications continue to expand, and the reporting of multiple RCI models has grown, it is incumbent on clinicians and researchers to obtain a conceptual grasp of the fundamentals of individual change assessment and its applications. This is the focus of our chapter.

Reliable change indices not only provide a metric for determining statistically significant change in an individual, they also can effectively dichotomize the outcome for the individual as "changed" or "unchanged." The change can be evaluated using a two-tailed analysis, assessing for significant change in a positive or negative direction, or (as is done more commonly) reported as a one-tailed analysis. The reliable-change approach provides the clinician with the opportunity to report treatment or insult effects, not just as an average difference observed in an RCT or observational study (e.g., information processing decreased by 5 points on average, with an effect size 0.33), but as a summary of effect for each individual (e.g., 45% of individuals had significantly reduced information processing). Once "change" is established at an individual level, RCI scores can be further analyzed in the same manner as single-point-in-time scores. For example, risk-reduction analyses and odds ratios are popular and generalizable approaches to evaluating the efficacy of clinical outcomes in group studies, where change can be used as a binary or dichotomous outcome. Such techniques provide a universal means for communicating the outcomes of treatment. Recently, the CONSORT statement (Schulz et al., 2010) suggested that reporting binary outcomes was the exemplary approach for summarizing patient-relevant effect sizes. In RCTs and systematic reviews of RCTs, the effects of new treatments on dichotomous outcomes (e.g., death vs. survival) can be expressed in several ways, including relative risk, absolute risk, odds ratio, and hazard ratio. These analytic techniques help determine whether the new treatment has an advantage over other treatments or placebo. If a treatment is effective in reducing the risk of an unwanted event, we see a reduction in risk, which can be expressed in relative or absolute terms (Suissa, Brassard, Smiechowski, & Suissa, 2012).

As an example, consider the situation when a new drug is designed to reduce cardiovascular stress, and thus hopefully reduce the incidence of myocardial infarction or heart attack. A sample of patients who are at risk for a heart attack are randomized to receive the new drug or a placebo, thus creating a treatment and a control group. The incidence of heart attack over five years is the outcome measure of interest, and is dichotomous with "presence" or "absence" of heart attack recorded. Now consider that, after five years, the control group has a heart attack rate (control event rate) CER = 0.20, or 20%. The treatment group has a heart attack rate (experimental event rate) EER = 0.10, or 10%. The absolute risk reduction (ARR) is the difference between rates observed for the control group and the drug group, that is, ARR = (CER – EER) = 0.20 – 0.10 = 0.10. The drug reduced the risk of heart attack by 10%. The relative risk reduction (RRR) is the absolute risk reduction divided by the control event rate, or ARR/CER = 0.10/0.20 = 0.50. This means the drug led to a 50% reduction in the control event rate, as the rate was cut in half. It is perhaps more meaningful to report the number needed to treat (NNT), which is the inverse of the absolute risk reduction, or 1.0/ARR = 1.0/0.10 = 10.0. In other words, the drug would need to be given to at least 10 at-risk patients, on average, for five years, in order to avoid one episode of heart attack. The reader can hopefully appreciate the uniformity and generalizability of this index as an effect size in treatment-directed studies (see Chapter 12 of this volume for additional details of risk-reduction statistics). If the treatment was directed towards the analysis of harm, such as development of kidney failure whilst on the drug, then we would expect the treatment group to have a higher rate of the event compared to the control group. Accordingly, a risk-increase analysis can be conducted, again calculating absolute and relative risk increase statistics, followed by a number needed to harm (NNH). The application of these statistics in psychological assessment, where constructs such as depression, intelligence, and memory are measured on continuous scales, is that individual significance of change can be determined using an RCI. Once individuals have been categorized following a treatment, a risk analysis can be performed.

When a prospective cohort study is conducted, two groups are measured serially, over time, with an event or process affecting one group—the clinical group, but not the other—the control group. An example of this would be the potential influence of cigarette smoking on lung cancer. Two groups, those who smoke and those who do not, are monitored over a period of time for the development of lung cancer. In this uncontrolled, longitudinal, observational study design, there is no treatment per se, so the reporting of a relative risk ratio or odds ratio is more appropriate than an NNT or NNH statistic. Relative risk and odds ratios are often confused and inappropriately used interchangeably. Relative risk is conceptually easier to understand. If 30% of smokers developed lung cancer over five years and only 5% of non-smokers did, the relative risk ratio would be the

EER/CER = 0.30/0.05 = 6.0. In other words, smokers were six times more likely to develop lung cancer than non-smokers. However, relative risk ratios are not as analytically versatile as odds ratios, with the latter being amenable to prediction using logistical regression. For example, if 30% of 100 smokers developed lung cancer after 10 years, then 30 smokers developed cancer, and 70 smokers did not. Thus, the odds of a smoker developing cancer become 0.30/0.70, or 0.43:1. Of 100 non-smokers, five developed cancer and 95 did not. Thus, the odds for a non-smoker are 0.05/0.95 or 0.053:1. The odds ratio then becomes the ratio of the clinical group odds to the control group odds, or 0.43/0.053 = 8.11. Therefore, the odds of a smoker developing cancer are around eight times that of a non-smoker. The odds ratio is often more impressive than the relative risk value, however, whenever possible, the latter is usually preferred. The difference between relative risk and odds ratios is far more complex than can be discussed here, so the interested reader is directed to a contemporary introductory discussion (see Viera, 2008). As with all inferential statistics, NNT, relative risk, and odds ratios can be reported with a confidence interval and statistical significance (see Straus, Glasziou, Richardson, & Haynes, 2010).

The use of reliable change statistics and risk-reduction techniques is increasingly recognized as the preferred approach for evaluating change at the level of the individual. However, there are several methods of evaluating reliable change and clinically meaningful change available within clinical psychology, and at present there is no clear consensus as to which model is preferable. Though sharing a fundamental structure, reliable change models vary in how they derive predicted retest scores and standard error terms. This variety can present a challenge to clinicians when deciding which approach to use to assess change. There is no universally sensitive or conservative reliable change model, and classification bias will vary depending on the individual case and the nature of the control test–retest parameters. We illustrate in this chapter that selection of measures with high reliability, in part, reduces the variation in the prediction of outcomes amongst models, thus, when utilizing reliable change indices, highly rigorous assessment methodology should be the goal for clinicians (see Chapter 5 of the current volume). Our aim in this chapter is to provide an overview of the methods and issues pertinent to implementing reliable change, followed by a consideration of extended applications for change scores in clinical outcome assessment.

This chapter will first consider the origins and fundamentals of reliable change, including an exploration of commonalities and key differences between models. In particular, the manner in which different RCI models account for practice effects and regression to the mean is evaluated. The opportunities for multiple regression-based RCI models are highlighted. Specific attention is given to the comparison of RCI models, and ultimately, to the choice of which model to interpret. Potential applications for using RCI scores for clinical outcome summary statistics are presented with worked examples, including effect sizes, responsiveness and ROC curves, number needed to treat, relative risk, and odds ratios. The chapter concludes with a discourse on the limitations of RCI and a summary of key practice points.

HISTORY OF RELIABLE CHANGE

Reliable change as a concept was first introduced by Jacobson, Follette, and Revenstorf (1984), and modified after a correction suggested by Christensen and Mendoza (1986). Reliable change techniques replaced earlier rudimentary approaches such as the "20% change score" that arbitrarily suggested that a change of 20% or more from a baseline score could be considered significant, and the "standard deviation method," which suggested that a retest score greater than one standard deviation from a baseline score should be considered significant. These approaches have since been, or at least should be, abandoned. They typically fail to consider important psychometric principles such as practice effects, measurement error, or test–retest reliability (Collie et al., 2004).

Jacobson and Truax (1991), in their landmark paper, laid the foundations for the concept of reliable change. RCIs were originally developed to demonstrate the effect of psychotherapy on measures of marital satisfaction. The Jacobson and Truax model was proposed for use in situations when there was no practice effect, and it only used baseline variance of test performance as the error estimate. In the Jacobson and Truax model (RCI_{JT}), a statistically significant change in scores for an individual was considered to have occurred when a change in test scores from baseline (X) to retest (Y) exceeded the change expected due to measurement error or "unreliability" of the test. (A worked example of the RCI_{JT} is presented in the following section.) Since RCI_{JT}, a litany of modifications has been proposed. A detailed discussion on various RCI models was presented by Hinton-Bayre (2010).

Although many RCI models exist, they can be reduced to the following expression:

$$\begin{aligned} \text{RCI} &= (Y - Y')/SE \\ &= (\text{Actual Retest Score } - \text{ Predicted Retest Score})/\text{Standard Error} \end{aligned}$$

Computationally, RCIs represent a ratio in which the numerator represents an observed difference score between two measurements, and the denominator is some form of standard error of measurement of the difference. Generally, RCI models differ in how the estimated retest score (Y') and standard error (SE) are determined. Subsequent RCI developments have sought to make the RCI more accurate, consequently becoming more sophisticated. These models can be conceptually divided into mean-practice models and regression-based models. At present, there is no clear consensus about which of these is the preferred method. Recommendations and considerations for selecting models will follow, after we provide an overview and discussion of the fundamental elements of reliable change models.

BASICS OF RELIABLE CHANGE METHODOLOGY

It is easy to become lost in the complexity and mathematics of RCI calculation. So, some time spent on the fundamentals is probably not wasted. It is also pertinent to note that all the calculations that follow are presented to provide an understanding of the mechanics behind RCI models and relevant concepts. It is not intended that researchers or clinicians be expected to use the expressions that follow: an Excel spreadsheet has been designed that automatically calculates many of the RCI scores we present and is available from the authors upon request (Hinton-Bayre, 2010). Alternatively, individual RCIs can be calculated online (www.uccs.edu/bgavett/psychocalc.html).

To explore the concepts of RCI methodology, take the case of a 75-year-old male referred by a neurologist with concerns regarding memory loss and forgetfulness. Medical investigations, including computed tomography (CT) and magnetic resonance imaging (MRI), were non-contributory. A presumptive diagnosis of Alzheimer's was made and medication started. The patient underwent neuropsychological assessment at initial referral (baseline) and six months later (retest). Table 6.1 presents the test–retest data for the described case.

Once a basic difference score has been calculated, the challenge is to determine whether this value represents a statistically significant difference. As mentioned, numerous methods have been utilized over the years. The original RCI model proposed by Jacobson and Truax (1991) is the most basic. Under the RCI_{JT}, the numerator is simply the difference score between baseline and retest. For the case example on Full Scale IQ, the difference between retest (Y) and baseline score (X) was −8.0, suggesting an 8-IQ-point decrease over the six months. The RCI_{JT} does not account for practice effects, so the predicted retest score (Y') is actually the baseline score (X), thus $Y - X$ is the same as $Y - Y' = -8.0$. The difference score between Y and Y' always forms the numerator of any RCI expression. The denominator, or error term under the RCI_{JT}, was referred to as "the standard error of the difference" (SE_{diff}). Any standard error is supposed to represent the amount of variability that can be attributed to chance. Thus, the standard error

Table 6.1 BASELINE AND RETEST RAW DATA FOR CASE A ON WECHSLER INDICES

Wechsler Scale	Baseline (X)	Retest (Y)	Difference ($Y - X$)
Full Scale IQ	104	96	−8
Processing Speed Index	92	71	−21
Working Memory Index	105	97	−8
Perceptual Reasoning Index	104	96	−8
Verbal Comprehension Index	110	105	−5
Auditory Memory Index	89	70	−19
Visual Memory Index	86	71	−15
Visual Working Memory Index	97	91	−6
Immediate Memory Index	86	69	−17
Delayed Memory Index	82	66	−16

of the difference is the amount of error expected for individual difference scores. It is dependent on the amount of variability in difference scores and the test–retest reliability of the measure. Jacobson and Truax initially determined this value, in the absence of test–retest normative data, according to the following expression:

$$SE_{diff} = \sqrt{2S_X^{\,2} * \left(1 - r_{XY}\right)}$$

It should be recognized that the $2S_X^2$ (or $S_X^2 + S_X^2$) component of the expression represented the "pooling" or addition of baseline and retest variances, assuming they were equivalent ($S_X^2 = S_Y^2$). But this assumption of equal variances is not always met, a circumstance that will be considered later in this chapter. When retest data are available, a better estimate of the denominator can be used (Abramson, 2000). Thus, with baseline and retest variability estimates, the following expression can be used:

$$SE_{diff} = \sqrt{\left(S_X^{\,2} + S_Y^{\,2}\right) * \left(1 - r_{XY}\right)}$$

The values of variability (S_X and S_Y) and retest reliability (r_{XY}) are taken from appropriate test–retest data. Consider Table 6.2, which shows published test–retest data for the Wechsler Adult Intelligence Scale–IV (WAIS-IV; Wechsler, 2008) and Wechsler Memory Scale–IV (WMS-IV; Wechsler, 2009) for a sample of healthy individuals.

For Full Scale IQ (FSIQ), the pooled standard error or SE_{diff}

$$SE_{diff} = \sqrt{\left(S_X^{\,2} + S_Y^{\,2}\right) * \left(1 - r_{XY}\right)}$$

$$SE_{diff} = \sqrt{\left(13.8^2 + 15.0^2\right) * \left(1 - 0.95\right)}$$

$$SE_{diff} = 4.56$$

Table 6.2 Baseline and Retest Normative Data for WAIS-IV (*N* = 298) and WMS-IV (*N* = 173)

Scale	M_X	M_Y	S_X	S_Y	r_{XY}
FSIQ	99.7	104.0	13.8	15.0	0.95
PSI	100.2	104.6	13.5	14.9	0.84
WMI	99.5	102.6	14.0	14.7	0.87
PRI	100.4	104.3	14.3	14.3	0.85
VCI	99.3	101.8	14.4	15.0	0.95
AMI	100.1	111.6	14.1	14.4	0.81
VMI	100.0	112.1	14.8	16.6	0.80
VWMI	99.5	103.8	14.4	15.6	0.82
IMI	99.9	112.3	14.9	15.6	0.81
DMI	100.4	114.1	15.0	15.0	0.79

Thus, according to RCI_{JT} for Case A on FSIQ:

$$RC_{JT} = (Y - Y')/SE$$
$$RC_{JT} = (Y - X)/SE_{diff}$$
$$RC_{JT} = (96 - 104)/4.56$$
$$RC_{JT} = -1.75$$

INTERPRETING SIGNIFICANCE OF RCI SCORES

One of the assumptions of reliable change methodologies is that the underlying distribution of scores approximates a normal distribution. Therefore, RCI should be considered a parametric statistic, along with *Z* tests, *t* tests, *F* tests, and the like. This is important, as the "normality" of the distribution is essential for making probability statements. RCI significance can be interpreted using normal distribution–based inferences. Thus, it follows that, under a standard normal or "Z" distribution, a score of + 1.96 cuts off the top and bottom 2.5%, or 5% two-tailed, yielding a 95% confidence interval. For the FSIQ in Case A, an RCI equal to – 1.75 should be considered non-significant, as it fails to exceed the cut score. Thus, from a statistical perspective, FSIQ remained stable over six months using a 95% confidence interval ($p > .05$, two-tailed). In clinical research utilizing the RCI methodology, it has been common to report significance using a more relaxed standardized cut score of *Z* exceeding ±1.645, or 10% two-tailed representing a 90% confidence interval. Alternatively, a one-tailed significance test could be considered using $p < 0.05$ one-tailed. This, again, would yield a cut score of <–1.645, assuming a deterioration of scores was strongly expected. In either case, the reader will immediately note that the RCI score obtained by Case A now becomes statistically significant, as –1.75 exceeds –1.645. Thus, simply by changing the cut score or confidence interval, sensitivity to change appears to be improved. However, as will be explored in detail later, relaxing cut scores for improved sensitivity will come at the expense of reduced specificity. Nonetheless, in the RCI literature a cut score using 90% confidence intervals is common. Occasional reports have been made using 80% and even 70% confidence intervals.

The astute reader will notice that cut scores derived from the *Z* distribution assume that population data have been collected. However, in many circumstances only sample data is available, particularly when test–retest normative data is concerned. When sample retest data are used, one must consider the use of a *t* distribution (Crawford & Garthwaite, 2006). The *t* distribution is also normally distributed, but the cut score to yield a 2.5% or 5% probability changes with degrees of freedom ($df = n - 1$). The smaller the sample size or degrees of freedom, the higher the cut score is, that needs to be exceeded to label the results a reliable change. For the sake of clarity, it is worth reminding the reader that when $df = \infty$, which in inferential statistics means the whole population was measured, the cut score for the *t* distribution and the *Z* distribution are identical (see Howell, 2011). For the WAIS-IV data, the retest normative sample had a sample size of 298 subjects. Alternatively, if this sample had been 30 subjects, then the underlying distribution would best be described using a t distribution with $df = n - 1 = 30 - 1 = 29$. The corresponding 95% and 90% confidence intervals would yield cut scores for RCI exceeding +2.045 and +1.699, respectively. Thus, when the retest normative sample is much smaller ($n = 30$), the confidence interval chosen would have still altered the interpretation of outcome on FSIQ RCI = −1.75, being significant with a 90% confidence interval, but not a 95% confidence interval. It is common that a confidence level of at least 90% is used, and a t distribution considered, when the retest sample is smaller ($n < 50$).

Once the distribution and cut score have been selected, a decision regarding statistical significance can be made. However, effectively, three outcomes can occur: (1) no change, (2) significant improvement, or (3) significant deterioration. For the purposes of further analyses requiring a dichotomous or binary outcome—e.g., risk or odds ratios—a one-tailed test can be interpreted as either option (2) or (3). Individuals can be thus classified as "improved" or not, or alternatively as "deteriorated" or not. The usual caveats of one-tailed testing need to be acknowledged when interpreting change in this manner.

Interpretation of significant "improvement" or "deterioration" also needs to consider the metric of the measure under investigation. In the example used, the Wechsler scales are all based on a metric such that higher scores represent better performance. All of the examples that follow are interpreted in such a way. However, when the metric is reversed, such that a higher score represents worse performance and a lower score represents better performance, RCI interpretation can become confusing. This phenomenon will be seen in measures when the metric is time—e.g., the Stroop Color-Word Test—or reaction time. In this situation, all that needs to change is that the sign of the RCI score is reversed so that a negative score becomes positive, and vice versa.

PRACTICE EFFECTS AND NEUROPSYCHOLOGICAL MEASURES

A great number of measures used by clinical neuropsychologists are performance based. As such, they are susceptible to learning effects, more commonly referred to as "practice effects" (Mitrushina, Boone, Razani, & D'Elia, 2005; Calamia, Markon, & Tranel, 2012). If performance can change simply due to repeated exposure to test items, this change may confound or exaggerate any interpretation of the influence of an independent variable. Moreover, a failure to demonstrate practice may be interpreted as cognitive decline or impairment, if a benefit from practice was seen in appropriately matched controls. If practice effects are present, then RCI_{JT} is likely to be biased in its estimation of change, and thus not be an appropriate statistic in such settings. Numerous techniques have been described and commonly used in practice to attempt to mitigate or at least minimize practice effects (Duff, 2012; Heilbronner et al., 2010). Strategies include the use of different measures of similar constructs, such a substituting Symbol Digit Modalities for Digit Symbol Substitution on retesting. The use of alternate or parallel forms may mitigate practice effects in some instances, and such forms are available for an increasing number of measures (Strauss, Sherman, & Spreen, 2006). It is worth noting that practice effects can still occur despite the use of alternate forms (Beglinger et al., 2005). While the content may vary from one form to the next, the learning process of how to complete the task is difficult to remove, with studies indicating that those with higher IQs are more likely to benefit from practice (Calamia et al., 2012; Rapport, Brines, Axelrod, & Theisen, 1997). Some authors have advocated prolonging the interval between assessments. However, this is not always possible or practical. If a clinical trial expects to see a change early, then brief test–retest intervals are required. If methodological strategies fail to reduce practice, then statistical methods are always available. Therefore, statistical control of practice effects in RCI models has received considerable attention (Hinton-Bayre, 2010).

Test–retest control data can be derived from published norms or from published or newly acquired control samples. The practice effect (*PE*) is indexed as a difference between the baseline control mean (M_X) and retest control mean (M_Y), or $PE = (M_Y - M_X)$. This value will be the same whether the mean difference score for individual controls ($Y - X$) is used, or the difference between means is calculated. For example, for the normative retest data on FSIQ (see Table 6.2), the difference between means at baseline and retest ($M_Y - M_X$) was a 4.3-IQ-point increase. A repeated measures *t*-test on the FSIQ retest norms data confirms that this change was statistically significant, $t\ (297) = 15.8$, $p < 0.01$. Failure to consider, and in some way correct for, practice effects, can bias subsequent interpretation of reliable change. Chelune and colleagues (1993) modified the RCI_{JT} to incorporate a correction for mean practice. It is worth noting that mean practice effects are exceedingly common in published retest data (Strauss et al., 2006). When the repeated measures *t* tests are performed on the published test–retest normative data, all five composite measures of the WAIS-IV and all five composite measures of the WMS-IV showed evidence of a significant practice effect ($p < .05$). Correction for practice effects should be mandatory for any performance-based RCI methodology employed.

RCI AND MEAN PRACTICE EFFECTS

In their original description, Chelune et al. (1993) effectively altered the numerator of the RCI formula so that the individual difference score ($Y - X$) was also modified by the control-group difference score or the practice effect ($M_Y - M_X$). Another way of conceptualizing this is to derive the predicted retest score Y' by adding the control-group practice effect ($M_Y - M_X$) to the individual baseline score (X). Such that $Y' = X + (M_Y - M_X)\ or\ X + PE$, and for the FSIQ case example:

RCI Chelune

$$
\begin{aligned}
&= (Y - Y')/SE \\
&= [Y - (X + PE)]/SE_{diff} \\
&= [96 - (104 + 4.3)]/4.56 \\
&= [96 - 108.3]/4.56 \\
&= -2.69
\end{aligned}
$$

One can clearly see that the expected score for an individual on retesting went from 104 to 108.3, and thus a larger RCI value was obtained under the Chelune model. An RCI score of –2.69 would be significant with either 90% or 95% confidence intervals, when cut scores are ±1.645 and ±1.96, respectively. Remember that, as the sample size of $n = 298$ is large enough to approximate a population from a statistical perspective, a Z distribution may be employed. It should be appreciated that failure to correct for a practice effect has the potential of underestimating any change score obtained over test sessions. To clarify, the error term used is identical to that used by RCI_{JT}, noting that in the original description by Chelune, SE was based on baseline variability only (S_X). However, a pooled estimate using baseline (S_X) and retest (S_Y) variability is again preferred, $SE_{diff} = \sqrt{(S_X^{\,2} + S_Y^{\,2}) * (1 - r_{XY})}$ (see Iverson et al., 2003). It must be noted that, in using the RCI Chelune, the same adjustment for practice effect is made for all individuals. Also, the same standard error is also applied for all individuals, assuming both the baseline and retest variance are equal. In other words, a uniform practice effect and standard error are applied to all individuals under the RCI Chelune. The mean practice approach can be contrasted to the regression-based models, which make further adjustments to both the prediction of retest scores (Y') and the standard error (SE).

RCI AND REGRESSION TO THE MEAN

The concept of regression to the mean is probably familiar to most readers (see discussion of predicted true scores in Chapter 5 of this volume). Regression to the mean results from imperfect reliability, which in RCI calculations is the test–retest reliability (r_{XY}). Essentially, when a measure is repeated and the instrument reliability is less than 1.00, on average, the retest score is expected to be less extreme or closer to the group mean. Scores falling above the mean at baseline will become lower on retesting, and scores falling below the mean at baseline will move up towards the mean on retesting. In other words, the more extreme a score is at baseline, the less it will be on retesting. The magnitude of correction for regression to the mean is inversely related to the test–retest reliability, such that the greater the reliability, the less the correction for regression to the mean. Several RCI models have sought to account for regression to the mean, however, the RCI model proposed by McSweeny et al. (1993) is by far the best known and most widely used. McSweeny's RCI method is a regression-based model, sometimes referred to as "RCI_{SRB}," where SRB is the standard regression-based model. Under the RCI McSweeny model, Y' is the predicted retest score calculated using a standard least squares regression technique, where the retest score could be derived from knowledge of the linear relationship between the baseline and retest scores, and calculated from $Y' = bX + a$, where b is the slope of the line, a is the intercept, and X is the baseline score. Using McSweeny's version of the RCI, not only was the mean practice effect accounted for, but also regression to the mean, due to less than perfect reliability. Computationally, the linear regression model corrects for imperfect reliability by adjusting the predicted retest score according to the deviation of the individual from the control mean at baseline. In this way, scores falling further from the control mean at baseline have a greater correction for regression to the mean when estimating retest scores. If the baseline score for the individual (X) falls below the control baseline mean (M_X), a change greater than the control mean practice effect must be observed to reach statistical significance. In contrast, if the value of X falls above the control mean, then a change less than the control mean practice effect must be exceeded to reach significance. For example, applying the McSweeny RCI method to the case example using FSIQ, the predicted retest score (Y') can be obtained using the least squares regression formula, $Y' = bX + a$. The slope of the line (b) can be calculated using FSIQ control test–retest statistics (see Table 6.2), such that:

$$\begin{aligned} b &= r_{XY} * (S_Y / S_X) \\ &= 0.95 * (15 / 13.8) \\ &= 1.03 \end{aligned}$$

The Y intercept of the regression line (a) can then be calculated as follows:

$$\begin{aligned} a &= M_Y - bM_X \\ &= 104 - (1.03 * 99.7) \\ &= 1.05 \end{aligned}$$

Once b and a have been calculated, the predicted retest score (Y') can be calculated:

$$\begin{aligned} Y' &= bX + a \\ &= (1.03 * 104) + 1.05 \\ &= 108.2 \end{aligned}$$

The reader will note that the predicted FSIQ retest score (Y') for McSweeny's RCI (Y' = 108.2) is close to, but not the same as, Chelune's RCI method (Y' = 108.3). This is because the test–retest reliability is excellent, r_{XY} = 0.95. Lesser reliability usually leads to greater discrepancy between RCI Chelune and RCI McSweeny (Hinton-Bayre, 2010). To continue, once Y' for RCI McSweeny is known, the generic RCI expression can be once again employed, RCI = $(Y - Y')/SE$. When using RCI McSweeny, the compatible standard error (*SE*) term is the standard error of estimate (*SEE*). The *SEE* is effectively the standard deviation of the regression residuals or error in the control retest data. The value is generated automatically in any regression analysis software, and is available in the aforementioned spreadsheet, but can be calculated using the expression:

$$\begin{aligned} SEE &= S_Y * \sqrt{(1 - r_{XY}{}^2)} \\ &= 15 * \sqrt{(1 - 0.95^2)} \\ &= 4.68 \end{aligned}$$

Thus, to continue the case example from Table 6.1 for FSIQ, RCI McSweeny:

$$\begin{aligned} RCI &= (Y - Y')/SEE \\ &= \left[Y - (bX + a)\right]/SEE \\ &= \left[96 - (108.2)\right]/4.68 \\ &= -2.61 \end{aligned}$$

Again, irrespective of the confidence interval or cut score used, 90% or 95%, the case example FSIQ RCI will be significant. The reader will notice that the score obtained under RCI McSweeny (–2.61) is less than that obtained under RCI Chelune (–2.69). The reason for this discrepancy is regrettably quite complicated, but nonetheless predictable, and will be touched on in a later section. It should be appreciated that RCI McSweeny also adjusts for mean practice effect as is done by RCI Chelune. However, the simplest way of conceptualizing the difference between the two models is to see that the degree of practice effect is adjusted depending on the individual's relative position at baseline and test–retest reliability.

THE CONCEPT OF DIFFERENTIAL PRACTICE

It would be incomplete to state that the predicted retest score (Y') of the RCI McSweeny only differs from RCI Chelune based on adjustments to the McSweeny expression for imperfect test–retest reliability. RCI McSweeny also adjusts for a quantity referred to as "differential practice," as coined by Maassen (2004). This concept has received limited attention in the RCI literature, but nonetheless has a bearing on RCI McSweeny (see Hinton-Bayre, 2010). The concept of differential practice suggests that individuals do not benefit equally from a practice effect. If all individuals did benefit equally, then baseline (S_X) and retest (S_Y) variability would be equivalent. Maassen (2005) suggested that differential practice can be assessed by testing for a statistically significant difference between S_X and S_Y, in a similar manner in which mean practice is evaluated, $M_Y - M_X$. To expand on this, Maassen reported an inferential statistic to determine whether S_X and S_Y are statistically different in the setting of repeated measures, again using a t distribution with $df = n - 2$.

$$t = \left[\left(S_X^{\,2} - S_Y^{\,2}\right) * \sqrt{(n-2)}\right] \Big/ \left[2 * S_X * S_Y * \sqrt{(1 - r_{XY})}\right]$$

Again, referring to the FSIQ example, a statistically significant difference was seen between S_X and S_Y in the normative retest data for FSIQ (see Table 6.2):

$$\begin{aligned} t &= \left[\left(13.8^2 - 15.0^2\right) * \sqrt{(298-2)}\right] \Big/ \left[2 * 13.8 * 15.0 * \left(\sqrt{1 - 0.95}\right)\right] \\ &= -4.60 \end{aligned}$$

Using a regular *t* distribution, this result is statically significant ($p < .001$, two-tailed) and suggests a significant increase in the retest variability when compared with baseline variability. In the analysis of WAIS-IV, FSIQ, Processing Speed Index (PSI), Working Memory Index (WMI), and Verbal Comprehension Index (VCI) all demonstrated differential practice with significant increases in retest variability ($p < .01$, two-tailed). On WMS-IV, only Visual Memory Index (VMI) and Visual Working Memory Index (VWMI) demonstrated differential practice, again with retest variability exceeding baseline variability (see Table 6.2). There remains a paucity of consideration of the underlying causes of differential practice and its implications for clinical-outcome interpretation. Nonetheless, the RCI McSweeny and its derivatives all make a mathematical correction to the predicted score based on mean practice, differential practice, and test–retest unreliability. Several authors have jointly presented outcomes using both RCI Chelune and RCI McSweeny, yet the understanding of actual differences between the models is yet to be fully explicated (see Hinton-Bayre, 2016).

SOPHISTICATION OF THE RCI REGRESSION MODEL

Perhaps the single greatest challenge when using RCI methods for clinical outcome research is the limited reliability of many neuropsychological measures, particularly if considered for decision making in individuals. Classic teaching has often suggested a reliability of $r = 0.90$ as the minimum requirement for statistical decisions regarding individuals (Cohen & Swerdlik, 2009: see also Chapter 5 of the current volume). The reader is again directed to Table 6.2, noting that only FSIQ and VCI composite scores have test–retest reliabilities greater than or equal to $r_{XY} = 0.90$. It should also be noted that none of the WMS-IV composite scores had a reliability coefficient >0.90. Evaluation of the individual Wechsler scales indicates that very few reach this criterion, despite being perhaps the most well-known and researched test batteries in clinical psychology and clinical neuropsychology. Although it has not been rigorously examined, a more relaxed figure of $r_{XY} \geq 0.70$ would be generally acceptable (for practical implications, see Chapter 5 of current volume). Moreover, it is important to recognize that reliability is not an innate feature of a measure, but is also influenced by how the measure is used. The retest reliability for a measure after a two-week time interval is likely to be significantly better than after a two-year time interval. This observation reiterates that the control statistics used need to take into account, not only patient demographics, but also testing schedule.

MULTIPLE REGRESSION RCI

In the setting of RCI, particularly with regression-based models, rather than lamenting the lack of test–retest reliability, one can make efforts to determine whether other factors significantly contribute to the prediction of retest scores. The extension from simple linear regression to multiple linear regression permits the use of more than just baseline scores to predict retest scores. To this end, Temkin and colleagues (1999) described a multiple regression RCI model. Although baseline performance was invariably the best predictor of retest performance, some measures also had statistically significant contributions from other factors like age and the duration of the test–retest interval. In effect, any extra significant contribution to prediction under the multiple regression model is equivalent to improving the test–retest reliability through a greater explanation of retest variance. For example, if the baseline score correlates with retest scores $r_{XY} = 0.70$, the coefficient of determination $r^2 = 0.70^2 = 0.49$. This means that baseline scores only account for 49% of retest score variability. If $r_{XY} = 0.90$, then $r^2 = 0.81$, and baseline scores predict 81% of retest score variability in the control group. If age, independent of baseline scores, correlates $r_{XY} = 0.20$ with retest scores, then age would predict 4% of retest variance. If test–retest interval independently correlated $r_{XY} = 0.35$ with retest scores ($r^2 = 0.123$), then the retest interval accounts for 12.3% of retest scores. Unique variance attributable to independent variables can be directly summed, such that the baseline score ($r^2 = 0.90^2 = 0.81$), age ($r^2 = 0.20^2 = 0.04$), and retest interval ($r^2 = 0.35^2 = 0.123$) can be combined such that $0.81 + 0.04 + 0.123 = 0.973$, or 97.3% of retest variance, might be explained. If the percentage of variance explained were equal to $r^2 = 0.973$, then the effective reliability coefficient would be $\sqrt{r^2} = \sqrt{0.973} = 0.986$ or nearly perfect reliability. Thus, whenever possible, a multiple regression approach to predicting retest scores is encouraged. Indeed, this is the methodology employed in Advanced Solutions package attached to the Wechsler scales (see Holdnack, Drozdick, Weiss, & Iverson, 2013).

INDIVIDUALIZED ERROR TERM RCI

The reader should begin to appreciate that the RCI Chelune makes a uniform adjustment when predicting the retest score (Y'), based on the mean practice effect observed in an appropriate retest control group. The RCI McSweeny individualizes the predicted retest score (Y') based on test–retest reliability and differential practice (difference between baseline and retest variance). Both of the approaches use a different, but uniform, error term for any individual. Crawford and Howell (1998) went further, to suggest that not only the predicted retest score, but also the error term, can be individualized. The premise here was that cases with more extreme scores at baseline under a normal distribution will have error terms derived from fewer individuals, and thus a greater degree of error in any estimation of change. This is reflected in the accompanying Standard Error of Prediction (*SEP*):

$$SEP = SEE * \sqrt{1 + (1/n) + \left\{(X - M_X)^2\right\} / \left\{S_X{}^2 * (n-1)\right\}}$$

It should be appreciated that the individualized error term *SEP* is an extension of the standard error of estimate (*SEE*) used in the RCI McSweeny expression as the denominator. The reader should also note the *SEP* will always exceed the *SEE*. The degree to which the SEP exceeds *SEE* will increase with a smaller sample size (n), and when the individual baseline score (X) differs more from the baseline control group mean (M_X). Thus, the *SEP* will be different for individuals, unless they have the same baseline score. To continue with the recurring case example using the Wechsler FSIQ (see Table 6.1):

$$
\begin{aligned}
SEP &= SEE * \sqrt{1+(1/n)+\left\{(X-M_X)^2\right\}/\left\{S_X{}^2 *(n-1)\right\}} \\
&= 4.68 * \sqrt{1+(1/298)+\left\{(104-99.7)^2\right\}/\left\{13.8^2 *(298-1)\right\}} \\
&= 4.68 * \sqrt{1+0.0033+(18.5/56560)} \\
&= 4.68 * \sqrt{1.066} \\
&= 4.83
\end{aligned}
$$

Thus, the RCI Crawford accounts for mean practice effect, differences between baseline and retest variance, measurement error due to test–retest unreliability, and extremeness of the individual case at baseline, by constructing both individualized predicted retest scores (Y') and standard error scores (*SEP*). As such, it may be considered the most complete RCI model.

CHOOSING THE RCI MODEL

At present, there is no clear consensus on which is the preferred model, and this can present a challenge for clinicians in deciding which approach to use when assessing for change. There is no universally sensitive or conservative reliable change model, and as will be discussed, the classification bias will vary depending on the individual case and the nature of the control test–retest parameters.

To recapitulate, all popular reliable change models share a fundamental structure. The individual's predicted retest score can be subtracted from their actual retest score and then divided by a standard error. This will yield a standardized score, which may be interpreted via a standard Z distribution or t distribution. With knowledge of test–retest means (M_X and M_Y), test–retest standard deviations (S_X and S_Y), and a test–retest reliability coefficient (r_{XY}), essentially any RCI model can be implemented—except the multiple regression RCI (Hinton-Bayre, 2010). Reliable change models vary in how they derive predicted retest scores (Y') and standard error (SE) values. It has also been shown that knowledge of an inferential statistic, such as t or F, can be also be manipulated to derive a test–retest reliability coefficient and thus expand the selection of RCI models available (Hinton-Bayre, 2011). This finding means that the interested researcher or clinician can choose which RCI model they wish to implement, rather than being constrained by the model provided by the test manual or reference study.

On review of current techniques, the multiple regression RCI with the individualized error term seems the most complete model and is probably preferred. However, it is important to note that, just because the RCI Crawford model is the most sophisticated, it is not necessarily the most sensitive. It has been shown that RCI models are not equivalent (Hinton-Bayre, 2012). Preliminary work further suggests an individual's relative position at baseline compared to controls (Z_X), and the discrepancy between baseline (S_X) and retest (S_Y) variability, can dramatically influence the magnitude and even direction (positive or negative change) of RCI scores (Hinton-Bayre, 2016).

COMPARISON OF RCI MODELS

To highlight how RCI models can be influenced by individual score values, two case examples, B and C, will be provided. In Case B, the individual baseline level of performance is less than the control mean, in Case C, it is greater than the control mean. The relative position of an individual to the baseline control mean can be expressed as a Z score [$Z_X = (X - M_X)/S_X$], with positive values reflecting above-average performance and negative values, below-average performance. This approach presumes that a greater score is associated with better performance, and the interpretation can be reversed if the scale is reversed.

Case B—Individual Baseline Performance BELOW Control Baseline Performance

Individual relative position at baseline: Case B scored 85 at baseline on the VMI scale of WMS-IV and 80 on retest. Note the control test–retest data for VMI are in Table 6.2, and the mean practice effect ($M_X - M_Y$) and differential practice effect ($S_X - S_Y$) were both significant, with increased retest variance. The relative position (Z_X) for this individual is as follows:

$$\text{VMI}: Z_X = (X - M_X)/S_X = (85 - 100)/14.8 = -1.01$$

Thus, Case B was just over one standard deviation below the control group mean VMI score at baseline.

RCI Chelune—Mean Practice model:

$$\text{VMI}: Y' = [X + (M_X - M_Y)] = 85 + 12 = 97$$

$$\text{VMI}: \text{ RCI Chelune} = (Y - Y')/SE = (80 - 97)/9.95 = -1.72$$

RCI McSweeny—Standard linear regression model:

$$\text{VMI}: Y' = bX + a = 0.90 * 85 + 22.4 = 98.6$$
$$\text{VMI}: \text{RCI McSweeny} = (Y - Y')/SE = (80 - 98.6)/9.96 = -1.87$$

RCI Crawford—Individualized linear regression model:

$$\text{VMI Crawford}: Y' = bX + a = 0.90 * 85 + 22.4 = 98.6$$
$$\text{VMI: RCI Crawford} = (Y - Y')/SE = (80 - 98.6)/10.03 = -1.86$$

Using a 90% confidence interval, all three RCI models produced scores exceeding + 1.645 and would be interpreted as a significant deterioration on VMI.

It is pertinent to note that the RCI Chelune produced a less negative score when the individual started below the control baseline mean, and retest variability was significantly greater than baseline variability. Clearly, the choice of RCI model would not have affected the ultimate interpretation, as the result suggested significant deterioration with any of the presented RCI models. However, the reader can appreciate the potential for the discrepant results depending on the RCI model chosen, which will be considered in the next example.

Case C—Individual Baseline Performance ABOVE Control Baseline Performance

Individual relative position at baseline: Case B scored 115 at baseline on the VMI scale of WMS-IV and 110 on retest. The raw difference score (X – Y) was deliberately made identical for cases B and C. The relative position (Z_X) for this individual is as follows:

$$\text{VMI}: Z_X = (X - M_X)/S_X = (115 - 100)/14.8 = 1.01$$

Case C was just over one standard deviation above than the control-group mean VMI score at baseline.

RCI Chelune—Mean Practice model:

$$\text{VMI}: Y' = [X + (M_X - M_Y)] = 115 + 12 = 127$$
$$\text{VMI: RCI Chelune} = (Y - Y')/SE = (110 - 127)/9.95 = -1.72$$

RCI McSweeny—Standard linear regression model:

$$\text{VMI}: Y' = bX + a = 0.90 * 115 + 22.4 = 98.6$$
$$\text{VMI: RCI McSweeny} = (Y - Y')/SE = (80 - 98.6)/9.96 = -1.56$$

RCI Crawford—Individualized linear regression model:

$$\text{VMI}: Y' = bX + a = 0.90 * 85 + 22.4 = 98.6$$
$$\text{VMI: RCI Crawford} = (Y - Y')/SE = (80 - 98.6)/10.03 = -1.55$$

Again, using a 90% confidence interval, the RCI Chelune for Case C was identical to that of Case B. This would be expected, given that a uniform practice effect and error term is utilized. However, despite the same raw-score difference ($X - Y$), a reversal in the relative position to a baseline score above the control mean subsequently revealed a non-significant result for the regression based models. It must be recognized that the choice of RCI model can readily effect interpretation of individual change statistical significance. The examples made of cases B and C should not be taken to suggest that when baseline scores are above the mean, RCI Chelune will be more sensitive (giving the most negative score), or that when baseline scores are below the mean, RCI McSweeny will be more sensitive. In fact, this pattern would be reversed if all factors remained equal and the direction of differential practice were changed. To elaborate: on VMI, the retest variance exceeded baseline variance ($S_X < S_Y$), as occurred with many Wechsler composite scales. However, this will not always be the case, as many subtests show differential practice in the opposite direction, with retest variance being less than the baseline variance ($S_X > S_Y$). Under such circumstances, the most sensitive RCI will also be reversed. Such concepts are complicated and take some digesting. The interested reader is directed to Hinton-Bayre (2016) for a brief introduction to this phenomenon. Further elaboration of this finding is in progress. For the present time, the user of any RCI model needs to appreciate that not all RCIs are equivalent. They cannot be used interchangeably, and they should not be averaged thinking this provides a more stable or valid estimate of change. The complexity of the situation is compounded when one realizes that selecting an RCI model based on presumed sensitivity will potentially lead to interpreting different RCI models depending on where the individual fell at baseline and the differential practice seen on the measures of interest. It is far more tenable, as well as more conceptually and practically justifiable, to select one RCI model for all interpretation.

It has already been demonstrated all RCI models are influenced by one or more of four factors: (1) mean practice effect ($M_X - M_Y$), (2) differential practice effect ($S_X - S_Y$), (3) test–retest reliability (r_{XY}), and (4) relative position of the individual compared to the mean of controls at baseline (Z_X). Knowledge of these parameters enables the reader to derive whichever RCI model they wish. Practically, the discrepancy between RCI models can be minimized through taking several steps. First, the individual case at hand should match the control group as closely as possible. It has been suggested that the individual's baseline score (X) fall within one standard deviation of the control group baseline mean (M_X) (Hinton-Bayre, 2005). However, as was seen in comparison of cases B and C, the interpretation can still be altered under these circumstances. Second, only use measures with adequate test–retest reliability in that context. Desirable reliability for measures being tested to determine if the change is significant are often quoted as needing to be $r_{XY} > 0.90$ (see Chapter 5 in the current volume). It is important to note that even the most well-standardized cognitive performance test batteries, WAIS-IV and WMS-IV, have the majority of composite measures failing to reach this benchmark, despite the relatively short retest intervals. Longer retest intervals on these measures have been associated with reduced mean practice effects along with reduced reliability (Calamia, Markon, & Tramal, 2013). Recall that reliability depends on how a test is used and is not an intrinsic property of the test. Moreover, if there are significant predictors of retest performance over and above baseline performance, a greater explained variance is equivalent to greater test–retest reliability and can be incorporated into a multiple regression–based RCI. Third, the extent to which normative baseline and retest standard deviations approach equality will influence the extent to which alternative RCI models will also converge. While no one model is more sensitive to change, there regrettably remains no consensus or guideline on which RCI model is preferable. However, the multiple regression RCI model accounts statistically for all of the factors known to affect individual change interpretation. In our opinion, the multiple regression RCI model with the individualized error term, or the multiple regression version of RCI Crawford, is preferred. Bear in mind that not all test–retest data will have multivariate predictors of retest performance, in which case the regular univariate RCI Crawford should be considered.

Given the complexity of the preceding discussion, a series of summary points are provided:

- There is a fundamental generic expression applicable to all RCI models
  - RCI = $(Y - Y')/SE$ = (Actual retest score – Predicted retest score)/ Standard Error
  - Models differ only in how they calculate Y' and SE
- Most RCI models can be can calculated with knowledge of basic test–retest parameters from a suitable control group, including the baseline mean and standard deviation (M_X, S_X), retest mean and standard deviation (M_Y, S_Y), and test–retest reliability (r_{XY}). These parameters do not allow calculation of the multiple regression RCI model, but the principles are the same.
- Differences between RCI models are a result of how the different models deal with the following concepts:
  - ($M_X - M_Y$) Mean practice effect, or difference between baseline and retest control means
  - (r_{XY}) Test–retest reliability
  - ($S_X - S_Y$) Differential practice, or inequality of baseline and retest variability
  - (Z_X) The individual's relative position to the control group at initial testing
- A test with lesser reliability will increase the error for all RC methods. When control baseline and retest variances are equal, agreement between methods will converge to a maximal point, making the matter of choice less concerning.
- Differential practice ($S_X - S_Y$) affects the predicted retest score in regression based RCI McSweeny and RCI Crawford models, with the magnitude depending on initial test performance relative to controls.

- There is no universally sensitive or conservative RC model. The classification bias will vary, depending on the individual case data and the nature of the control test–retest parameters.
- When the individual (X) starts below the control baseline mean (M_X), or $Z_X < 0$, regression based RCI models will be more responsive to negative change. The RCI McSweeny will always be more responsive to change than RCI Crawford, as the standard error (*SE*) will always be larger for the latter model.
- Conversely, when the individual (X) starts above the control baseline mean (M_X), or $Z_X > 0$, RCI Chelune will be more responsive to negative change.
- We currently believe the multiple regression RCI Crawford is the preferred model for individual change.
- Pragmatically, it is important that the individual match the control sample well. This not only includes performance at initial testing, but also the interval of retesting. Variations in the retest interval will probably lead to differences in practice effect, test–retest reliability, and possibly even differential practice. All of these may have significant bearing on RCI estimates. Retest norms are subject to the same limitations as regular norms, and clinicians are responsible for selecting both so as to match the individual and setting as closely as possible. Failure to do so could result in potentially biased predicted scores when individuals fall at the extreme ends on baseline testing. It is incumbent on researchers and clinicians to use their assessment tools in the most reliable manner possible. Using measures in a reliable and valid manner is perhaps the single best way to ensure a dependable result, irrespective of formula used (Hinton-Bayre, 2005).

REPORTING GROUP ANALYSES FOR INTERPRETATION OF CHANGE

RCI provides an index of relative change, regardless of the model used. The change, whether it be positive or negative, is relative to any change seen in the control or normative group. If the control or normative group shows no practice effect, interpretation of change is straightforward and intuitive. A change in the individual's raw score in the negative direction may be sufficient to become significantly "deteriorated." Conversely, a change in the positive direction may be sufficient to be considered significantly "improved." However, if there is a mean practice effect in the control or normative group, then it is important to consider this in the interpretation of reliable change. Consider a situation where the control group demonstrates a significant mean practice effect, such that raw scores increase, for example with FSIQ. The individual may demonstrate a significant deterioration on RCI score, but there may be minimal difference between the individual's raw scores at baseline and retest. Thus, an absence of practice may be interpreted as deterioration. Moreover, a simple increase in an individual's raw scores from baseline to retest will not indicate significant improvement if it does not exceed the practice effect seen in the control or normative group. For this reason, RCI analyses should always be interpreted in the context of the mean difference seen in the comparison group.

INDIVIDUAL STATISTICAL SIGNIFICANCE WITH MULTIPLE MEASURES

It is rare to conduct repeated assessment on only one measure. More typically, a selection or battery of measures is utilized at repeated assessment, as a single measure is unlikely to be sufficiently reliable or sensitive on its own. Once an RCI model has been selected, further analyses can be conducted when more than one measure has been used. In the following example, the RCI Crawford was implemented. To continue, both Wechsler scales have five composite scales (see Table 6.2). If every measure is tested with a 5% type 1 error rate, a greater number of measures tested will lead to an inflation of the type 1 or family-wise error rate. The actual degree of inflation will depend on the degree of association between the measures and their sensitivity to an altering event such as drug effect or dementia. There are many corrections that can be made for family-wise error (e.g., the Bonferroni procedure), all of which effectively reduce the alpha-level or p value for any one measure (Howell, 2010). Such corrections will naturally reduce the power and sensitivity of the analysis. Alternatively, the actual rates of significant change can be observed in the control and experimental or clinical group. Significant deterioration on a single measure may be suspicious, but knowledge of false positive rates is essential. As with measures taken at a single time point, reliable change outcomes can be interpreted in a similar manner.

Consider Case A, suffering from Alzheimer's (see Table 6.1). The index scores for Case A were as follows for the WAIS-IV (FSIQ = –2.65, PSI = –3.21, WMI = –1.46, Perceptual Reasoning Index [PRI] = –1.52, VCI = –1.52) and the WMS-IV (Auditory Memory Index [AMI] = –3.82, VMI = –2.85, VWMI = –1.18, Immediate Memory Index [IMI] = –3.42, Delayed Memory Index [DMI] = –3.49). Using a 90% confidence interval ($p < .05$, two-tailed), a significant deterioration was seen on FSIQ and PSI from WAIS-IV, and AMI, VMI, IMI, and DMI from WMS-IV. Significant deterioration on so many measures would argue strongly that a change in memory and processing speed had occurred. However, if only one index had been significant, would this be considered sufficient evidence to say overall that deterioration had occurred? For this interpretation, knowledge of control rates of change is necessary (Holdnack et al., 2013).

To reconsider the interpretation of significant change due to an event (e.g., traumatic brain injury [TBI] or Alzheimer's) or intervention (e.g., surgery or drugs), RCI scores from control and clinical or experimental data should be considered. As an example, suppose a cohort study was designed to track memory decline following cardiac surgery with baseline and retest scores obtained on the WMS-IV. The clinical (generically referred to as "experimental") group consisted of 25 patients who were tested before and six months cardiac surgery. A control group of 25 suitably matched individuals was also retested at a six-month interval. Of the 25 experimental-group patients, 20 performed significantly worse than their baseline on any one measure. Thus, it may be concluded that the surgery negatively affected memory in 20/25, or 80% of the treated patients. Using a similar criterion—significant decline on any one measure—only five of the control patients could be classified as deteriorated, equivalent to 5/25, or a 20% rate of change. If a significant deterioration in scores on two or more measures was used as a criterion, only six of the experimental patients had "deteriorated," whereas none of the control patients demonstrated decline on two or more measures. In summary, using significant reliable change on any one measure as a criterion for memory decline post–cardiac surgery yielded an 80% Experimental Event Rate (EER) and 20% Control Event Rate (CER). However, if the criterion were set as a decline in memory by change on two or more measures, EER would be reduced to 24%, yet CER would be 0%. While a prescription for EER and CER is not essential, there will almost always be a tradeoff.

Another approach is to derive a composite (averaged) score. Consider the performance of Case A on WMS-IV (AMI = –3.82, VMI = –2.85, VWMI = –1.18, IMI = –3.42, DMI = –3.49). An unweighted composite or average of these values (M_{RCI} = –2.95) could also be used to interpret significance. However, the composite score cannot be interpreted in the same manner as a single score. Because the averaged score does not follow the same distribution as a single score, an RCI score exceeding ±1.645 cannot be consistently associated with a probability such as $p < .05$ or 90% confidence. However, it is possible to use a composite score for sensitivity analysis, such as the Receiver Operator Characteristic (ROC) curve analysis, which will be covered in a later section. It is important to be aware that the process of averaging RCI scores only makes interpretive sense if the measures being combined assess a similar construct, such as information-processing speed (see Chapters 2 and 3 of the current volume), or share an association with the criterion, such as being affected by dementia.

RCI AND GROUP-BASED ANALYSES

The preceding sections have focused on the use of RCI when single or multiple measures are taken for an individual. However, RCI methodology also lends itself to analysis of groups and is thus useful in randomized control trials and cohort studies. The following section further explores the opportunities for RCI scores, again using RCI Crawford as an example statistic.

RELIABLE CHANGE AND EFFECT SIZE

Most readers will be familiar with the concept of effect size as means of quantifying and standardizing the magnitude of influence of the independent variable on a dependent variable. Many such indices exist, and most readers will be familiar with Cohen's *d* used to quantify the difference between two groups, and r^2 the coefficient of determination, which describes the percentage of shared variance between two linearly related continuous variables. Effect sizes should be considered mandatory, as statistical significance alone does attest to the importance of the result (Schulz et al., 2010). Reporting of effect size is easy to reconcile when one recalls that, with a sufficiently large sample size, essentially any difference or association can be made statistically significant. As RCI standardizes the difference score for an individual after a designated effect, the average of such scores may be considered an effect size for change in repeated-measures clinical outcome studies.

To continue the cardiac surgery and memory cohort study example, the average RCI score of the 25 surgery patients can be calculated for each of the five WMS-IV indices (see Table 6.3). The DMI and VWMI appeared to be most affected by surgery, demonstrating the most negative scores. If the average RCI score in the surgical group approximates zero, this indicates that on that index they do not differ from the average RCI change score seen in the control group. Thus, the surgical group RCI mean serves as a point-estimate for a treatment effect. Interval-estimates can also be calculated using a standard error of the mean with subsequent confidence intervals. The standard deviation (*SD*) of the clinical group RCI scores is calculated in the usual manner, with the standard error of the mean (*SEM*) being calculated as follows: $SEM = SD\sqrt{n}$. When *SEM* is multiplied by ±1.96, it will yield a 95% confidence limit, assuming an underlying normal distribution. A multiplication factor of 1.645 provides a 90% confidence limit. The mean RCI, plus and minus the relevant limit, yields a confidence interval for the effect size. The use of RCI to yield an effect size is a novel application and requires further validation. It does, however, provide the potential to report a generalizable standardized index for comparison across measures and studies of clinical outcome on continuous variables where individual change is the ultimate focus.

RELIABLE CHANGE AND RESPONSIVENESS

If a single test or test battery is being utilized to make clinical decisions regarding outcome, an index of sensitivity to change, or "responsiveness," is required. One approach to assessing this responsiveness is to report the percentage of

Table 6.3 RCI Statistics for a Group *N* = 25 Cardiac Surgery Patients

Measure	Mean	*SD*	*SEM*	95% Limit	95% CI
AMI	−0.38	0.93	0.18	± 0.35	−0.73 to −0.03
VMI	−0.17	1.24	0.03	± 0.07	−0.24 to −0.10
VWMI	−0.76	1.61	0.31	± 0.61	−1.37 to −0.15
IMI	−0.29	1.16	0.22	± 0.44	−0.73 to 0.15
DMI	−1.11	0.97	0.19	± 0.42	−1.53 to −0.69

SD = standard deviation, *SEM* = standard error of measurement; 95% limit = 1.96**SEM; CI* = confidence interval

clinical cases recording a statistically significant reliable change. A commonly used metric is an RCI score of less than −1.645 denoting deterioration, and an RCI score of greater than +1.645 denoting improvement. Suppose, for example, of the 25 cardiac surgery patients, two significantly deteriorated on AMI (8%), five on VMI (20%), seven on VWMI (28%), two on IMI (8%), and eight on DMI (32%). In the example data set (Table 6.3), the study was intended to determine if cardiac surgery was associated with deterioration in memory, as indexed through negative change in WMS-IV scores six months after surgery. In this example, the inability of a single measure to successfully identify even a third of patients as deteriorated suggests that cardiac surgery might have limited influence on memory decline. Either the majority of patients did not actually deteriorate, or the measures were not sufficiently sensitive to change. In any event, the percentage of individuals impaired (or improved) provides a metric of sensitivity and potential clinical utility. It should be recalled that, by definition, the control false-positive rate approximates 5% in the positive and negative direction when a 90% confidence level is implemented.

An alternative approach to examining the potential clinical utility of a measure is to employ a Receiver Operator Characteristic (ROC) curve. ROC curves traditionally plot sensitivity against specificity using the continuous variable of interest. ROC curves can also be used to evaluate EER and CER when examining the clinical utility of a measure. RCI scores from an individual or composite measure can be examined using such curves. ROC curves provide the ability to closely examine the classification accuracy through the sensitivity/specificity tradeoff. This is particularly useful in the case of composite RCI scores where the score itself does not intrinsically reflect a probability. RCI scores derived for individual measures can be interpreted as unusual using traditional *Z*-scores or confidence intervals. Composite scores, on the other hand, are not standardized in such a way that a score is reflective of an underlying probability, for example, a composite score $Z > 1.645$ does not necessarily equate to a probability less than 5%. Figure 6.1 presents an ROC curve for the averaged composite Memory score of the five WMS-IV indices assessed from baseline to retest for cardiac surgery and control groups. The straight diagonal line represents the classification of individuals according to chance. A curve above the diagonal suggests classification better than chance, and area under the curve (AUC) analysis can determine whether the measure classifies significantly better than chance (Streiner & Cairney, 2007).

When an ROC curve is generated, any criterion score on the continuum (e.g., WMS-IV composite scores) is given an associated Sensitivity estimate (based on the experimental or clinical group) and Specificity estimate (based on the control group). A cut score can be chosen so as to define a desired level of sensitivity (or EER) and specificity (or 1-CER). For example, a WMS-IV composite score of <-0.4 for the data in Figure 6.1 represents an EER of 63% and a CER of 19%. A more negative criterion score reduces CER (akin to improving specificity), but it will lead to a corresponding decline in EER (or sensitivity). Using a more positive cut score will have the opposite effect, by increasing EER and CER.

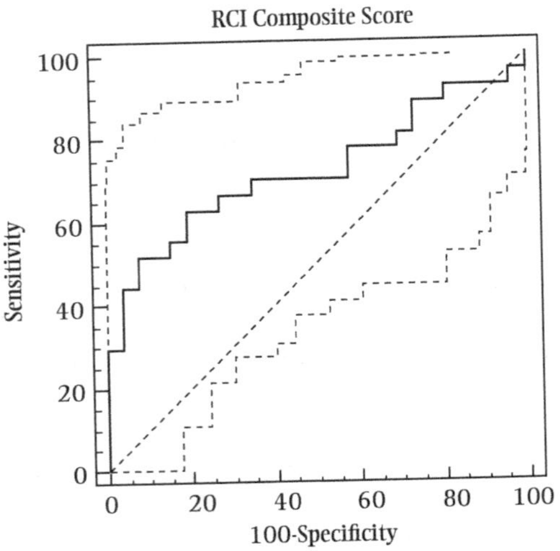

Figure 6.1 Receiver Operating Characteristic (ROC) curve for Wechsler Memory Scale-IV (WMS-IV) Reliable Change Index (RCI) composite scores in cardiac surgery and control patients. Straight diagonal line represents the chance classification. The heavy line represents the actual ROC curve, with the lighter dotted lines representing 95% confidence intervals.

Such estimates are only as stable or reliable as the sample and its corresponding size. A classic method to summarize the usefulness of a single or composite measure to classify individuals is the Youden Index, or the maximal difference between true-positive and false-positive rates (also known as the Youden *J* statistic = Sensitivity + Specificity − 1). Scores range from 0 to 1, with scores close to zero suggesting that the cut score is not able to classify better than chance, and a score of one suggesting a perfect classification, that is, no false positives or false negatives. For the clinical dataset, a Youden Index $J = 0.44$ was found, with an associated criterion of RCI <−0.61 (Sensitivity 52%, Specificity 92%).

Alternatively, the utility of a measure can be expressed in terms of likelihood ratios (LRs). LRs typically assist in the determination of post-test probabilities of the condition of interest (e.g., cardiac surgery), and can be positive or negative. Like Sensitivity and Specificity estimates, the LR will change as the criterion changes. A Positive LR is the ratio of the proportion of patients who have the target condition (surgery) and test positive (memory decline) to the proportion of those without the target condition (controls) who also test positive (memory decline). In the current example, with an example criterion of <−0.4, the positive LR was 3.27. In other words, using the WMS-IV RCI composite cut score <−0.4, those having undergone surgery were 3.27 times more likely to be labelled "deteriorated" than controls. A Negative LR is the ratio of the proportion of patients who have the target condition (surgery) who test negative (memory stable) to the proportion of those without target condition (controls) who also test negative. Again, using the WMS-IV RCI composite score <−0.4 cut score, the negative

LR was 0.46. In other words, those who underwent surgery were 0.46 times, or almost half as likely, to show stable memory function.

ROC curves can also be used to make comparisons between measures. For example, a composite index may be significantly more accurate than the most accurate single measure (DMI). Such analyses can also be useful for "value added" studies, where the new measure should demonstrate a significant improvement in classification over the existing standard.

NUMBER NEEDED TO TREAT

RCI methodology provides an index for change that can be analyzed as a continuous variable as above, or alternatively as a dichotomous outcome, for example, improved or not. Dichotomous outcomes are common in biomedical outcome studies: diseased or not, cured or not, alive or not. Once a dichotomy has been established, numerous analyses less common in psychological literature are available. A popular and generalizable approach to quantifying treatment efficacy is the Number Needed to Treat (NNT) statistic (Suissa et al., 2012; see also Chapters 7 and 12 of this volume). Classically, the value represents the number of individuals that were "treated" to avoid a specified negative outcome. For example, if the NNT = 8 in the assessment of a new treatment to reduce the risk of a myocardial infarction, eight patients would have to be treated on average before a single negative result (myocardial infarction) could be avoided. As such, a low score represents better treatment efficacy. The NNT is the inverse of the "absolute risk reduction" or 1.0/ARR. ARR represents the difference between the CER and EER of the designated outcome. This methodology can be extended to situations where the treatment effect seeks to provide a positive result, as opposed to the classic reduction of a negative result. The interpretation fundamentally depends on the direction of the outcome, however, a lower result is always associated with a greater likelihood of the outcome, positive or negative.

It is also worth noting that a related index can be derived when the event is expected to have a negative outcome, such as our example of deteriorating memory following cardiac surgery. Correspondingly, the Number Needed to Harm (NNH) is a related index where the intervening or treatment effect results in a negative outcome, rather than avoiding one. Using the example data described above, using deterioration on one or more WMS-IV index scores as the criterion, the EER was 80% or 0.8, and the CER was 20% or 0.2. The Absolute Risk Increase (ARI) due to surgery would be ARI = 0.8 – 0.2 = 0.6, yielding a NNH = 1/ARI = 1/0.6 = 1.67. Thus, for every 1.67 individuals undergoing cardiac surgery, one would be expected to show memory decline, as indexed by deterioration on at least one WMS-IV composite score. When NNT or NNH = 1.0, this suggests the intervention or event has a guaranteed effect, in that all treated or affected individuals would have significantly changed. It should now become apparent to the reader that the NNT/NNH statistic provides a potentially more universal index for reporting treatment or injury effects with dichotomous outcomes (see also Chapter 12).

RELATIVE RISK AND ODDS RATIOS

The efficacy of a treatment can also be expressed in terms of relative risk or an odds ratio (Viera, 2010). However, as alluded to in the introduction to this chapter, these analyses are well suited to uncontrolled repeated-measure designs such as prospective cohort studies. To provide a further example of these analyses, consider the same example where 80% of those undergoing cardiac surgery demonstrated a significant deterioration in memory scores at six months post-surgery, compared to 20% of non-operated at-risk controls. The experimental (or clinical) event rate (EER) would be 0.80, and the control event rate (CER) would be 0.20. The relative risk (for cognitive impairment) would be RR = EER/CER = 0.80/0.20 = 4.0. This suggests that those undergoing heart surgery had a four times greater risk of demonstrating cognitive impairment at six months.

To work out the odds ratio, we need to know the odds of memory impairment recorded in the surgery group and the odds of memory impairment recorded in the controls. If there are 20 patients in each group, the odds of memory impairment in the surgery group can be calculated thus: 80% of 20 or 0.80 * 20 = 16 impaired, thus 0.20 * 20 = 4 not impaired, giving odds of 16:4 or 4:1. The odds of memory impairment for the control group will be 20% of 20 or 0.20 * 20 = 4 impaired, thus 0.80 * 20 = 16 not impaired, thus odds of impairment for the control group would be 4:16 or 0.25:1. Therefore, the odds ratio for impairment would be 4:0.25 = 16. Thus, the odds of a surgical patient's recording memory impairment are 16 times greater than that of controls. Note that the odds ratio provides a larger value. Nonetheless, the relative risk (RR) is often preferred as a descriptive statistic and is easier to understand. The odds ratio, however, is more versatile in that it can be utilized in more sophisticated analyses, including logistical regression.

It can be confusing to the uninitiated, but the number needed to treat (NNT), relative risk (RR), and odds ratios (OR) are all viable methods of reporting treatment efficacy (Straus et al., 2010). However, we feel that, for ease of interpretation, NNT should be used when an actual therapeutic intervention has been conducted. When an uncontrolled event has occurred with either negative or positive potential influence, RR is preferable wherever possible. However, ORs may be acceptable, provided they are presented and interpreted appropriately.

LIMITATIONS TO RELIABLE CHANGE ANALYSES

There are numerous important caveats to consider in the use of RCIs, not only when monitoring individual change, but also when evaluating the effects of treatment or injury. First, the decision on statistical significance relies on the accuracy of the probability statement, for example, does RCI <–1.645 equate to a probability of <5%? The underlying distribution must approximate normality in order to substantiate this assertion. The normality of the baseline and retest distributions can be tested, as can the normality of the difference scores of the control group. Numerous methods have been described to test normality, including the Kolmogorov-Smirnoff test (Howell, 2010). Second, RCIs are a measure of statistical change, not clinical change. A significant RCI can only be truly interpreted as a difference between baseline and retest scores, once relevant systematic and error variances have been considered. In essence, RCI provides a result like a repeated measures *t*-test, but for the individual rather than a group. Clinically meaningful change is a different, but related, concept that has historically been difficult to define. In their original description of RCI, Jacobson and Truax (1991) considered not just the significance of change, but also the transition from the "clinical" to the "control" group. This "meaningful change" index was operationalized as moving over the midpoint between the two distributions. Clinically important change has also been operationalized as the difference score associated with subjective or clinician judgement of change, which heavily depends on the outcome measure of interest, the accuracy of the patient's subjective judgements, or the expertise of the clinician-judge.

There remains no consensus on what constitutes clinically meaningful change. However, it should be considered that a clinically meaningful change cannot be viewed as reliable unless it exceeds the corresponding statistical change score, or RCI. In other words, the RCI provides the minimal change score required to be potentially meaningful. A significant RCI score is thus not equivalent to clinically meaningful change, but a precursor to it. It is also worth considering that the concept of minimally important difference or change is actually synonymous with a reliable change index that looks at the simple difference between baseline and retest scores, not accounting for mean practice or regression to the mean, but pooling baseline and retest variances in the estimate of error variance. Third, there is no consensus for which RCI is most valid, and it has been demonstrated that no one model is more sensitive than another (Hinton-Bayre, 2012). In fact, sensitivity of RCI models is determined by how the particular model accounts (or does not) for the relative position of the clinical case to controls at baseline (viz., above or below the mean), the presence of a mean practice effect or differential practice effect, and also the test–retest reliability. Essentially, it is possible that a different RCI model will be more or less sensitive across different individuals and different tests. It seems theoretically untenable to consider an ad hoc approach to RCI model-selection.

The slowness of clinical outcome research to adopt RCI models is perhaps in part due to the lack of consensus, which is further probably due to the lack of understanding of how RCI models systematically differ. This latter topic is of considerable further research interest and would help guide further recommendations for RCI usage. Fourth, the RCI methodology was originally designed for a pre–post scenario where individuals started at an abnormal level (Jacobson & Truax, 1991). Using a control group that was also starting at an abnormal level, the RCI was used to determine whether an individual significantly improved following a therapeutic intervention. A beneficial effect can be demonstrated by a significant increase in retest score, using non-treated individuals as a control group. In contrast, individuals can start at "normal" level prior to a negative intervening event such as surgery or traumatic brain injury, and then be reassessed to determine whether there has been a statistically significant deterioration in functioning. The similarity of these two methodologies is that the individual or clinical group and corresponding control group start at the same level, either both "abnormal," or both "normal." Thus, it should be recognized that the use of RCI methodology when the clinical individual or group starts at a different level to the control group has not been well validated. An example of this would be examining recovery in those suffering from a traumatic brain injury where baseline data does not exist. When retesting to examine for recovery from an abnormal starting point, the use of an RCI based on an uninjured control group with retest normative data is not well validated. An option worthy of further consideration in this setting is to use an estimate of premorbid functioning as the baseline score. The potential validity of this approach will lie in how accurate is the premorbid estimate of functioning.

CONCLUSION AND PRACTICE POINTS

In order to conclude such a mathematically laden chapter, we thought it best to present a checklist of important points to consider in order to assist the prospective RCI user:

- RCI scores are essentially standardized change scores. Providing that relevant assumptions are met, RCI scores can be interpreted in the same way as a *Z* score—where +1.645 corresponds to a 90% confidence interval. When an RCI score exceeds the nominated level, it can be considered a statistically significant individual change.
- There are several RCI models in existence, however, the RCI Chelune and RCI McSweeny are the most widely reported.
- RCI models all share a fundamental structure: RCI = $(Y - Y')/SE$. Models differ only in how they estimate the predicted retest score (Y') and the standard error (SE).
- Most RCI models can be derived from basic test–retest parameters, namely, baseline (M_X) and retest (M_Y) means and standard deviations (S_X and S_Y), and test–retest reliability (r_{XY}).
- No one RCI model is universally more responsive to change. Responsiveness of models is determined on test–retest parameters and the individual's relative position at baseline (Z_X). If an individual starts below the control baseline mean, the regression RCI models described will be more responsive to negative change. If the individual starts above the baseline mean, the RCI Chelune will more responsive to negative change. If positive change is of interest, then RCI model responsiveness will be reversed. If the direction of differential practice changes, RCI model responsiveness will also be reversed.
- Many steps can be taken to ensure a reliable estimate of change can be made, irrespective of model used. Models will converge in estimates of change when the individual matches the control group mean, there is minimal differential practice, and test–retest reliability is adequate.
- RCI models assume that a suitable retest control or normative group in terms of demographics, setting, and retest interval is selected.

- RCI scores can essentially change a continuous outcome to a dichotomous outcome.
- Interpretation of RCI scores needs to made with the consideration that RCI is a statistic relative to the practice effect seen in the comparison group. Therefore, an evaluation of comparison-group practice effects should always be reported.
- The direction of RCI scores, positive or negative, must be interpreted with reference to the underlying metric. If the measure is time-based, or a lower score represents better performance, then the RCI value needs to be reversed prior to interpretation.

RELIABLE CHANGE IN INDIVIDUALS

- Select a suitable test–retest normative data set. The demographics and retest interval should correspond to the individual being evaluated. The relative position of the individual (Z_X) to the baseline control or normative mean should be clear.
- Examine the test–retest data for mean practice effect ($M_X - M_Y$), differential practice effect ($S_X - S_Y$), and test–retest reliability (r_{XY}). Measures with suboptimal reliability should not be used for clinical assessment of individual change. A r_{XY} of 0.90 or better would seem overly onerous, an $r_{XY} > 0.70$ may be considered.
- If the test–retest normative group is $n < 50$, then a t-distribution should be considered.
- A cut score based on a 90% confidence interval is commonly used in clinical settings.
- Several RCI models exist, with no consensus on which is most valid. We currently advise the use of RCI Crawford with multiple predictors if relevant data are available.
- Calculations are complex. However, there are several Internet-based RCI calculators. The authors have a spreadsheet available on request for automated calculation of several RCI models and the ability to save test–retest normative data.
- In the common setting where multiple measures are used, a knowledge of false positive rates can be helpful when determining if an overall effect of a treatment or event has led to significant change

RELIABLE CHANGE IN GROUPS

- RCI is calculated as above for each individual.
- An effect size can be derived by averaging the clinical or experimental RCI scores. Corresponding confidence intervals can also be derived in the traditional manner. This effect size can be used for randomized control studies for treatment effects, or cohort studies for influence of an event

or process (e.g., TBI, dementia). The effect size automatically corrects for systematic and random variability as afforded by the RCI model.

- If the outcome is correct patient selection or diagnostic accuracy, and change is kept on a continuous scale, ROC curves can be employed. ROC curves importantly take into account aspects of sensitivity and specificity and allow direct examination of the tradeoff. Cut scores can be derived for maximizing sensitivity or specificity or overall group separation, for example, with Youden's *J* index or likelihood ratios.
- If the outcome is the influence of a treatment on reliable change measured as a dichotomy (changed or not), then NNT or NNH can be used. NNT and NNH values can also be expressed as point and interval estimate statistics, for example, as a point-estimate, an NNT = 8 suggests on average 8 individuals would need to be treated in order for one significant reliable change to occur. Interval-estimates can also be derived, for example, with a 95% confidence level, between 6.5 to 9.5 individuals would need to be treated for significant reliable change to occur.
- If the outcome is measured before and after an uncontrolled event, then RR or OR can be presented. Although RR is preferable, it will usually give a lower estimate of influence. OR should be reserved for instances where RR cannot be calculated, or the OR is the outcome produced through logistical regression.

REFERENCES

Abramson, I. S. (2000). Reliable Change formula query: A statistician's comments. *Journal of International Neuropsychological Society, 6*, 365.

Beglinger, L. J., Gaydos, B., Tangphao-Daniels, O., Duff, K., Kareken, D. A., Crawford, J., . . . Siemers, E. R. (2005). Practice effects and the use of alternate forms in serial neuropsychological testing. *Archives of Clinical Neuropsychology, 20*, 517–529.

Calamia, M., Markon, K., & Tranel, D. (2012). Scoring higher the second time around: Meta-analyses of practice effects in neuropsychological assessment. *The Clinical Neuropsychologist, 26*, 543–570.

Calamia, M., Markon, K., & Tranel, D. (2013). The robust reliability of neuropsychological measures: Meta-analyses of test–retest correlations. *The Clinical Neuropsychologist, 27*, 1077–1105.

Christensen, L., & Mendoza, J. L. (1986). A method assessing change in a single subject: An alteration of the RC index. *Behavior Therapy, 12*, 305–308.

Chelune, G. J., Naugle, R. I., Luders, H., Sedlak, J., & Awad, I. A. (1993). Individual change after epilepsy surgery: Practice effects and base-rate information. *Neuropsychology, 7*, 41–52.

Cohen, R. J., & Swerdlik, M. (2009). *Psychological Testing and Assessment* (7th ed.). Boston, MA: McGraw-Hill.

Collie, A., Maruff, P., Makdissi, M., McStephen, M., Darby, D. G., & McCrory, P. (2004). Statistical procedures for determining the extent of cognitive change following concussion. *British Journal of Sports Medicine, 38*, 273–278.

Crawford, J. R., & Howell, D. C. (1998). Regression equations in clinical neuropsychology: An evaluation of statistical methods for comparing predicted and obtained scores. *Journal of Clinical and Experimental Neuropsychology, 20*, 755–762.

Crawford, J. R., & Garthwaite, P. H. (2006). Comparing patients' predicted test scores from a regression equation with their obtained scores: A significance test and point estimate of abnormality with accompanying confidence limits. *Neuropsychology, 20*, 259–271.

Duff, K. (2012). Evidence-based indicators of neuropsychological change in the individual patient: Relevant concepts and methods. *Archives of Clinical Neuropsychology, 27*, 248–261.

Heilbronner, R. L., Sweet, J. J., Attix, D. K., Krull, K. R., Henry, G. K., & Hart, R. P. (2010). Official position of the American Academy of Clinical Neuropsychology on serial neuropsychological assessment: The utility and challenges of repeat test administrations in clinical and forensic contexts. *The Clinical Neuropsychologist, 24*, 1267–1278.

Hinton-Bayre, A. D., Geffen, G. M., Geffen, L. B., McFarland, K., & Friis, P. (1999). Concussion in contact sports: Reliable change indices of impairment and recovery. *Journal of Clinical and Experimental Neuropsychology, 21*, 70–86.

Hinton-Bayre, A. D. (2005). Methodology is more important than statistics when determining reliable change. *Journal of the International Neuropsychological Society, 11*, 788–789.

Hinton-Bayre, A. D. (2010). Deriving reliable change statistics from test–retest normative data: Comparison of models and mathematical expressions. *Archives of Clinical Neuropsychology, 25*, 244–256.

Hinton-Bayre, A. D. (2011). Calculating the test–retest reliability co-efficient from normative retest data for determining reliable change. *Archives of Clinical Neuropsychology, 26*, 76–77.

Hinton-Bayre, A. D. (2012). Choice of reliable change model can alter decisions regarding neuropsychological impairment after sports-related concussion. *Clinical Journal of Sports Medicine, 22*, 105–108.

Hinton-Bayre, A. D. (2016). Detecting impairment post-concussion using Reliable Change indices. *Clinical Journal of Sports Medicine, 26*, e6–e7.

Holdnack, J. A., Drozdick, L. W., Weiss, L., G., & Iverson, G. L. (2013). *WAIS-IV, WMS-IV, and ACS: Advanced Clinical Interpretation*. Waltham, MA: Academic Press.

Howell, D. C. (2010). *Statistical Methods for Psychology* (8th ed.). Belmont, CA: Wadsworth, Cengage Learning.

Iverson, G. L., Lovell, M. R., & Collins, M. W. (2003). Interpreting change on ImPACT following sport concussion. *The Clinical Neuropsychologist, 17*, 460–467.

Jacobson, N. S., Follette, W. C., & Revenstorf, D. (1984). Psychotherapy outcome research: Methods for reporting variability and evaluating clinical significance. *Behavior Therapy, 15*, 336–352.

Jacobson, N. S., & Truax, P. (1991). Clinical significance: A statistical approach to defining meaningful change in psychotherapy research. *Journal of Consulting and Clinical Psychology, 59*, 12–19.

Kneebone, A. C., Andrew, M. J., Baker, R. A., & Knight, J. L. (1998). Neuropsychologic changes after coronary artery bypass grafting: Use of reliable change indices. *Annals of Thoracic Surgery, 65*, 1320–1325.

Maassen, G. H. (2004). The standard error in the Jacobson and Truax reliable change index: The classical approach to the assessment of reliable change. *Journal of the International Neuropsychological Society, 10,* 888–893.

Maassen, G. H. (2005). Reliable change assessment in the sport concussion research: A comment on the proposal and reviews of Collie et al. *British Journal of Sports Medicine, 39,* 483–488.

Martin, R., Sawrie, S., Gilliam, F., Mackey, M., Faught, E., Knowlton, R., & Kuzniecky, R. (2002). Determining reliable cognitive change after epilepsy surgery: Development of reliable change indices and standardized regression-based change norms for the WMS-III and WAIS-III. *Epilepsia, 43,* 1551–1558.

McSweeny, A. J., Naugle, R. I., Chelune, G. J., & Luders, H. (1993). "T scores for change": An illustration of a regression approach to depicting change in clinical neuropsychology. *The Clinical Neuropsychologist, 7,* 300–312.

Mitrushina, M., Boone, K. B., Razani, J., & D'Elia, L. F. (2005). *Handbook of Normative Data for Neuropsychological Assessment* (2nd ed.). New York: Oxford University Press.

Rapport, L. J., Brines, D. B., Axelrod, B. N., & Theisen, M. E. (1997). Full scale IQ as mediator of practice effects: The rich get richer. *The Clinical Neuropsychologist, 11,* 375–380.

Schulz, K. F., Altman, D. G., & Moher, D. (2010). CONSORT 2010 statement: Updated guidelines for reporting parallel group randomized trials. *Annals of Internal Medicine, 152,* 1–7.

Straus, S. E., Glasziou, P., Richardson, W. S., & Haynes, R. B. (2010). *Evidence-Based Medicine: How to Practice and Teach It* (4th ed.). Edinburgh: Churchill Livingston.

Strauss, E., Sherman, M. S., & Spreen, O. (2006). *A Compendium of Neuropsychological Tests: Administration, Norms and Commentary* (3rd ed.). New York: Oxford.

Streiner, D. L., & Cairney, J. (2007). What's under the ROC? An introduction to receiver operating characteristic curves. *Canadian Journal of Psychiatry, 52,* 121–128.

Suissa, D., Brassard, P., Smiechowski, B., & Suissa, S. (2012). Number needed to treat is incorrect without proper time-related considerations. *Journal of Clinical Epidemiology, 65,* 42–46.

Temkin, N. R., Heaton, R. K., Grant, I., & Dikmen, S. S. (1999). Detecting significant change in neuropsychological test performance: A comparison of four models. *Journal of the International Neuropsychological Society, 5,* 357–369.

Viera, A. J. (2008). Odds ratios and risk ratios: What's the difference and why does it matter? *Southern Medical Journal, 101,* 730–734.

von Elm, E., Egger, M., Altman, D. G., Pocock, S. J., Gotzsche, P. C., & Vandenbroucke, J. P. (2007). Strengthening the reporting of observational studies in epidemiology (STROBE) statement: Guidelines for reporting observational studies. *British Medical Journal, 335, 806–808.*

Wechsler, D. (2008). *Wechsler Adult Intelligence Scale–Fourth Edition.* San Antonio, TX: Pearson.

Wechsler, D. (2009). *Wechsler Memory Scale–Fourth Edition.* San Antonio, TX: Pearson.

7

Evidence-Based Practices in Neuropsychology

GORDON J. CHELUNE

Evidence-based medicine (EBM) is a relatively new concept in health care, with the term first being introduced in the literature by David Sackett and Gordon Guyatt and their colleagues at McMaster University in 1992 (Evidence-Based Medicine Working Group, 1992). As initially conceived, it was a call for clinicians to place less emphasis on intuition and unsystematic clinical experiences and to make greater use of empirical clinical research to guide clinical decision making. As thinking on the subject evolved, Sackett and colleagues (Sackett, Rosenberg, Gray, Haynes, & Richardson, 1996) later described EBM as "the conscientious, explicit, and judicious use of current best evidence in making decisions about the care of individual patients" (p. 71).

Although neuropsychology has a strong tradition of empirical research, widespread use of evidence-based practices in clinical neuropsychology has lagged behind other professions (Chelune, 2010). In part, this may be due to the disconnection between how the findings of neuropsychological studies are reported in the literature and their direct applicability to individual patient care, that is, our research often fails to achieve its implicit if not explicit intent—to better inform the clinical decision-making process at the level of the individual patient. The problem of translation between science and practice is not new, nor unique to neuropsychology (Rosenberg & Donald, 1995). In 1983, Costa (Costa, 1983) remarked that patients

> deserve decisions and recommendations that are founded increasingly upon empirical validation. The instruments chosen to produce data to resolve questions in a valid fashion should be selected for their power to reduce uncertainty with respect to those questions, not primarily because they fit into a diagnostic battery. (p. 7)

While not new, this problem has become acute within current value-driven, evidence-based health care systems where outcomes accountability and the management of individual patients on the basis of epidemiological information regarding outcomes has become increasingly critical to the practice of medicine (Johnson, 1997). The standard of care, almost by definition, is now "evidence-based."

This chapter is intended to provide readers with the knowledge to engage in the five basic steps involved in evidence-based practice: (1) assess the patient, (2) ask appropriate questions, (3) acquire relevant data, (4) appraise the data, and (5) apply the results. We will first briefly review the context within which EBM arose, taking into account its core components. We will then expand these components to provide a definition of evidence-based practice in clinical neuropsychology, with an emphasis on its "value" to patient care in terms of reducing uncertainity. We will conclude by working through the five steps in the evidence cycle, with special attention to the use of test operating characteristics to inform clinical decisions at the level of the individual case.

HISTORICAL ANTECEDENTS

Although EBM is a relatively recent movement in health care, its historical antecedents can be traced back to antiquity. In their excellent review of the history and development of EBM, Claridge and Fabian (Claridge & Fabian, 2005) note that perhaps the first report of a rudimentary controlled study appeared in the biblical Book of Daniel (Holy Bible, 2011):

> [8] But Daniel resolved not to defile himself with the royal food and wine, and he asked the chief official for permission not to defile himself this way. . .. [11] Daniel then said to the guard whom the chief official had appointed over Daniel, Hananiah, Mishael and Azariah, [12] "Please test your servants for ten days: Give us nothing but vegetables to eat and water to drink. [13] Then compare our appearance with that of the young men who eat the royal food, and treat your servants in accordance with what you see." [14] So he agreed to this and tested them for ten days. [15] At the end of the ten days they looked healthier and better nourished than any of the young men who ate the royal food. [16] So the guard took away their choice food and the wine they were to drink and gave them vegetables instead. (Daniel 1:8–16)

The evolution of modern EBM resulted from a coalescence of factors. Present-day EBM had its scientific beginnings in the late twentieth century with the work of Archie Cochrane in the United Kingdom and David Sackett in Canada (Claridge & Fabian, 2005). Cochrane was a staunch proponent of the randomized controlled trial (RCT) for evaluating the effectiveness of medical treatments and interventions, and his book *Effectiveness and Efficiency: Random Reflections on Health Services* (Cochrane, 1972) is considered a cornerstone of modern EBM. It was his lifelong dedication to using empirical research to guide clinical practice that led to the foundation of the Cochrane Collaboration in 1993 and the development of the Cochrane Database of Systematic Reviews (Hill, 2000). Across the

Atlantic, David Sackett and his colleagues in Canada are credited with coining the term "evidence-based medicine" (Evidence-Based Medicine Working Group, 1992) and providing the first succinct definition for its use in the field (Sackett et al., 1996). Sackett and associates (Sackett, Straus, Richardson, Rosenberg, & Haynes, 2000) have subsequently refined the definition of EBM further in their book *Evidence-Based Medicine: How to Practice and Teach EBM* as simply "the integration of best research evidence with clinical expertise and patient values" (p. 1) with the goal of maximizing clinical outcomes and quality of life for the patient. Note that the authors do not advocate the blind application of research data to guide patient care, but give equal importance to the clinical acumen of the practitioner and to the values of the individual patient. This tripartite composition of EBM is at the heart of virtually all descriptions of evidence-based practice, and its core elements can be seen in the definition of evidence-based practice adopted by the American Psychological Association (APA Presidential Task Force on Evidence-Based Practice, 2006): "Clinical decisions [should] be made in collaboration with the patient, based on the best clinically relevant evidence, and with consideration for the probable costs, benefits, and available resources and options" (p. 285).

Like all successful movements, evidence-based practices in health care did not arise in a social vacuum. Financial considerations were also a major impetus for the rapid adoption of evidence-based practices in the 1990s (*Encyclopedia of Mental Disorders*, 2016). Until the middle of the twentieth century, in the United States, health care services were provided primarily on a fee-for-service basis or covered by private indemnity insurance plans, which generally paid for any medical service deemed necessary by a physician. There were few controls on overuse of expensive and often unnecessary treatments and diagnostic procedures. In 1965, the United States government amended the Social Security Act and introduced Medicare (Title XVIII) and Medicaid (Title XIX) as national insurance policies for the elderly and individuals who have inadequate income to pay for medical services. It quickly became apparent that a significant portion of health care expenditures in the United States was being wasted on redundant and often unproven or ineffective tests and treatments (Horwitz, 1996), giving rise to an urgent need for health-care reform. In 1973, the U.S. Congress passed the Health Maintenance Organization (HMO) Act, and in 1978, Congress increased federal spending to further develop HMOs and other forms of managed-care payment systems in an effort to contain costs through largely administrative control over primary health care services (*Encyclopedia of Mental Disorders*, 2016). Fortunately, one model of managed care to emerge was "outcomes management," a system that proposed the use of epidemiological information about patient outcomes to assess and identify medical and surgical treatments that could be objectively demonstrated to have a positive impact on a patient's condition in a cost-effective manner (Segen, 2006). Outcomes management rather than administrative management called for a more value-driven, evidence-based health care system in which procedures and treatments were seen as having "value" if they could be objectively demonstrated to have a positive impact on a patient's condition in a cost-effective manner. This provided the perfect backdrop for EBM to emerge.

The final element that helped move EBM to the forefront of current health care was modern "informatics"—the digital collection, classification, storage, retrieval, and dissemination of recorded knowledge. Although electronic databases such as the Cochrane Library, an electronic database of RCTs produced by the Cochrane Collaboration, and MEDLINE, the online portal to the Medical Literature Analysis and Retrieval System (MEDLARS) database maintained by the U.S. National Library of Medicine, were available in the 1980s and early 1990s, access was primarily available only through institutional facilities such as university libraries. It was not until personal computers became widely available and the release of Web-based search engines such as PubMed in 1996 that the era of free, public, home- and office-based access to vast sources of published clinical research became a reality (National Library of Medicine, 2006-10-05). Today, practitioners have access to a wide array of databases (see Table 7.1 for examples) they can search for published information relevant to their specific patient-related questions.

EBM AS A PARADIGM SHIFT

When Sackett and colleagues introduced EBM as a new method of practicing medicine, they described it as a "paradigm shift," a new set of assumptions about

Table 7.1 Common Web-Based Electronic Research Databases

Database	**Content**
Medline/PubMed	General medical database; many journals not referenced
PsychINFO	General psychological literature, including book chapters
CINAHL	Nursing/Allied Health
Embase	Pharmacological and biomedical database including international entries
BIOSIS	Biological and biomedical sciences; journal articles, conference proceedings, books, and patents
HSTAT	Health Sciences Technology and Assessment; clinical guidelines, Agency for Healthcare Research and Quality (AHRQ) and National Institutes of Health (NIH) publications
CCRCT	Cochrane Central Register of Controlled Trials
CDSR	Cochrane Database of Systematic Reviews
DARE	Database of Abstracts and Reviews of Effects; critically appraised systematic reviews
Campbell Collaboration	Systematic reviews in education, criminal justice, and social welfare

patient care and the fundamental principles and methods for providing that care (Evidence-Based Medicine Working Group, 1992). They described the traditional paradigm of clinical practice as resting on four assumptions:

1. Unsystematic observations acquired in the course of clinical practice were a valid basis of building and maintaining one's knowledge of such things as prognosis, validity of test procedures, and treatment,
2. Simply understanding the pathophysiology and mechanisms of disease is sufficient to guide clinical practice,
3. Basic training and common sense are sufficient to evaluate new tests and interventions, and
4. Clinical expertise and general knowledge of a content area are a sufficient basis for generating guidelines for practice.

If one reflects for a moment, one can begin to question how much of our current day-to-day neuropsychological practice is based on clinical lore and the uncritical adoption of new cognitive tests and treatment procedures on their face-value alone (Dodrill, 1997).

The emerging paradigm that Sackett's group espoused rested on new assumptions. First, while acknowledging the value and necessity of clinical experience, the practice of EBM stresses the importance of making systematic observations in a clear and reproducible manner to increase confidence about patient outcomes, the value of diagnostic tests, and efficacy of treatments. Second, understanding of basic disease mechanisms is important but not sufficient for clinical practice, as one must understand symptoms within the context of the individual patient. Finally, understanding the rules of evidence is necessary to critically appraise the methods and results of published clinical research. With these assumptions, a new model of health care emerged in which the clinician's proficiency and expertise were called upon to integrate a patient's preferences, values, and circumstances with critically appraised external research evidence (Haynes, Devereaux, & Guyatt, 2002).

EVIDENCE-BASED CLINICAL NEUROPSYCHOLOGICAL PRACTICE (EBCNP): A WORKING DEFINITION

Chelune (2010) has noted that any definition of evidence-based practice in clinical neuropsychology will undoubtedly contain the same core elements found in EBM, namely, the integration of the clinician's experience and proficiency with the best available outcomes research, within the context of the unique characteristics and circumstances of the patient. In addition, because neuropsychological services are often rendered as a consultative service to other health care providers who have primary responsibility for managing the care of the patient, neuropsychologists must also integrate the specific concerns and needs of these referral sources into their evidence-based practices. With these considerations in mind, the following working definition of evidence-based clinical neuropsychology can be articulated:

> "Evidence-based clinical neuropsychological practice" (EBCNP) is a value-driven pattern of clinical practice that attempts to integrate the "best research" derived from the study of populations to inform clinical decisions about individuals within the context of the provider's expertise and individual patient values with the goal of maximizing clinical outcomes and quality of life for the patient in a cost-effective manner while addressing the concerns and needs of the provider's referral sources.

There are several elements of this definition that are worthy of comment. First, EBCNP is presented, not as a discrete action or body of knowledge, but as a process—an ongoing "pattern" of routine clinical practice. This pattern of practice is "value-driven," which is distinct from "cost-effective." "Value-driven" is used here to indicate that the practitioner's goal is to provide a service that uniquely enhances the clinical outcomes of patients in terms of the diagnosis, management, care, and ultimately quality of life for the patients (Chelune, 2002, 2010), and hence warrants reimbursement. In the context of most patient evaluations, the value of a neuropsychological test or the assessment as a whole can be judged in terms of its ability to reduce diagnostic uncertainty (Costa, 1983).

As in other areas of evidence-based practice, clinical expertise is paramount. The evidence-based neuropsychologist uses "best research" to guide his or her clinical decision-making process. However, the idea of "best" research implies that the clinician has the knowledge and expertise to first acquire relevant clinical research and then to critically appraise the information for its validity and applicability to the questions s/he has about the patient (Rosenberg & Donald, 1995). Often research findings are based on group data and group comparisons, and again the evidence-based practitioner must have skills to transform data derived from group comparisons into statements that can be directly applied to specific patients. Thus, as shown in Figure 7.1, EBCNP is an integrative process

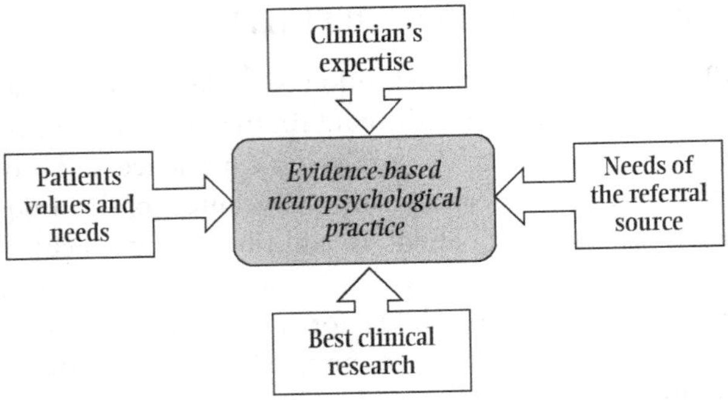

Figure 7.1 Evidence-based practice as an integrative process.

that starts with the clinician's expertise, which encompasses his or her clinical knowledge and experience, as well as skills in asking answerable patient-focused questions, acquiring relevant clinical research through informatics, critically appraising this research, and then applying the information in a way that respects the patient's needs and values. When functioning as consultant, the evidence-based neuropsychologist must also apply the information in ways that answer the referral source "need to know" in order to best manage the patient's care.

The process of EBCNP should be familiar to all of us, as it parallels that of the scientific method: hypothesis formation, literature review, study design, and data collection, analysis, and conclusions. Consider the example of a 59-year-old college-educated woman who has been working in middle management at a technology firm. She suffers an ischemic left middle cerebral artery stroke and presents to the Emergency Room with symptoms of slurred speech, confusion, and right hemiparesis. She is treated with tissue Plasminogen Activator (tPA) within two hours of symptom onset and appears to make a good recovery over the course of two months. This patient may be referred for neuropsychological evaluation by her outpatient neurologist to determine if she has any significant residual language or memory deficits that might benefit from speech therapy. The same patient maybe referred by the Employee Assistance Program at her company to determine whether to let the patient come back to work or move her from sick-leave to short-term disability. In both situations, the neuropsychologist needs to:

1. Convert the patient's presenting complaints and problems into answerable questions (i.e., "Does the patient have cognitive deficits that would benefit from speech therapy?" or "Is the patient fit for returning to work?"),
2. Gather relevant background information from the patient's social, vocational, and medical history and integrate this with the best available research specific to the referral question,
3. Critically appraise the acquired information,
4. Design a relevant test protocol that will generate data to answer the specific referral question regarding the patient, and
5. Evaluate the data and answer the referral question.

FIVE KEY STEPS IN EVIDENCE-BASED PRACTICE

Depending on the source, there are essentially five basic steps in evidence-based practice, each requiring a specific set of skills (Akobeng, 2005; Rosenberg & Donald, 1995).

These steps are as follows:

1. Assessing the patient is the starting point of every clinical evaluation, and the basics of patient interviewing and deconstructing neuropsychological referral questions are commonly taught (Lezak, Howieson, Bigler, & Tranel, 2012; Schoenberg & Scott, 2011) and are not unique to evidence-based

practice. For the purposes of this chapter, we will focus on steps 2 to 5, as follows.

2. Ask answerable clinical questions based on the patient's problem, that is, convert our need for information regarding diagnosis, prognosis, causation, or therapy into an answerable question.
3. Acquire the "best" evidence to address our question.
4. Appraise the evidence for its validity, applicability, and impact for our patient.
5. Apply the evidence.

Asking Answerable Questions

Just as every journey begins with the first step, patient evaluations always begin by presenting us with a need for some information regarding the patient's diagnosis, prognosis, or management. Translating this clinical need to know into a focused and answerable question is not always as straightforward as it might seem, and it often can be quite challenging (Akobeng, 2005). For example, a patient is referred for neuropsychological evaluation for suspected frontotemporal lobar degeneration (FTD), and I want to know if there are specific neuropsychological tests or test patterns that can help me differentiate FTD from other neurodegenerative conditions such as Alzheimer's disease (AD). In my general reading, I believe that patients with AD perform differently on semantic and phonemic fluency tests than patients with AD. Sackett and colleagues suggest first breaking my clinical question into a general background question and then a focused foreground question (Sackett et al., 2000). The general background question has two components: a "question stem" (such as "can," "why," "how," "when") followed by some aspect of the disorder. In our FTD example, the background question might simply be, "Can neuropsychological tests differentiate FTD from AD?" To focus this question so that it can be empirically answered, we would employ the PICO model (Patient/Population/Problem, Intervention/Indicator, Comparison, and Outcome). In our example, the foreground question becomes:

- Patient: with frontotemporal dementia
- Intervention: fluency tests
- Comparison: compared to patients with Alzheimer's disease
- Outcome: are compared (sensitivity, specificity)?

In more recent years, others (Heneghan & Badenoch, 2006) have extended the PICO model of formulating answerable clinical questions to include Type of Question and Type of Study (PICO-TT).

As seen in Table 7.2, clinical questions can fall into a several categories, including questions about etiology, diagnosis, prognosis, therapy, cost-effectiveness, and quality of life. Knowing the type of question we want to ask tells us "what" to look for, "where" to look, and "what" to expect. In our example, if we have a

Table 7.2 Common Types of Clinical Questions and the Types of Study Designs That Can Address Evidence-Based Questions (adapted from Heneghan & Badenoch, 2006)

Type of Question	Type of Study Designs
Etiology: Disease causes and modes of operation	Case-control or cohort studies
Diagnostic: Signs, symptoms, or tests for diagnosis of a disorder	Diagnostic validations studies
Prognosis: The probable course of disease over time	Inception cohort studies
Therapy: Selection of effective treatments that meet patient values	Randomized controlled trials
Cost-effectiveness: Comparison of efficacy/cost of interventions	Economic evaluation
Quality of Life: What will QoL of the patient be?	Qualitative study

patient presenting with possible FTD, and our question is primarily diagnostic, we might use PubMed to look for diagnostic validity studies that provide information on the sensitivity and specificity of fluency procedures in discriminating FTD from other neurodegenerative conditions such as AD. On the other hand, if we were interested in the efficacy of using cholinesterase inhibitors to treat FTD, we might look for treatment studies in the Cochrane Report for randomized clinical trials that have attempted to use these medications to treat FTD compared to AD.

Acquire Relevant Information

Once a focused clinical question has been articulated, it is time to acquire the relevant evidence that will help answer the question. One might turn to traditional sources such as textbooks or journals that are on hand, but that information is likely to be dated and randomly organized. One could also do a simple Google search, but this is likely to produce spurious citations and may not reflect "the best available research." Depending on the question and patient, Akobeng suggests using secondary sources of well-summarized evidence that may provide quick, evidence-based answers to specific questions (Akobeng, 2005). Examples of such secondary sources include *Archimedes* (http://adc.bmjjournals.com/cgi/collection/archimedes), *BestBets* (http://www.bestbest.org/index.html), and *Clinical Evidence* (http://www.clinicalevidence.com/ceweb/conditions/index.jsp). However, use of an online electronic bibliographic database such as MEDLINE is apt to be the most productive in terms of quickly identifying relevant research with respect to our clinical question. The terms generated from the PICO question can be readily used as the key search terms. In our example, we might use *Frontotemporal* or *Frontal Temporal Dementia, Alzheimer's disease, verbal fluency*, and *compare* or *differentiate*.

The ability to search databases efficiently is a skill that develops through frequent searches on a regular basis, and there are many shortcuts that one can learn. Use of Boolean operators such as AND, OR, and NOT, and nesting terms within parentheses can make searches more precise (APUS Librarians, 2015). If one expands the PICO question to incorporate the Type of question and/or Type of study, even more refined advanced searches are possible.

For those who do frequent searches, one might anticipate that our specific search question might get different results depending on whether we use "Frontotemporal" versus "Frontal Temporal" dementia or whether we use Alzheimer's "Disease" versus "Dementia." To simplify our search, we could use the Boolean operator "OR" to capture both "Frontotemporal" and "Frontal Temporal" subjects, whereas we might simplify our search for subject groups labeled Alzheimer's "Disease" or "Dementia" by simply using "Alzheimer's," without specifying *disease* or *dementia*. For example, in the case of our PICO question where we are interested in diagnostic studies that use verbal fluency to differentiate FTD and AD, one could put our various terms into the search bar of a research database such as PsycINFO, using Advanced Search, designating our subject (SU) fields as (*frontal temporal* OR *frontotemporal*) AND *Alzheimer's*, AND the keyword (KW) *fluency*, to generate a list of eight primary references. Alternately, we could go to the home page of PubMed (http://www.ncbi.nlm.nih.gov/pubmed/) and use the PubMed tool "Clinical Queries" (in the center column of options) to do a more focused search. Here we can put in our search terms, and when we enter "Search" we are then prompted with options for Category (Etiology, Diagnosis, Treatment, Prognosis, or Clinical prediction guidelines) and Scope of search (Broad or Narrow), with the results segregated into Clinical Studies and Systematic Reviews. In our example, we would select "Diagnostic" and perhaps "Broad." For our search statement, we are interested in both AD and FTD as variably used in the literature, so nesting terms is helpful, with the search entry being—"(Frontal temporal OR frontotemporal) AND Alzheimer's AND fluency, compare." This search generated six primary clinical studies and one meta-analysis, a very manageable number of papers to appraise in our next step.

Appraise the Evidence

While systematically identifying potentially relevant clinical research is a necessary step in evidence-based practice, it is not, in itself, sufficient. The studies acquired by our systematic searches must still be appraised as to their merits and limitations. The popular adage "you are what you eat," which can be traced to the nineteenth-century philosopher Brillat-Savarin (Gooch, 2013), stresses the relationship between a healthy diet and a healthy body. By analogy, one could argue that our knowledge and ability to practice as neuropsychologists are likewise dependent on the quality of the research we consume. While neuropsychology has a robust research literature, many research studies fail to provide key details that can inform the consumer about the quality and applicability of the investigational findings to individual clinical decision making. The evidence-based neuropsychological practitioner must not only develop the skills to acquire relevant clinical research, but also have the skills to critically appraise its validity, reliability, and applicability once obtained.

There are many ways to consider the quality of evidence acquired by our systematic searches. As a starting point, one can use the *levels of evidence pyramid*, which looks at different types of evidence in terms of their rigor, study design, and generalizability. As seen in Figure 7.2, the lowest level of evidence consists of *editorials, expert opinions,* and *chapter reviews* such as this one. Evidence at this level is personally filtered by the author(s) and thus subject to the biases of the writer. This may be a good starting point to gain an appreciation of a topic, but the information may be dated and seldom should be the sole basis of evidence-based clinical decisions. As we move up the evidence pyramid, we encounter empirical studies that are unfiltered, that is, peer-reviewed studies that report data from specific investigations. *Case series and case reports* are typically considered weak evidence, as they generally have no control groups for comparison, or provide limited statistical analyses of the findings. Although weak by comparison to large group studies, case series and qualitative reports can be useful, however, when the condition of interest is rare in the population, and case series provide some degree of replication.

Case controlled studies provide a stronger level of evidence and are quite common in the neuropsychological research literature. These are retrospective studies in which the investigator compares one or more patient groups that already have known conditions of interest or exposures, and looks for factors that differentiate the groups. For example, an investigator may wish to determine if cognitive impairment is related to severity of chronic kidney disease (CKD) by comparing the neuropsychological performances of non–dialysis-dependent patients (CKD Stages III and IV) with those on hemodialysis for end-stage renal disease (Kurella, Chertow, Luan, & Yaffe, 2004). Groups are often large, and the

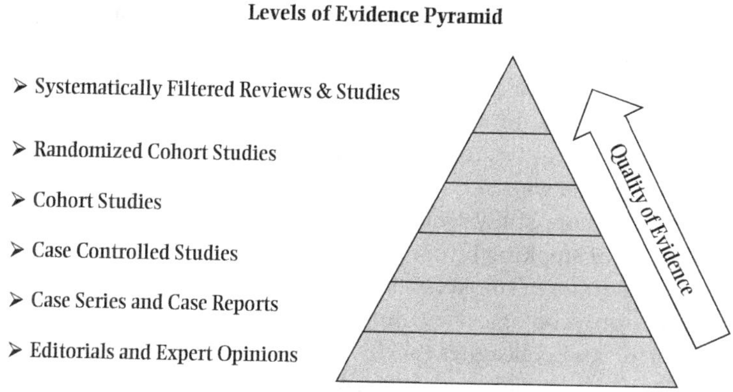

Figure 7.2 Levels of the Evidence Pyramid. EBM Pyramid and EBM Page Generator, (c) 2006 Trustees of Dartmouth College and Yale University. All rights reserved. Produced by Jan Glover, David Izzo, Karen Odato, and Lei Wang.

statistical analyses can be quite eloquent. However, selection bias can be a significant problem in case-controlled studies, and the evidence-based researcher should look to see if there other studies that provide convergent findings. The astute reader also needs to review the *Participants* section of the research reports very carefully. Incomplete or inadequate reporting of subject-selection procedures and research findings can hamper the assessment of the strengths and weaknesses of studies, possibly leading to faulty conclusions. Take, for example, one of our early epilepsy-surgery studies (Hermann et al., 1999), where we examined changes in visual confrontation among 217 patients with intractable left temporal lobe seizures who underwent one of four surgical approaches (tailored resections with intraoperative mapping, tailored resections with extraoperative mapping, standard resections with sparing of the superior temporal gyrus, and standard resections including excision of the superior temporal gyrus). Changes in naming were standardized against a group of 90 patients with complex partial seizures who were tested twice but who did not undergo surgery. The abstract for the paper reported: "Results showed significant decline in visual confrontation naming following left ATL, regardless of surgical technique. Across surgical techniques, the risk for decline in visual confrontation naming was associated with a later age of seizure onset and more extensive resections of lateral temporal neocortex" (p. 3). At first glance, it would appear that any of the four surgical approaches would be reasonable for a patient with intractable left temporal lobe seizures. However, on closer examination of the *Participants* section, we find that the patient selection was restricted to those without neocortical lesions and who did not have evidence on MRI of lesions other than hippocampal atrophy. Hence, the equipoise among the surgical approaches in terms of visual confrontation naming morbidity does not extend to patients whose seizures were related to tumors, cortical dysplasias, hamartomas, or other structural lesions. Also, because this was a retrospective case-controlled study in which patients were not randomized to different surgical approaches, we do not know whether the four surgical approaches were truly equivalent, or whether the apparent equivalency was due to unsuspected factors such as the skill of the neurosurgeons to select appropriate patients for a given approach.

Higher on the evidence pyramid are *cohort studies*, which involve a prospective design. Here the investigator compares a group of individuals with a known factor (condition, treatment, or exposure) with another group without the factor to determine whether or not outcomes are different over time. A classic example of a cohort study would be one designed to study the long-term deleterious effects of smoking by comparing differences in the incidence of lung disease between a group of smokers and a comparable group of nonsmokers after 10 years. A neuropsychological example of a prospective cohort study is one reported by Suchy and colleagues (Suchy, Kraybill, & Franchow, 2011) in which 50 community-dwelling older adults were assessed for reactions to "novelty" and then followed for over 1.5 years using a comprehensive mental status exam. Those who displayed a novelty effect at baseline were found to be four times more likely (LR+ = 3.98) of showing a reliable cognitive decline on the mental status exam than those who did not have the novelty effect. Because cohort studies are essentially observational studies, they are not as robust as randomized controlled studies since the groups under consideration may differ on variables other than the one under investigation.

The most rigorous, unfiltered study design is that of a *randomized controlled trial* (RCT). By using randomization and blinding, these studies are carefully designed, planned experiments in which a treatment, intervention, or exposure is introduced in a random order to one patient group (the intervention group) but not the other (no-intervention group) to study its clinical impact. Differences in outcomes are measured between the two groups and subjected to quantitative analysis to determine cause and effect. The recent Systolic Blood Pressure Intervention Trial (SPRINT)—Memory and Cognition in Decreased Hypertension (MIND) trial sponsored by the National Institutes of Health (SPRINT Research Group, 2015) is an example of a two-arm, multicenter RCT designed to test whether a treatment program aimed at reducing systolic blood pressure to a lower goal (120 mm Hg) than the currently recommended target (140 mm Hg) would reduce cardiovascular disease risk and decrease the rate of incident dementia and cognitive decline in hypertensive individuals over the age of 50. Follow-up of the 9,361 patients randomized in the trial was stopped early after three and a half years because the risk of cardiovascular death and morbidity was dramatically lower in the intensive treatment arm. The longitudinal cognitive outcome data are still being collected.

At the top of the evidence pyramid, we find *critically appraised topics, systematic reviews,* and *meta-analyses*. These are filtered studies, that is, they are selected by the author on the basis of clearly defined criteria. Critically appraised topics (CATs) are brief summaries of systematically acquired evidence deemed by the author to represent the best available research evidence on a specific clinical topic of interest. CATs are patient-centered and designed to answer explicit clinical questions that arise repeatedly in clinical practice (e.g., "Will my elderly patient benefit from a computerized 'brain-training' program?"). Individual CATs often have a limited scope and can become outdated as new evidence emerges in the literature. However, for the busy clinician, CATs can be a reasonable substitute for the more extensive gold standard—the systematic review. For in-depth treatments of CATs, see the chapters by D. Berry (Chapter 11) and J. Miller (Chapter 12) in this volume, and the paper by Bowden and associates (Bowden, Harrison, & Loring, 2014).

Systematic reviews are more comprehensive and rigorous versions of CATs, and also more labor-intensive to construct. Like CATs, systematic reviews are focused on specific clinical topics and designed to answer well-defined questions. However, unlike CATs that may be based on as little as a single, critically appraised research report, systematic reviews represent extensive literature searches, often involving multiple databases such as those shown in Table 7.1. They typically have an explicit and well-articulated search strategy with clear inclusion and exclusion criteria, and after assessing the quality of the papers located, the authors present their findings in a systematic fashion to address the predetermined clinical question. For examples of systematic reviews, the interested reader may refer to the systematic review published by Karr and associates (Karr, Areshenkoff, & Garcia-Barrera, 2014), *The neuropsychological outcomes of concussion: A systematic review of meta-analyses on the cognitive sequelae of mild traumatic brain injury*, or the one reported by Spector and colleagues (Spector, Orrell, & Hall, 2012), *Systematic review of neuropsychological outcomes in dementia from cognition-based psychological interventions*, which has been included in the *Database of Abstracts of Reviews of Effects (DARE): Quality-Assessed Reviews*. The reader may also refer to the journal *Neuropsychology Review*, which is now dedicated to publishing quality systematic reviews and meta-analyses in neuropsychology (Loring & Bowden, 2016). For those interested in developing their own systematic reviews for publication, guidelines and checklists can be found on the website of PRISMA (Preferred Reporting Items of Systematic Reviews and Meta-Analyses), http://www.prisma-statement.org/Default.aspx.

Meta-analyses are often based on the results of systematic reviews and represent a statistical extension in which the results of studies identified in the systematic review are combined and reported as if they were a single large study. For example, Rohling and colleagues (Rohling, Faust, Beverly, & Demakis, 2009) performed a meta-analysis of the literature systematically reviewed by Cicerone et al. (Cicerone et al., 2000; Cicerone et al., 2005) involving 2,014 patients from 115 studies, and in doing so, they were able to provide empirical support for the effectiveness of attention training after traumatic brain injury and for language and neglect symptoms after strokes.

As we stated at the onset of this section, the evidence pyramid is a good starting point in terms of appraising evidence. However, it is still incumbent on evidence-based practitioners to evaluate the relative merits of the individual studies that were identified in their systematic searches if they wish to use this information to guide their clinical decisions. While RCTs may represent a rigorous study design to answer questions about *effects*, not all RCTs are necessarily well designed. In the end, a very well-executed case-controlled study may be more useful and applicable to a given patient. It may seem obvious, but readers of the scientific literature need to be able to discern from a paper what the purpose or hypothesis of the paper was, what was planned in terms of executing the research design (and what was not), what the results were and whether the statistical procedures used were appropriate, and whether the conclusions are appropriate given the results. As most journal editors know well, it takes skill (and practice) to know how to read papers critically—in terms of both what is stated and what is missing due to inadequate reporting.

Because of the great variability in the quality of reporting of research studies, many journals are beginning to adopt standards for various types of reports that are designed to increase the transparency, accuracy, and completeness of reporting so that readers are better able to identify potential sources of bias that may limit the study generalizability. Chapter 9 by M. Schoenberg in this volume discusses some of these guidelines. While primarily meant to be used by researchers in preparing their reports for publication and not meant to judge quality, many of these guidelines are accompanied by checklists that readers may find useful to guide their appraisals of the articles while they are reading the papers. For our purposes here, I will only mention three guidelines: STROBE, CONSORT, and STARD.

STROBE stands for Strengthening the Reporting of Observational Studies in Epidemiology. The STROBE guideline was developed through an international collaboration of epidemiologists, methodologists, statisticians, researchers, and journal editors who were actively involved in the conduct and publication of observational studies (von Elm et al., 2007). The details of the STROBE guideline can be found on the website http://www.strobe-statement.org/, along with several downloadable checklists for case-controlled, cohort, and cross-sectional studies. While the checklists are intended for researchers who are preparing manuscripts for publication, they are useful guides for readers as well. In fact, the STROBE criteria have recently been reviewed by Loring and Bowden to show how they are applicable to neuropsychological research, and how adherence to these standards can promote better patient care and enhance the rigor of neuropsychology among the clinical neurosciences (Loring & Bowden, 2014).

The CONSORT (Consolidated Standards of Reporting Trials) statement of 2010 (Schulz, Altman, & Moher, 2010), like STROBE, is intended to alleviate some of the problems that arise from inadequate reporting, but specifically in clinical trials. CONSORT proposes a minimum set of recommendations for reporting RCTs, with the goals of improving reporting, and enabling readers to understand trial design, conduct, analysis, and interpretation, and to assess the validity of its results. The 2010 CONSORT statement contains a 25-item checklist and flow diagram that are available for review and download at the website: http://www.consort-statement.org/. Miller and colleagues have reviewed CONSORT criteria and have discussed how the individual criteria could be implemented in neuropsychological research paradigms (Miller, Schoenberg, & Bilder, 2014).

The final guideline to be mentioned here is STARD (Standards for the Reporting of Diagnostic Accuracy Studies). Because many neuropsychological studies have an implicit, if not explicit, intention to provide diagnostic information, STARD is especially relevant for the evidence-based clinical neuropsychologist. The objective of the STARD initiative is to improve the accuracy and completeness of reporting of studies of diagnostic accuracy so that readers can assess potential bias in a study and evaluate the generalizability of the findings (Bossuyt et al., 2003). The STARD guideline consist of a 25-item checklist and recommends the use of a flow diagram that describes the study design and selection of patients. Figure 7.3 provides an example of a STARD-inspired flow chart for a retrospective case-controlled study in which the investigators wanted to compare the diagnostic utility of verbal fluency patterns to distinguish patients with prototypical Alzheimer's versus frontotemporal dementia PET scans. The two groups each consisted of 45 patients, but to arrive at these groups, nearly 3,100 patients in a clinic registry needed to be considered.

The STROBE, CONSORT, and STARD guidelines can all be useful to have on hand when appraising evidence, but they are primarily meant for use in preparing

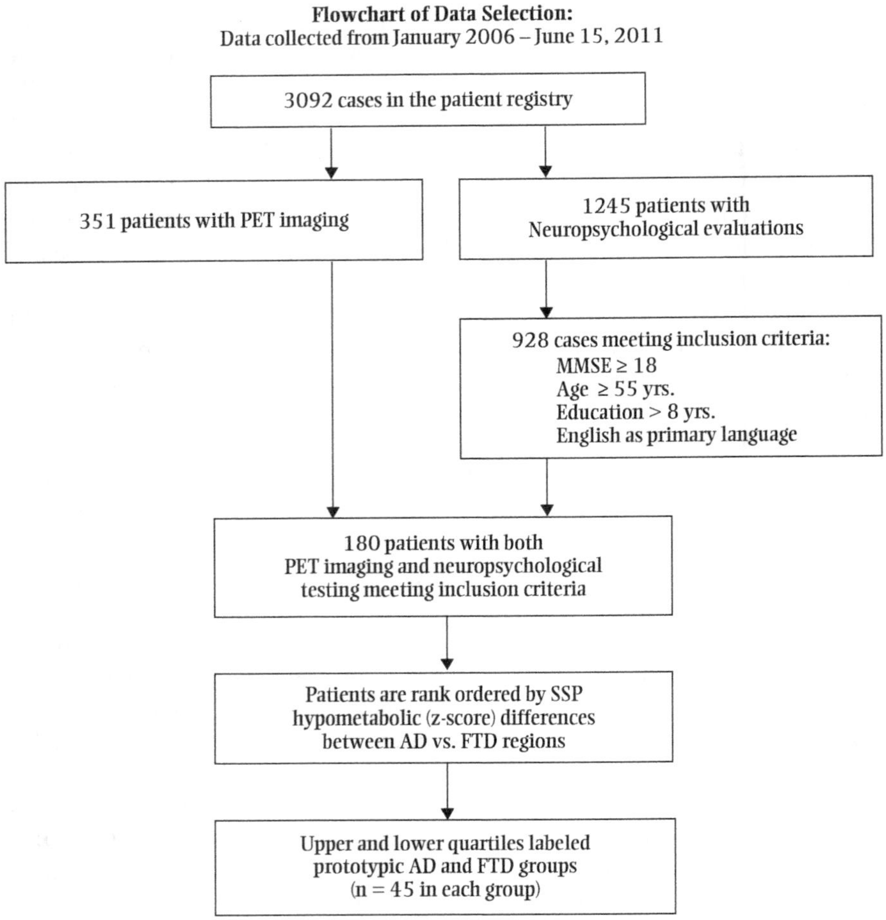

Figure 7.3 Example of a data-collection flowchart.

manuscripts for publication. The small volume *How to Read a Paper: The Basics of Evidence-Based Medicine* (Greenhalgh, 2006) is specifically intended for the consumer, and it is an extremely useful guide. The text not only guides the evidence-based reader on how to set up literature searches, but guides the reader through different sections of a typical research report, providing a checklist to accompany each of the chapters. Since most neuropsychological evaluations are designed to reduce diagnostic uncertainty (Costa, 1983) and rely heavily on the diagnostic validity of neuropsychological tests (Ivnik et al., 2001), Chapter 7, "Papers That Report the Results of Diagnostic or Screening Tests," is especially relevant for appraising the quality of diagnostic studies and their applicability to patient decision making. Common Test Operating Characteristics (TOC) such as sensitivity, specificity, odds ratio, and, importantly, the likelihood ratio are discussed. These Bayesian-based indices reflect how a given test operates in clinical situations, and will form the empirical basis of our discussion of the final step in evidence-based practice, namely, applying research evidence.

Apply the Evidence

After our clinical assessment of the patient, we have taken our need for information, translated it into an answerable question, searched the research literature to acquire relevant information, and critically appraised it in terms of its validity and applicability to our patient's problem. Now we must apply what we have found to guide our clinical decision making about the patient. For example, our search to answer the question of whether differences in semantic and phonemic fluency could help us differentiate patients with AD from those with FTD yielded several papers of interest, including a meta-analysis (Henry, Crawford, & Phillips, 2004). The meta-analysis collapsed 153 studies involving 15,990 patients and concluded that "semantic, but not phonemic fluency, was significantly more impaired . . ." and that "semantic memory deficit in Dementia of the Alzheimer's Type [DAT] qualifies as a differential deficit . . ." (p. 1212). This adds to our clinical confidence that poor semantic versus phonemic fluency in a patient suspected of AD may, in fact, have AD. However, it does not tell us how big a discrepancy is needed to be confident that the patient has AD. Herein lies the rub. In our working definition of EBCNP, we proposed that one of the defining features of evidence-based practice was the ability to *integrate the "best research" derived from the study of populations to inform clinical decisions about individuals.* To move from group data to data that are applicable at the level of the individual, the evidence-based practitioner in neuropsychology needs to shift how she or he interprets and uses data.

Most case-controlled studies, and even many cohort studies, report statistical differences between aggregate or mean levels of performance, with the probability (*p*-value) level denoting whether the difference is reliable and repeatable and not due to measurement error or chance fluctuations in the test scores. In what was truly a seminal paper, Matarazzo and Herman pointed out that there is a difference between *statistical significance* and *clinical significance*, with the latter referring to whether an observed finding is *sufficiently rare* in a reference population (e.g., normal population) such that it is more likely to have been obtained in a population external to the reference group (e.g., "abnormal"—a group with a condition of interest: Matarazzo & Herman, 1984). This distinction between "how much" of a difference is needed to be statistically significant versus "how many" to be rare and clinically meaningful (an issue of base rates) is important in outcomes research (Smith, 2002), and central for moving from group data to data that can be applied at the level of the individual.

For illustration, let us consider the comparison of patients with presumed mild cognitive impairment (MCI; the condition of interest or COI) and cognitively normal individuals (reference population: RP) on a mental status test such as the Montreal Cognitive Assessment or MOCA (Nasreddine et al., 2005). The idealized distributions of MOCA scores for both groups are depicted in Figure

7.4. It is clear that the average performance of the COI group is much lower than that of the RP (M = 22.1 vs. 27.4), although there is some overlap between the distributions. Besides looking at the mean level of performance between the groups, we can also look at the diagnostic efficiency of the MOCA in terms of base rates. At the point of overlap between the two distributions (position "A"), we have placed a heavy dotted line representing the optimal cutoff below which most individuals with the COI score, and above which most of the RP group scores. For the MOCA, this cutoff score is ≤25 (Nasreddine et al., 2005). Those with the COI who fall below the cutoff are "True Positives," and those in the RP group who score above the cutoff are "True Negatives." There are some individuals with the COI who fall above the cutoff, and they represent "False Negatives," and some in the RP group that fall below the cutoff and are considered "False Positives." Knowing the number of individuals who fall below and above the cutoff in each group allows us to calculate, among many other things, the sensitivity (percentage of true positives in the COI group) and the specificity (percentage of true negatives in the RP group), given the stated cutoff score.

In our example of the MOCA, Nasraddine and colleagues (2005) reported a sensitivity of 90% and a specificity of 87% when comparing individuals with MCI versus cognitively normal controls and using a cutoff of ≤25, that is, 90% of individuals in their MCI group scored below the cutoff, and 87% of in the normal group scored above this cutoff. Of course, individuals in each group showed a range of performance on the MOCA. We could use a more stringent cutoff of ≤23, shown as position "B" in Figure 7.4. At this cutoff, there would be fewer true positives identified in the COI group (resulting in lower sensitivity), but more true negatives in the RP group (increased specificity). This is not necessarily a bad thing. In their volume on evidence-based medicine, Sackett and colleagues (Sackett, Straus, Richardson, & Haynes, 2000) describe cutoffs with very high specificity as a *SpPin*—a score with high specificity such that a positive result (a

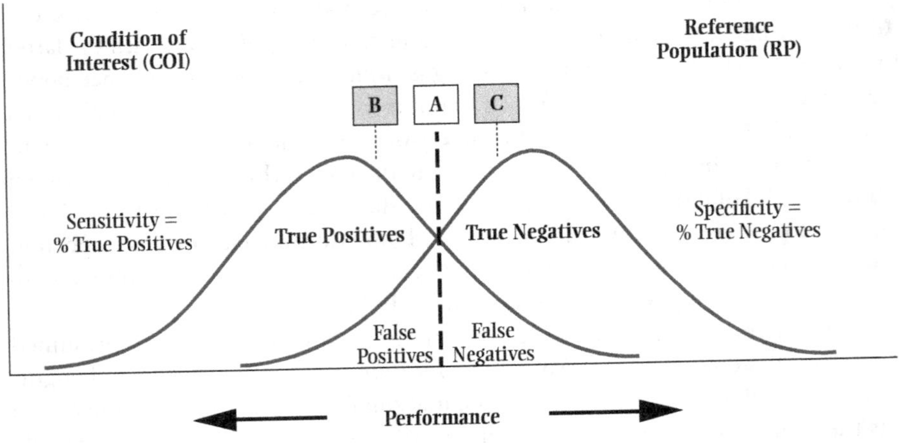

Figure 7.4 A base-rate approach to looking at group differences.

score below the cutoff) rules the COI "in." We may want to have at cutoff score that is a SpPin if we were relying heavily on the test for diagnostic purposes, since we want to be confident in capturing as many individuals as possible with the COI. Conversely, we could use a more liberal cutoff score such as ≤28, shown as position "C" in Figure 7.4. At this cutoff, we would misclassify more of the RP group (false positives), but very few of the COI group would be expected to score above this cutoff. This cutoff results in a SnNout—a cutoff with high sensitivity where a negative result (scores above the cutoff) rules the COI "out" (Sackett et al., 2000). Cut-off scores that result in a SnNout may be useful for screening purposes since most RP cases are ruled out, and those that remain will be expected to go on for further evaluation.

It is clear from the discussion above that "tests" themselves do not have sensitivity and specificity. Rather, it is the specific test scores that have sensitivity and specificity, and these are specific to how the test operates within the context of the specific samples examined. Plotting the sensitivity and specificity of each score, we could generate a receiver operating curve (ROC) as well as the likelihood of the COI with each score. Because the operating characteristics of a test depend on the samples within which they are used, it is incumbent on the evidence-based practitioner to critically evaluate the characteristics of the patient groups to determine their representativeness and adequacy.

When we compare groups in terms of base-rate information, we can cast the data into a simple 2 x 2 matrix as shown in Figure 7.5, typically with the true positive cases with the COI placed in the upper left corner. Then, by combining the cells in different ways, we can calculate a number of useful indexes that can inform our clinical decision making. Table 7.3 summarizes a number of these base-rate indexes, and many online calculators are available to calculate these and other indexes automatically (e.g., http://statpages.info/ctab2x2.html). For the purpose of our discussion here, we will focus on six common diagnostic indexes: prevalence, sensitivity, specificity, likelihood ratio, pre-test probability, and post-test probability, and the online calculator located at http://araw.mede.uic.edu/cgi-bin/testcalc.pl is particularly helpful, as it allows one to adjust the expected prevalence of the COI to match local samples and produces a *nomogram*, a visual illustration of how test results change the post-test likelihood of detecting the COI, given the prevalence.

		Condition of Interest	
		Yes	**No**
Test Result	**Yes** +	True Positive A	False Positive B
	No –	False Negative C	True Negative D

Figure 7.5 The 2 x 2 diagnostic matrix for Bayesian analyses.

Table 7.3 Sample of Base-Rate Indexes That Can Be Derived from a 2 x 2 Classification Matrix

Index	Calculation	Description
% Prevalence (Base-Rate) of COI	[(A+C)/N]*100	% of cases with the COI in the sample (COI + RP)
% Overall Correct Hit Rate	[(A+B)/N]*100	% of True Positives and True Negatives
Sensitivity (% True Positives)	[(C+D)/N]*100	% of cases with the COI who test positive
Specificity (% True Negatives)	[(A+D)/N]*100	% of case without the COI who test negative
Positive Predictive Power	A/(A+C)	% of cases with a positive test score who have the COI
Negative Predictive Power	D/(B+D)	% of cases with negative test scores that are free of the COI
Odds Ratio	(A*D)/(B*C)	A measure of effect size; the odds of having the COI when tested positive, divided by the odds of having the COI when tested negative
Risk Ratio (cohort studies)	[A/(A+B)]/[C/(C+D)]	Like the odds ratio, but expressed as a proportion and used in cohort studies
Likelihood Ratio (LR+)	Sensitivity/ (1-Specificity)	Likelihood of testing positive with the COI vs. likelihood of positive results without the COI; i.e., how likely is the COI given a positive result?
Pre-Test Odds	Prevalence/ (1-Prevalence)	Odds of having the COI before a test is given
Post-Test Odds	Pre-Test Odds*LR	Odds of having the COI after a test is given
Pre-Test Probability	(A+C)/N	Probability of having the COI before a test is given
Post-Test Probability	Post-test Odds/(Post-test Odds+1)	Probability of having the COI after a test is given

In diagnostic settings, the purpose of giving a test is to reduce uncertainty, or conversely, to increase diagnostic certainty (Costa, 1983). The degree that a given test accomplishes this goal reflects its "value." Recall that from our working definition, EBCNP is a "value-driven pattern of practice." Statistically, one way of thinking about "value" can be deduced by applying Bayes Theorem, which loosely translated (Mayer, 2010) states that what we know after giving a test (i.e., post-test probability) is equal to what we knew before doing the test (i.e., pre-test probability or prevalence of the COI) times a modifier (based on the test results). Test results are used to adjust a *prior distribution* to form a new *posterior distribution* of scores (post-test probabilities). The more that a test result changes the pre-test probability (what we knew before giving the test), the greater value or contribution the test has in the diagnostic process, and potentially for contributing to treatment choices. This shift from pre-test to post-test probabilities is captured by the positive Likelihood Ratio (LR+), which is the ratio of sensitivity divided by the quantity (1 minus specificity), or the ratio of the percentage of "true positives" to percentage of "false positives." (The negative Likelihood Ratio [LR–] represents the decrease in likelihood of the COI with a negative test result.) Because sensitivity and specificity are properties of how a test performs in specified populations, they are independent of prevalence, and by extension, so is the LR+. This is important because once research has established a LR+, it can be used in settings where the prevalence of the COI may be different from the one in which it was originally derived. Positive Likelihood Ratios of less than 1.0 are not meaningful, 2–4 are small, 5–9 are considered moderate, and 10 or greater are large and considered virtually diagnostically certain.

APPRAISING AND APPLYING THE EVIDENCE: WORKED EXAMPLES

It is time for a concrete example. Let us consider the paper by Filoteo and associates (Filoteo et al., 2009), who conducted a case-controlled study looking at differential patterns of verbal learning and memory among patients with autopsy-confirmed dementia with Lewy bodies (DLB) and Parkinson's disease with dementia (PDD). The patients were matched on demographics and performance on a comprehensive mental status exam, with 24 patients in each group. By study design, the PDD group was identified as the COI, and the DLB group was the RP. Using a statistically derived composite cutoff score, the authors report an overall hit rate of 81.3% and a sensitivity for classifying the PDD patients of 75% and a specificity of 87.5% (i.e., 18/24 of the PPD and 21/24 of the DLB cases were correctly classified by the cutoff score). We now have the four base-rate scores to put into a 2 x 2 diagnostic matrix (cell A = 18, B = 3, C = 6, and D = 21), and we can use the online calculator found at http://araw.mede.uic.edu/cgi-bin/testcalc.pl to calculate the positive and negative Likelihood Ratios, as well as the changes in pre- to post-test probabilities, given the results of the test. The LR+ was 6.0 or moderate, that is, a patient with a positive test result was six times more likely to have PPD than DLB. (When the test result was negative, the LR– was .29.) Because the sample sizes are equal, the prevalence or pre-test probability of the COI (PDD) in this study is 50%. Given the results of the learning and memory test, the post-test probability of PDD given a positive test is now 86%. If the test results were negative, the post-test probability of PDD would have decreased from 50% to 22%. These results are visually summarized in the nomogram depicted on the left side of Figure 7.6. The pre-test probability or prevalence of the COI (.50) is indicated along the left column, and the LR+ ratio of 6.0 is indicated in the middle column.

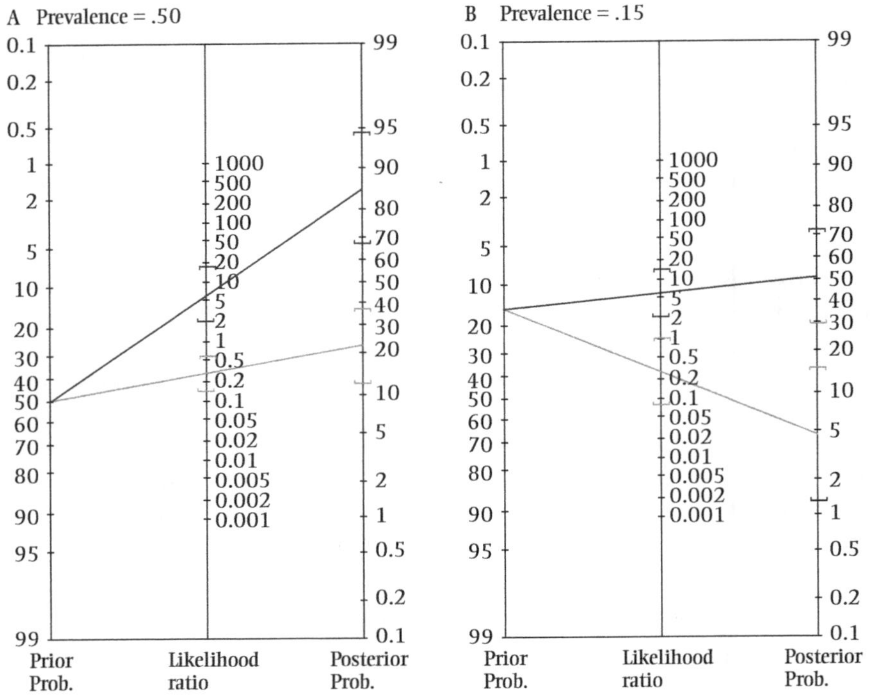

Figure 7.6 Nomograms depicting post-test odds based on two prevalence rates.

By drawing a line from the pre-test probability through the LR in the middle column, we see our post-test probability of .86 indicated along the right column. The results of a negative test (LR–) are shown in the bottom line.

The results of the above study (Filoteo et al., 2009) are based on an observed prevalence rate PDD of 50%. But what if I work in a specialized memory-disorders clinic where the majority of patients presenting with symptoms of Parkinsonism and dementia are the result of DLB, and cases of PDD are relatively rare—about 15%? As an evidence-based practitioner, I know that Likelihood Ratios are independent of prevalence. I therefore can use the LR+ finding from the Filoteo et al. study (2009) and apply it to my setting where I estimate the prevalence of PDD to be 15% compared to DLB. Again using the online calculator found at http://araw.mede.uic.edu/cgi-bin/testcalc.pl, I can adjust the local prevalence to be 0.15 and recalculate the pre-test and post-test probabilities, with the results depicted in the panel on the right side of Figure 7.6. Sensitivity and specificity are unchanged, as are the Likelihood ratios. However, because the pre-test probability (prevalence) is only 15% in my setting, the post-test probabilities are different. Given a positive test result in a setting where the prevalence of PDD is only 15%, an additional 35% of PDD cases (a post-test probability of 51%) can now be identified. Alternatively, a negative test result has a LR– of 0.29 and a post-test probability of 0.05, allowing me to now accurately rule out all but 5% of PDD cases.

Let me present one last example, with an emphasis on how evidence-based practices can guide individual patient care. In this scenario, I work in a university-based memory disorders clinic, and I am often faced with the challenge of differentiating AD from FTD. Our neurologists are quite keen on getting flurodeoxyglucose positron emission tomography or FDG-PET scans on our patients because they are aware of the reported diagnostic utility in differentiating AD from FTD on the basis of PET imaging (Foster et al., 2007). However, PET scans are very expensive procedures, and the nuclear medicine department at our university is reluctant to accept referrals out of concerns about reimbursement, unless neuropsychological assessment documents "appropriateness." As an evidence-based practitioner, I have a need to know if there are tests or test signs that might help me in making the differentiation between AD and FTD. I have heard talks at conferences and have read filtered review papers (Levy & Chelune, 2007) suggesting that patients with AD and FTD have different patterns of phonemic and semantic fluency, and I decide to explore this question more formally. I couch my question in PICO-format and go to PubMed where I do an Advanced Search under Clinical Queries to explore the sensitivity and specificity of verbal fluency tests to differentiate AD and FTD. My search generates a number of case-controlled studies and one meta-analysis. The meta-analysis (Henry et al., 2004) indicates that AD patients have more difficulty with semantic than with phonemic fluency. One of the unfiltered case-controlled studies appears particularly promising (Rascovsky, Salmon, Hansen, Thal, & Galasko, 2007), and I do a critical appraisal of the study, carefully examining the rationale, methods, patient-selection procedures, statistical analyses, and conclusion using the checklists in Greenhalgh's (2006) book. I feel I can use the data in this study as the patient samples mirror the patients I see in my practice.

The paper by Rascovsky et al. (2007) compared two groups of carefully matched, autopsy-confirmed cases of AD (n = 32) and FTD (n = 16) on a Semantic Index defined as: semantic fluency/(semantic + letter fluency). As predicted, the AD and FTD groups showed different patterns of semantic and letter fluency, and the ratio of semantic to total fluency significantly differentiated the two groups with a large effect size of $d = 1.28$. Using an optimal cutoff score, Rascovsky et al. (2007) report that 12 out of 16 of the FTD and 26 out of 32 AD cases were correctly classified, with an overall correct discrimination rate of 79.2%. If we define the COI in this study as FTD and the RP as AD, we can take the classification data and enter it into a 2 x 2 diagnostic matrix and determine the sensitivity, specificity, LR+, and change in pre-test to post-test probability associated with the cutoff score (use an online calculator to compute the data for yourself). The prevalence of FTD in this study is 33.3%, and the resulting LR+ was 4.0, meaning that patients having a semantic index above the cutoff score were four times more likely to be in the autopsy-confirmed FTD group than in the AD group. Given the prevalence rate of 0.333 and a LR+ of 4.0, the post-test probability of correctly identifying a FTD patient based on fluency measures alone was now 0.667, or double what it would have been without testing. Whether a positive finding on a semantic index composed of fluency measures is sufficient to warrant a referral for a PET scan is open to discussion, but it certainly strengthens the confidence of the neuropsychologist in making the recommendation for a PET scan. As in the previous example, if FTD were to be diagnosed in a different sample with different prevalence rates, post-test probability would need to be re-estimated accordingly.

The application of clinical research derived from the study of populations to guide individual clinical decision making is the essence of evidence-based practice. It basically amounts to answering the question, "If my clinical patient were in this study, what is the likelihood that they would have the COI, given their test score(s)?"

SUMMARY

Evidence-based practices in neuropsychology are not esoteric rituals performed by the academic elite. They represent basic skill sets designed for routine clinical practice with the goal of adding value to patient care and outcomes in an accountable manner. Assessing our patients and deconstructing referral questions, asking answerable questions about our patients, acquiring relevant clinical research information to answer these questions, critically appraising the information we gather, and applying this information in an informed and thoughtful way are the hallmarks of the evidence-based practitioner. These skills are not acquired overnight, nor are they mastered as discrete events. Evidence-based practice is an ongoing pattern of activity that becomes streamlined and improves with repetition and frequency. It is incumbent on us as clinicians to be good consumers of clinical science and to learn how to best apply this information in a patient-centered way. Clinical neuropsychology has always prided itself on being an applied science based on empirical research. Adopting evidence-based practices merely helps us realize this goal in everyday practice.

REFERENCES

Akobeng, A. K. (2005). Principles of evidence based medicine. *Archives of Disease in Childhood, 90*(8), 837–840. doi:10.1136/adc.2005.071761

APA Presidential Task Force on Evidence-Based Practice. (2006). Evidence-based practice in psychology. *American Psychologist, 61*(4), 271–285.

APUS Librarians. (2015). What are Boolean operators, and how do I use them? Retrieved June 27, 2016 from http://apus.libanswers.com/faq/2310.

Bossuyt, P. M., Reitsma, J. B., Bruns, D. E., Gatsonis, C. A., Glasziou, P. P., Irwig, L. M., . . . de Vet, H. C. (2003). Towards complete and accurate reporting of studies of diagnostic accuracy: The STARD Initiative. *Annals of Internal Medicine, 138*(1), 40–44.

Bowden, S. C., Harrison, E. J., & Loring, D. W. (2014). Evaluating research for clinical significance: Using critically appraised topics to enhance evidence-based neuropsychology. *Clinical Neuropsychology, 28*(4), 653–668.

Chelune, G. J. (2002). Making neuropsychological outcomes research consumer friendly: A commentary on Keith et al. (2002). [Comment]. *Neuropsychology, 16*(3), 422–425.

Chelune, G. J. (2010). Evidence-based research and practice in clinical neuropsychology. [Review]. *Clinical Neuropsychology, 24*(3), 454–467. doi:10.1080/13854040802360574

Cicerone, K. D., Dahlberg, C., Kalmar, K., Langenbahn, D. M., Malec, J. F., Bergquist, T. F., . . . Morse, P. A. (2000). Evidence-based cognitive rehabilitation: Recommendations for clinical practice. *Archives of Physical Medicine and Rehabilitation, 81*(12), 1596–1615.

Cicerone, K. D., Dahlberg, C., Malec, J. F., Langenbahn, D. M., Felicetti, T., Kneipp, S., . . . Catanese, J. (2005). Evidence-based cognitive rehabilitation: Updated review of the literature from 1998 through 2002. *Archives of Physical Medicine and Rehabilitation, 86*(8), 1681–1692.

Claridge, J. A., & Fabian, T. C. (2005). History and development of evidence-based medicine. [Historical Article]. *World Journal of Surgery, 29*(5), 547–553. doi:10.1007/s00268-005-7910-1

Cochrane, A. L. (1972). *Effectiveness and Efficiency: Random Reflections on Health Services.* London, United Kingdom, Nuffield Provincial Hospitals Trust.

Costa, L. (1983). Clinical neuropsychology: A discipline in evolution. *Journal of Clinical Neuropsychology, 5*(1), 1–11.

Dodrill, C. B. (1997). Myths of neuropsychology. *The Clinical Neuropsychologist, 11*(1), 1–17.

Encyclopedia of Mental Disorders. Managed Care. (2016). Available at www.minddisorders.com/Kau-NU/managed-care.html.

Evidence-Based Medicine Working Group. (1992). Evidence-based medicine. A new approach to teaching the practice of medicine. *Journal of the American Medical Association, 268*(17), 2420–2425.

Filoteo, J. V., Salmon, D. P., Schiehser, D. M., Kane, A. E., Hamilton, J. M., Rilling, L. M., . . . Galasko, D. R. (2009). Verbal learning and memory in patients with dementia with Lewy bodies and Parkinson's disease dementia. *Journal of Clinical and Experimental Neuropsychology, 31*(7), 823–834.

Foster, N. L., Heidebrink, J. L., Clark, C. M., Jagust, W. J., Arnold, S. E., Barbas, N. R., . . . Minoshima, S. (2007). FDG-PET improves accuracy in distinguishing frontotemporal dementia and Alzheimer's disease. *Brain, 130*(Pt 10), 2616–2635.

Gooch, T. (2013). Ludwig Andreas Feurebach. In E. N. Zalta (Ed.), *The Stanford Encyclopedia of Philosophy* (Winter 2013 ed.). Retrieved June 27, 2016 from http://plato.stanford.edu/archives/win2013/entries/ludwig-feuerbach/.

Greenhalgh, T. (2006). *How to Read a Paper: The Basics of Evidence-Based Medicine* (3rd ed.). Malden, MA: Blackwell Publishing.

Haynes, R. B., Devereaux, P. J., & Guyatt, G. H. (2002). Clinical expertise in the era of evidence-based medicine and patient choice. *Evidence-Based Medicine, 7*, 36–38.

Heneghan, C., & Badenoch, D. (2006). *Evidence-Based Medicine Toolbox* (2nd ed.). Maiden, MA: Blackwell Publishing.

Henry, J. D., Crawford, J. R., & Phillips, L. H. (2004). Verbal fluency performance in dementia of the Alzheimer's type: A meta-analysis. *Neuropsychologia, 42*(9), 1212–1222.

Hermann, B. P., Perrine, K., Chelune, G. J., Barr, W., Loring, D. W., Strauss, E., . . . Westerveld, M. (1999). Visual confrontation naming following left anterior temporal lobectomy: A comparison of surgical approaches. *Neuropsychology, 13*(1), 3–9.

Hill, G. B. (2000). Archie Cochrane and his legacy. An internal challenge to physicians' autonomy? *Journal of Clinical Epidemiology, 53*(12), 1189–1192.

Holy Bible. (2011). *New International Version*. Grand Rapids, MI: Zondervan.

Horwitz, R. I. (1996). The dark side of evidence-based medicine. *Cleveland Clinic Journal of Medicine, 63*(6), 320–323.

Ivnik, R. J., Smith, G. E., Cerhan, J. H., Boeve, B. F., Tangalos, E. G., & Petersen, R. C. (2001). Understanding the diagnostic capabilities of cognitive tests. *Clinical Neuropsychology, 15*(1), 114–124.

Johnson, L. A. (1997). Outcomes management a decade out: An interview with Paul Ellwood. *Group Practice Journal, 46*, 12–15.

Karr, J. E., Areshenkoff, C. N., & Garcia-Barrera, M. A. (2014). The neuropsychological outcomes of concussion: A systematic review of meta-analyses on the cognitive sequelae of mild traumatic brain injury. *Neuropsychology, 28*(3), 321–336.

Kurella, M., Chertow, G. M., Luan, J., & Yaffe, K. (2004). Cognitive impairment in chronic kidney disease. *Journal of the American Geriatric Society, 52*(11), 1863–1869.

Levy, J. A., & Chelune, G. J. (2007). Cognitive-behavioral profiles of neurodegenerative dementias: Beyond Alzheimer's disease. [Review]. *Journal of Geriatric Psychiatry and Neurology, 20*(4), 227–238.

Lezak, M. D., Howieson, D. B., Bigler, E. D., & Tranel, D. (2012). *Neuropsychological Assessment: Edition 5*. New York: Oxford University Press.

Loring, D. W., & Bowden, S. C. (2014). The STROBE statement and neuropsychology: Lighting the way toward evidence-based practice. *Clinical Neuropsychology, 28*(4), 556–574.

Loring, D. W., & Bowden, S. C. (2016). Editorial. *Neuropsychology Review, 26*(1), 1–2.

Matarazzo, J. D., & Herman, D. O. (1984). Base rate data for the WAIS-R: Test-retest stability and VIQ-PIQ differences. *Journal of Clinical Neuropsychology, 6*(4), 351–366.

Mayer, D. (2010). *Essential Evidence-Based Medicine* (2nd ed.). New York: Cambridge University Press.

Miller, J., Schoenberg, M., & Bilder, R. (2014). Consolidated Standards of Reporting Trials (CONSORT): Considerations for neuropsychological research. *Clinical Neuropsychology, 28*(4), 575–599.

Nasreddine, Z. S., Phillips, N. A., Bedirian, V., Charbonneau, S., Whitehead, V., Collin, I., . . . Chertkow, H. (2005). The Montreal Cognitive Assessment, MoCA: A brief screening tool for mild cognitive impairment. *Journal of the American Geriatric Society, 53*(4), 695–699.

National Library of Medicine. (2006-10-05). PubMed celebrates its 10th anniversary. *NLM Technical Bulletin*. Retrieved June 27, 2016 from United States National Library of Medicine website: https://www.nlm.nih.gov/pubs/techbull/so06/so06_pm_10.html.

Rascovsky, K., Salmon, D. P., Hansen, L. A., Thal, L. J., & Galasko, D. (2007). Disparate letter and semantic category fluency deficits in autopsy-confirmed frontotemporal dementia and Alzheimer's disease. *Neuropsychology, 21*(1), 20–30.

Rohling, M. L., Faust, M. E., Beverly, B., & Demakis, G. (2009). Effectiveness of cognitive rehabilitation following acquired brain injury: A meta-analytic re-examination of Cicerone et al.'s (2000, 2005) systematic reviews. *Neuropsychology, 23*(1), 20–39.

Rosenberg, W., & Donald, A. (1995). Evidence based medicine: An approach to clinical problem-solving. [Research Support, Non-U.S. Gov't]. *British Medical Journal, 310*(6987), 1122–1126.

Sackett, D. L., Rosenberg, W. M., Gray, J. A., Haynes, R. B., & Richardson, W. S. (1996). Evidence based medicine: What it is and what it isn't. [Editorial]. *British Medical Journal, 312*(7023), 71–72.

Sackett, D. L., Straus, S. E., Richardson, W., & Haynes, R. B. (2000). *Evidence-Based Medicine: How to Practice and Teach EBM* (2nd ed.). New York: Churchill Livingston.

Sackett, D. L., Straus, S. E., Richardson, W. S., Rosenberg, W., & Haynes, R. B. (2000). *Evidence-Based Medicine: How to Practice and Teach EBM* (2nd ed.). New York: Churchill Livingston.

Schoenberg, M. R., & Scott, J. G. (2011). *The Little Black Book of Neuropsychology: A Syndrome-Based Approach*. New York: Springer.

Schulz, K. F., Altman, D. G., & Moher, D. (2010). CONSORT 2010 statement: Updated guidelines for reporting parallel group randomized trials. *Annals of Internal Medicine, 152*(11), 726–732.

Segen, J. C. (2006). *McGraw-Hill Concise Dictionary of Modern Medicine*. New York: McGraw-Hill Companies.

Smith, G. E. (2002). What is the outcome we seek? A commentary on Keith et al. (2002). [Comment]. *Neuropsychology, 16*(3), 432–433.

Spector, A., Orrell, M., & Hall, L. (2012). Systematic review of neuropsychological outcomes in dementia from cognition-based psychological interventions. *Dementia and Geriatric Cognitive Disorders, 34*(3–4), 244–255.

SPRINT Research Group. (2015). A randomized trial of intensive versus standard blood-pressure control. *New England Journal of Medicine, 373*(22), 2103–2116.

Suchy, Y., Kraybill, M. L., & Franchow, E. (2011). Practice effect and beyond: Reaction to novelty as an independent predictor of cognitive decline among older adults. *Journal of the International Neuropsychology Society, 17*(1), 101–111. doi:10.1017/S135561771000130X

von Elm, E., Altman, D. G., Egger, M., Pocock, S. J., Gotzsche, P. C., & Vandenbroucke, J. P. (2007). The Strengthening the Reporting of Observational Studies in Epidemiology (STROBE) statement: Guidelines for reporting observational studies. *Annals of Internal Medicine, 147*(8), 573–577.

8

Evidence-Based Integration of Clinical Neuroimaging Findings in Neuropsychology

ERIN D. BIGLER

Without debate or dispute, neuroimaging represents the greatest breakthrough in modern science for studying *in vivo* brain structure and function (Gabrieli, Ghosh, & Whitfield-Gabrieli, 2015). The speed with which neuroimaging achieved this ascendancy is all the more astonishing when one views the timeline. Given that the concepts of modern neuroimaging were developed in the 1960s, with the first prototype computed tomographic (CT) scanner in development in the late 1960s and early 1970s, and the first clinical CT scanner installed at the Mayo Clinic in Rochester, Minnesota, in 1973, scanning technology is but half a century old. Prototype magnetic resonance (MR) scanners were developed a few years later, and the first clinical MR imaging (MRI) was performed in the early to mid-1980s. Given this timeline, neuropsychology had its origins prior to any modern neuroimaging techniques. For example, in 1976, in the first edition of Lezak's *Neuropsychological Assessment* textbook, there were no references to CT imaging, and that edition was published prior to any application of MRI methods in neuropsychology. As reviewed by Bigler (2015), not much was done with these technologies in neuropsychology until the end of the twentieth and beginning of the twenty-first century. When neuroimaging techniques were introduced in the 1970s and 1980s, there were limited quantitative methods that could be applied, and combined with the coarseness of the original brain image from early CT or MRI, only limited methods for image interpretation were available.

Given this historical setting, the fundamental principles of neuropsychological assessment and diagnostic inference-making occurred prior to any development where brain anatomy and potential neuropathology could be simultaneously viewed or investigated in the living individual undergoing some type of cognitive or neurobehavioral assessment. The first textbooks devoted to neuropsychological assessment that attempted to incorporate neuroimaging did not appear until 1980s (Bigler, Yeo, & Turkheimer, 1989; Kertesz, 1983). What this has meant for neuropsychology is that the assessment process mostly developed independently of any type of neuroimaging metric that potentially could be incorporated into neuropsychological diagnostic formulation.

In contrast, since neuropsychological assessment is all about making inferences about brain function, and given the exquisite anatomical and pathological detail that can now be achieved with contemporary neuroimaging, clinical neuropsychology *should* be using neuroimaging findings. Additionally, given the currently available technology, it would seem that neuroimaging information should be routinely incorporated into the neuropsychological metric in diagnostic formulation, treatment programming, monitoring, and predicting outcome. But where to start? This book is on evidence-based practices, so this chapter will review well-accepted clinical neuroimaging methods that have relevance to neuropsychological outcome. For example, in various diseases, especially neurodegenerative, as well as acquired disorders like traumatic brain injury (TBI), the amount of cerebral atrophy coarsely relates to cognitive functioning. Therefore, this review begins with clinical rating of cerebral atrophy, but we then will move into specific region of interest (ROI) atrophic changes or pathological markers.

Neuroimaging studies are routinely performed on most individuals with a neurocognitive or neurobehavioral complaint or symptom, at least in the initial stages of making a diagnosis. Incredibly sophisticated image-analysis methods are available, but all such techniques require sophisticated image-analysis hardware and software, as well as the expertise to analyze and interpret. For the typical front-line clinician, these resources may not be available, nor may they be available through the typical clinical radiology laboratory performing the neuroimaging studies. Thus, another compelling reason for neuropsychologists to use clinical rating schema for assessing neuroimaging studies is the ease with which these rating methods can be performed. Although the future is likely to involve routine advanced image-analysis methods that are fully automated with comparisons to normative databases (see Toga, 2015) performed at the time of initial imaging and integrated with neuropsychological test findings (see also Bilder, 2011, as to how this might be implemented), but this may still be a decade or two away from being clinically implemented.

The discussion that follows assumes that the reader has some fundamental understanding of basic neuroanatomy and neuroimaging, which can be obtained from multiple sources, including Schoenberg et al. (2011) and Filley and Bigler (2017). It is beyond the scope of this chapter to provide elaborate details of the various clinical rating methods that are available on the basics of CT or MR neuroimaging. It is recommended that the reader go to the original cited reference source for each clinical rating discussed in this chapter, should a particular type of rating be considered.

ETHICAL CAVEAT

While the Houston Guidelines (see http://www.theaacn.org/position_papers/houston_conference.pdf, or Hannay, 1998) for training in neuropsychology under Section VI, *Knowledge Base*, explicitly state that neuropsychologists are to possess training and knowledge in "functional neuroanatomy" and "neuroimaging and other neurodiagnostic techniques," such a background may not be sufficient for performing clinical ratings based on CT or MRI. We recommend that, before embarking on performing clinical ratings as discussed in this chapter, the individual clinician consult with a neuroradiologist who could provide such training and initial supervision to result in the highest accuracy of rating possible. Also, all clinical imaging will come with a radiological interpretative report. The purposes of the neuroimaging evaluation are to provide an overall statement about brain anatomy and potential neuropathology, along with whether any emergency medical circumstance may be present (e.g., neoplasm, aneurysm, vascular abnormality, etc.). Often the neurobehavioral questions to be addressed by the neuropsychologist are not necessarily the topic for the initial referral to obtain a brain scan. So the post-hoc clinical rating applied to the scan becomes important for neuropsychology when specific symptoms or problems can be explored in light of the neuroimaging findings.

THE NEURORADIOLOGICAL REPORT

Understanding the limits of what can be detected with CT or MRI is essential for understanding potential relationships between brain, behavior, and cognition. Since typical conventional neuroimaging will not detect abnormalities less than a cubic millimeter, contemporary neuroimaging only identifies the location and size of potential macroscopic abnormalities of the brain along with a general image of brain anatomy. Since neuroanatomy is the foundation for the emergence of cognition and behavior, for the neuropsychologist, this information provides the general backdrop as to the gross anatomical appearance of the brain. Typically, the neuroradiological report will identify where major lesions or abnormalities may reside, especially focal pathology like that from cerebrovascular accidents, neoplasms, or demyelinating disorders. If focal lesions are present, the neuroradiological report becomes the "clinical rating," because within the report, which lobe or lobes may be affected within which hemisphere and whether cortical and/or subcortical pathology is present will typically be reported. In this manner, the neuropsychologist may readily use the information for coarse categorization, such as left or right hemisphere damage, or which lobe(s) may be most affected. For the clinical ratings discussed in this chapter, it is assumed that a standard neuroradiological report already has been generated where the benefit of clinical rating comes with additional qualitative metrics of brain anatomy not provided in the clinical neuroradiological report, unless the neuroradiologist provides such ratings.

CLINICAL RATINGS

Brain Atrophy

Normal aging is associated with some brain volume loss, often best visualized as increased size of the lateral ventricles and greater prominence of cerebral spinal fluid (CSF) within the cortical subarachnoid space as shown in Figure 8.1, which compares the author's axial mid-lateral ventricle MRI cut at age 66 with that of his lab director at age 44, to that of an adolescent brain. Note the enlargement of the ventricular system in the author's brain compared to the younger brains. This increase in ventricular size occurs to compensate for the volume loss of brain parenchyma that occurs through the normal aging process, associated with neuronal loss. Concomitant with age-related brain volume loss is increased prominence of cortical sulci and the interhemispheric fissure (see white arrowhead in Figure 8.1 that points to visibly increased sulcal width in the author's older brain compared to the younger brains). Although this is the natural aging process, it does, in fact, produce cerebral atrophy. So, for cerebral atrophy to be clinically significant, it must exceed what is expected to be "normal" variation in brain volume associated with typical aging.

Wattjes and colleagues (2009) provide some important comparisons and guidelines for interpreting either CT or MRI in a memory clinic. This is shown in Figure 8.2. The important comparison here with CT imaging to MRI is that CT scanning is much faster, less expensive, and does not have restrictions like MRI in the case of heart pacemakers, other implanted medical devices, dental or facial bone implants, or any metal that may produce artifacts. While CT does not provide the exquisite anatomical detail achieved by MRI, it nonetheless has the ability to display ventricular size and white matter density along with sulcal and interhemispheric width. Knowing the anatomical relationship of certain cortical and subcortical structures to ventricular anatomy does permit inferences about

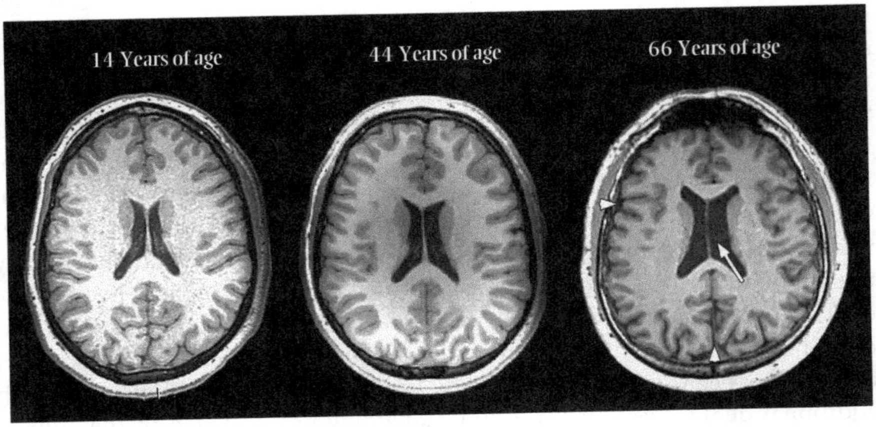

Figure 8.1 Age-related normal changes in ventricular size. The image on the right is the author's at age 66. Arrow points to ventricle. Arrowhead on the side points to more prominence of the cortical sulci, with the bottom arrowhead pointing to greater prominence of the interhemispheric fissure in the older brain.

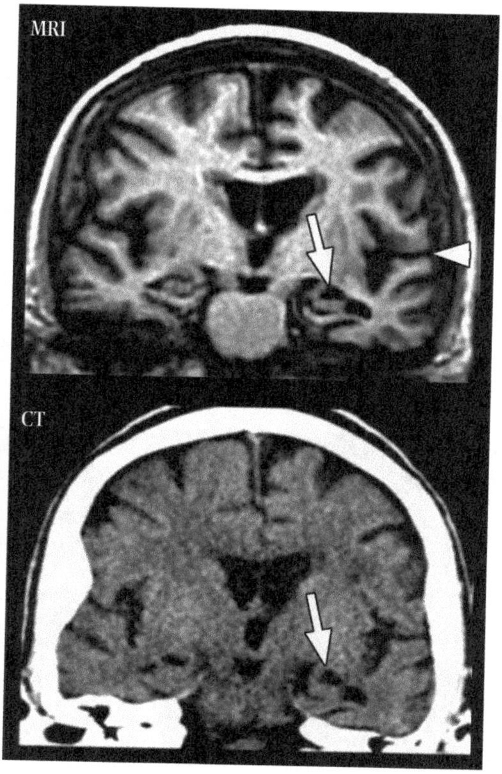

Figure 8.2 Comparison of coronal MRI (top) and CT (bottom) in the same subject, with the cutting plane perpendicular to the hippocampal formation. CT does not provide the kind of anatomical detail that MRI does, but note that the ventricular system morphology can be identified with either CT or MRI. White arrow in the MRI points to the reduced hippocampal volume and dilated temporal horn of the lateral ventricular system. The white arrow in the CT image points to the same region as the MRI. The distinct appearance of the hippocampus cannot be visualized in CT, but it may be inferred by the dilated temporal horn. Also, the prominence of the Sylvian fissure (white arrowhead points to the Sylvian fissure) and the temporal lobe gyri signifies temporal lobe atrophy.

Illustration used with permission from Wattjes et al. (2009) and the Radiological Society of North America, p. 176.

atrophic findings, even from CT. For example, in the illustration in Figure 8.2, the MRI clearly shows hippocampal atrophy in association with temporal horn dilation. The corresponding CT where the image plane is identical to MRI only shows the temporal horn dilation, as hippocampal anatomy is ill-defined with CT. Nonetheless, given CT-defined temporal horn dilation, an inference may be made that hippocampal size has been reduced. Both CT and MRI show the prominence of the Sylvian fissure (white arrowhead). Accordingly, qualitative analyses on both CT and MRI brain scanning may be performed.

From Wattjes and colleagues (2009), Figure 8.3 depicts the same transverse axial views of the same subjects comparing CT and MRI but in three different subjects with various levels of cerebral atrophy, from minimal to extensive. Note that the defining feature, whether CT or MRI, is prominence of the interhemispheric fissure and cortical sulci.

Some of the earliest and most widely used clinical rating methods were developed by Scheltens and colleagues (see Pasquier et al., 1996; Pasquier et al., 1997; Scheltens et al., 1993; Scheltens, Barkhof, et al., 1992; Scheltens, Launer, Barkhof, Weinstein, & van Gool, 1995; Scheltens, Leys, et al., 1992; Scheltens, Pasquier, Weerts, Barkhof, & Leys, 1997). In the Pasquier et al. (1996) study, four neuroradiologists rated the degree of cerebral atrophy on a 0–3-point scale. As with any

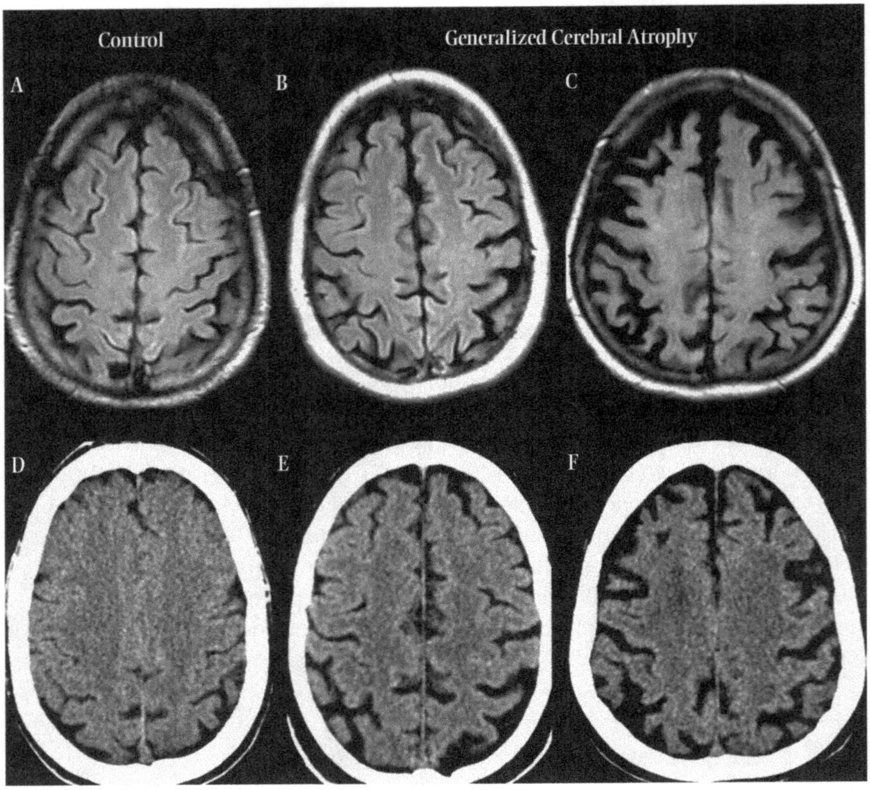

Figure 8.3 Top images are MRI with each subject's CT below cut in the same plane as the MRI. Note that both CT and MRI adequately and similarly depict cortical sulci, which increase in prominence as a reflection of cortical atrophy. These images are taken from Wattjes et al. (2009), where global cerebral atrophy or GCA was rated on a 4-point scale, where 0 was no atrophy, and 3 the highest rating. For these images, the control (a and c) was rated "0," with the subject in b and e rated a "1," and the subject in c and f rated a "2."
Illustration used with permission from Wattjes et al. (2009) and the Radiological Society of North America, p. 179.

rating system, inter-observer agreement (mean overall kappa = 0.48) was lower than intra-observer (mean overall kappa = .67) when comparing scan findings from the same neuroimaging studies interpreted one month apart. Nonetheless, these kinds of coarse ratings do provide general information about structural brain integrity with reasonably good agreement for clinical purposes between raters.

Figure 8.4, also from the Wattjes et al. (2009) publication on diagnostic imaging of patients in a memory clinic, shows images in the coronal plane from age-related "normal" appearance (A and E) to various levels of pathological display. Images on top are MRI, compared to the same plane coronal CT view on the bottom. Note that in the subject depicted in A and E, there is minimal cortical CSF visualized because the sulci are so narrow, such that most sulci cannot even be visualized on the CT image. Also note the small size of the lateral and third ventricle. Furthermore, in A and E, note the homogenous, symmetrical, and rather uniform appearance of brain parenchyma, characteristic of normal parenchyma. In contrast, beginning with the case presented in B and F, ventricular size begins to increase, associated with greater and greater prominence of cortical sulci. Also note in D and H that CT density and the MR signal around the ventricle also change, suggesting degradation in white matter integrity. In age-related disorders, this is typically considered to relate to vascular changes, where the MRI sequence referred to as *fluid attenuated inversion recovery* (FLAIR) is particularly sensitive to white matter abnormalities that may be incident to age and disease, as shown in Figure 8.5. On the FLAIR image sequence (as well as T2 weighted sequences), a white matter hyperintensity (WMH) shows up, as its

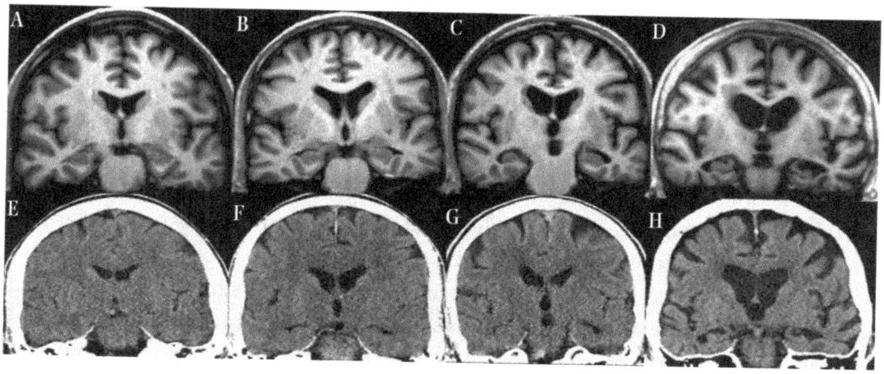

Figure 8.4 As in Figure 8.3, top images are coronal-slice MRI with corresponding identical slice-level CT from the same subject depicted below. Coronal images are best for rating medial temporal lobe atrophy, referred to as MTA, by Scheltens et al. (Scheltens, Leys, et al., 1992). Images are as if the patient were standing in front of the examiner, so patient's left is on the viewer's right. The MTA rating scale is a 5-point scale from 0 to 4. A and E represent the Control with a "0" rating, B and F "1," C and G "2," and D and H "3" (right side) and "4" left side.

Illustration used with permission from Wattjes et al. (2009) and the Radiological Society of North America, p. 180.

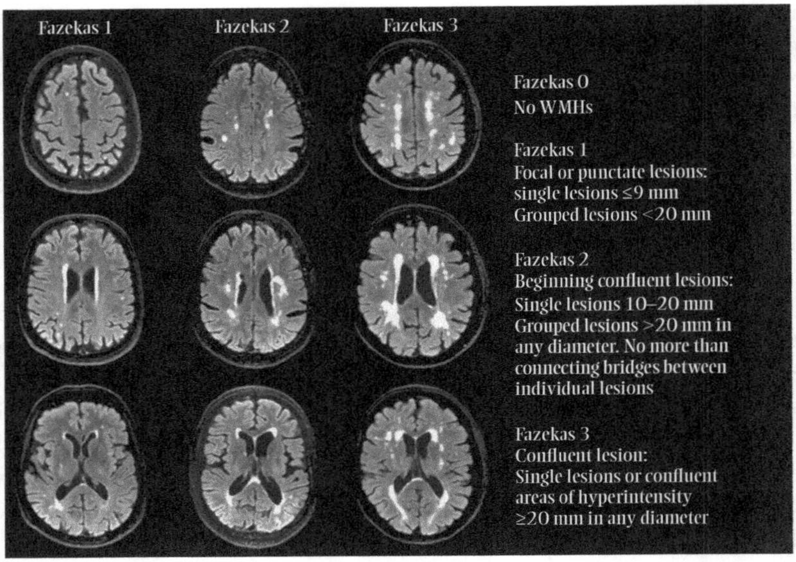

Figure 8.5 Fazekas ratings (see Fazekas et al., 1987) for classifying white matter hyperintensities. (WMHs).

Illustration adapted and used with permission from Prins and Scheltens (Prins & Scheltens, 2015) and with permission from *Lancet Neurology*, p. 160.

name implies, as a bright white region, distinctly different from the uniform signal intensity from surrounding white matter parenchyma. More will be discussed about white matter ratings in the next section and how changes are detected with CT and MRI.

Most rating scales for temporal lobe atrophy and hippocampal volume loss are based on images obtained in the coronal plane, as shown in Figure 8.4. Any number of studies have shown that, with the increasing presence of pathologically definable changes in brain structure adjusted for age, such as whole brain, temporal lobe, or hippocampal atrophy findings, relate to neuropsychological impairment (Jang et al., 2015; van de Pol et al., 2007), and are especially associated with memory impairment (DeCarli et al., 2007).

More recently, two more comprehensive rating methods have been proposed, both of which utilize aspects of what has been discussed above. Guo et al. (2014) introduced an elaborate rating method referred to as the Brain Atrophy and Lesion Index (BALI), and Jang et al. (2015) introduced the Comprehensive Visual Rating Scale (CVRS). What is important for neuropsychology about the BALI study is that a variety of raters were trained including non-physician Ph.D.s, with all raters capable of achieving a high degree of accuracy. Other studies have shown that the BALI approach was sensitive in discrimination of Alzheimer's disease from mild cognitive impairment and normal aging (Chen et al., 2010; Song, Mitnitski, Zhang, Chen, & Rockwood, 2013). The CVRS from Jang et al. (2015) utilizes prior rating methods as introduced by Scheltens and colleagues as previously described, but it incorporates atrophy and WMH ratings into a single scale based on either axial or coronal images, as shown in Figure 8.6. What

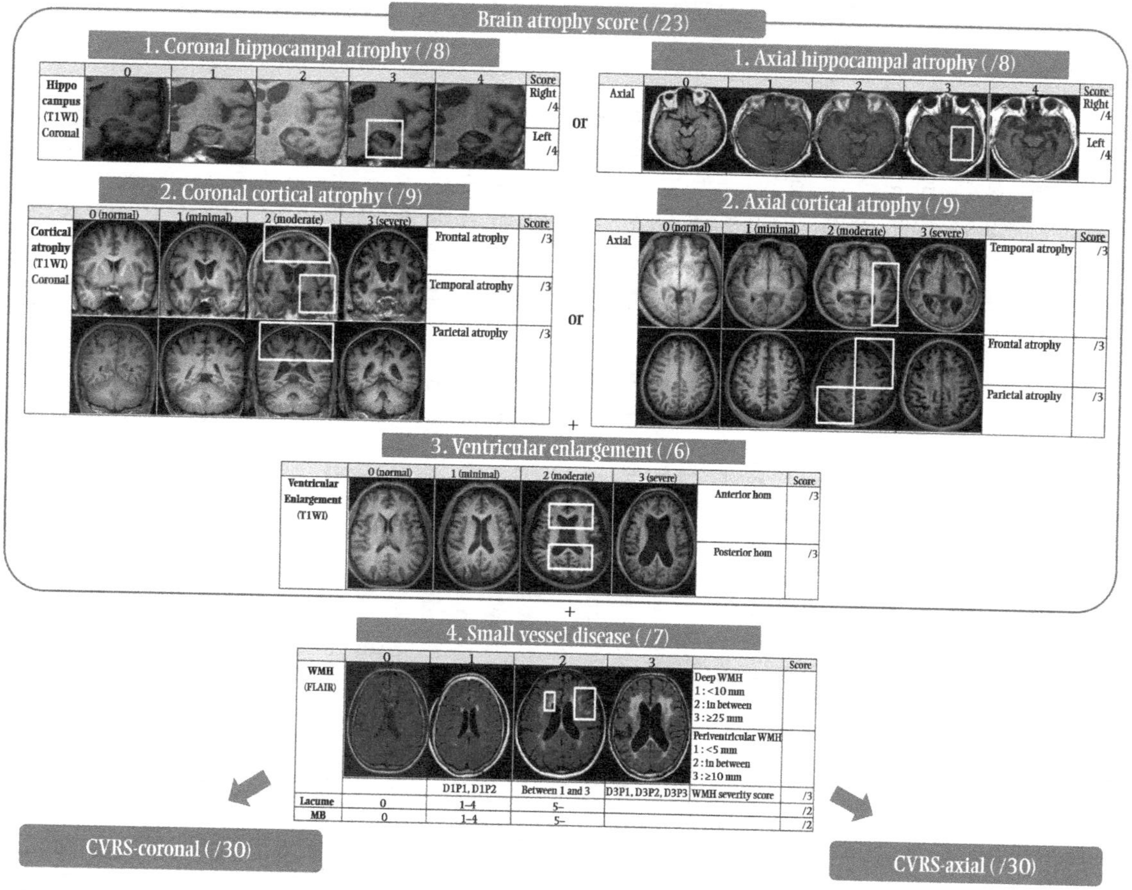

Figure 8.6 The scoring table of the Comprehensive Visual Rating Scale (CVRS). T1WI, T1-weighted images. The white rectangles are the brain regions that need to be focused on.

FLAIR, fluid-attenuated inversion recovery; WMH, white matter hyperintensity; D, deep; P, periventricular; MB, microbleeds.

From Jang et al. (2015), used with permission from the *Journal of Alzheimer's Disease* and IOS Press. For details on using this, please refer to the original publication as the details are lengthy, elaborate, and beyond the scope of discussion within this chapter, p. 1025.

is particularly important about the CVRS approach is that these investigators also compared CVRS findings in a subset of subjects who also had imaging that permitted advanced quantitative analyses, including voxel-based morphometry (VBM). VBM findings demonstrated that regional or whole brain atrophy demonstrated on clinical ratings corresponded to clinical ratings. This is a very important observation because it proves that useful clinical information is available within qualitative rating methods that matches what is found with lengthier and more time-consuming advanced imaging techniques.

Because of heterogeneity within any disorder or disease process, atypical cortical atrophy or degenerative changes may occur. For example, in Alzheimer's disease, a more posterior presentation as described by Koedam et al. (2011) may occur. Accordingly, with any clinical rating, considerable clinical experience and judgement is needed in performing the necessary clinical correlation of an imaging finding to a neuropsychological outcome. It is also true that certain lesions or abnormalities that may occur during neonatal development may not correlate well with neuropsychological outcome in adolescence or adulthood because of neurodevelopmental and plasticity issues (Dennis et al., 2014).

Lastly, all of the methods described above permit using a clinical rating method to establish a baseline and track the patient over time (DeCarli et al., 2007). This is particularly important in patients who initially present with mild complaints without a clear diagnosis and potentially no neuroimaging abnormalities. Such patients are typically longitudinally tracked over time, so comparing baseline information, both from a neuroimaging as well as a neuropsychological perspective, often becomes the key diagnostic procedure in eventually making the correct diagnosis. As shown by DeCarli et al. (2007), the neuroimaging clinical rating adds unique information, as do the neuropsychological findings, beyond what each may provide individually. Additionally, there are simple tracing programs that merely require outlining critical ROIs in comparison to a normative database, which reduces the arbitrariness of clinical ratings but does require obtaining images in an identical orientation and plane, which represents a limitation (Menendez-Gonzalez, Lopez-Muniz, Vega, Salas-Pacheco, & Arias-Carrion, 2014). Scan images come in Digital Imaging and Communication in Medicine (DICOM) file formats, with a variety of DICOM reading programs commercially available, all of which have simple linear measuring tools.

White Matter Hyperintensities (WMHs)

As introduced above, WMH ratings often go hand-in-hand with aging and cerebral atrophy. As Prins and Scheltens (2015) recently observed, "The underlying pathology of these lesions mostly reflects demyelination and axonal loss as a consequence of chronic ischaemia caused by cerebral small vessel disease (microangiopathy). The prevalence and severity of WMHs increase with age, and in association with arterial hypertension" (p. 157). Numerous WMH rating methods have been developed, but all in some fashion go back to Fazekas et al. (1987) as shown and described in Figure 8.5.

Following the development of the Fazekas scale, Scheltens and colleagues (see Scheltens et al., 1993) broadened the number of areas rated, as outlined in Figure 8.7. The Fazekas scale focuses on rating WMHs in the periventricular and subcortical region combined, on a 0–3-point scale. In contrast, the Scheltens scale (see Figure 8.7) separately rates WMHs in the periventricular region on a 0–6-point scale and in subcortical regions on a 0–24-point scale, based on size and number of the lesions, including a scale for rating for basal ganglia and infratentorial regions. Wahlund et al. (2001) modified these white matter ratings for use with CT, which also permits comparison of CT and MRI, should they be performed at different times in the clinical course of assessing a patient.

The burden of overall white matter pathology relates to the degree of neuropsychological impairment (Bigler, Kerr, Victoroff, Tate, & Breitner, 2002; Boone et al., 1992; Heo et al., 2009; Leaper et al., 2001; Lesser et al., 1996; Tuladhar et al., 2015), including coarse mental status ratings as shown in Figure 8.8. In Figure 8.8, greater cognitive impairment on the modified Mini-Mental State Exam (3MS; see Tschanz et al., 2002) is associated with higher levels of WMHs. What is also important about these very quickly performed WMH clinical ratings is that they accomplish accuracy similar to that of more time-consuming and labor-intensive quantitative methods, also shown in Figure 8.8, of global brain pathology. Often, ratings of WMHs are done in conjunction with global

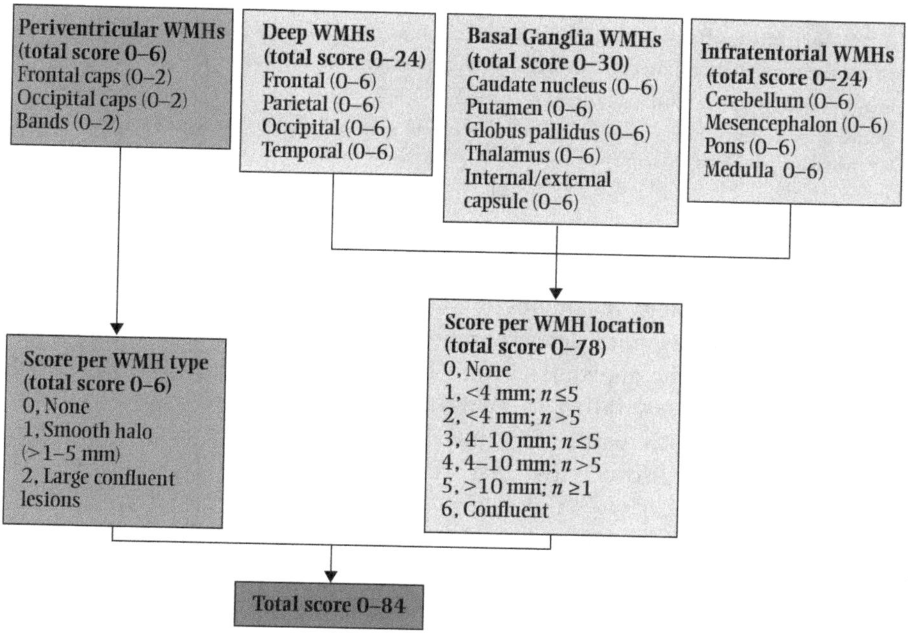

Figure 8.7 Visual ratings of white matter hyperintensities (WMHs) according to Scheltens.

Used with permission from Prins and Scheltens (2015) and *Lancet Neurology*, p. 159.

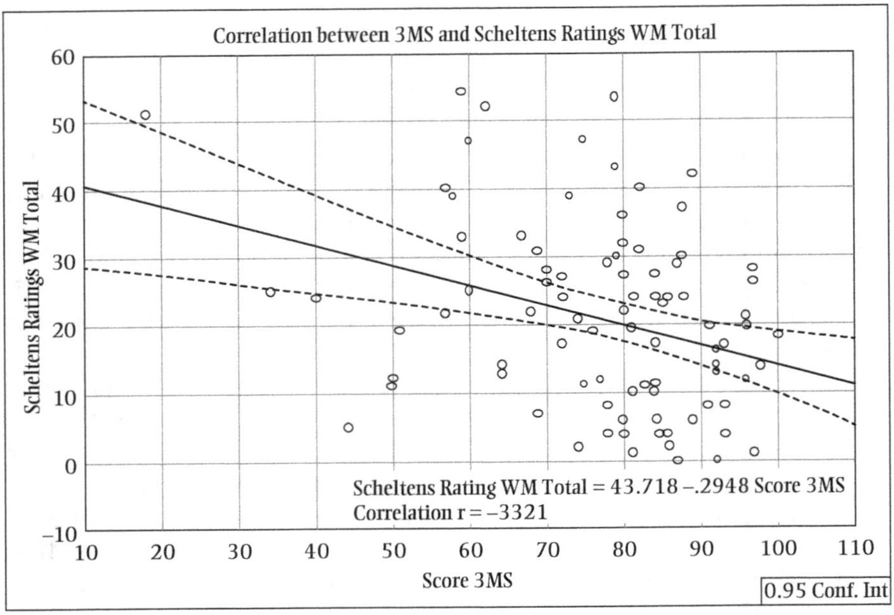

Figure 8.8 These scatter plots show that the WMH Scheltens et al. ratings (see Figure 8.7) inversely relate to cognitive status, based on a modified Mini-Mental State Exam, using a transformed score ranging from 0–100 (see Tsui et al., 2014). In this same study, increased WMHs were associated with generalized atrophy and volume loss, but WMH ratings had a more robust correlation associated with impaired cognitive functioning and associated with worse WMH rating.

Image adapted from Tsui et al. (2014), p. 154.

Dotted lines represent 0.95 confidence interval, with overall white matter Scheltens Rating Score positively correlated with modified Mini-Mental Status (3MS) test performance ($r = .32$, $p = 0.001$).

ratings of cerebral and hippocampal atrophy. The combination of increased white matter pathology in conjunction with cerebral atrophy, ventricular dilation, and reduced hippocampal size represents a very increased likelihood for dementia. While the above discussion has applied to aging and age-related degenerative diseases, rating of WMHs may be applied to other disorders like TBI, multiple sclerosis (MS), lupus erythematosus, poly-substance abuse, or any disease or disorder that may affect white matter (see Lindeboom & Weinstein, 2004).

An important nomenclature caveat in the neuroimaging of white matter of CT versus MRI needs to be made. Since CT is based on tissue density assessed by passing X-ray beams through brain parenchyma, compared to MRI, which is based on the MR signal intensity, how abnormal white matter findings are described differs between the two different imaging modalities. When white matter integrity is reduced as assessed by CT imaging, it is often referred to as diminished or reduced density. Reduced white matter integrity based on MR FLAIR imaging is referred to as a "*hyperintense signal.*" Although CT density relates to MR signal intensity, they are not the same, and MRI performs better in detecting and defining the extent of white matter pathology, especially on the subtle end of the spectrum. Nonetheless, a darker CT appearance of white matter reflects reduced tissue density, with T2-based MR "hyperintense" signal findings reflecting abnormal white matter, and both indicate underlying white matter pathology (Prins & Scheltens, 2015), as shown in Figure 8.9 comparing CT with FLAIR imaging with varying levels of white matter abnormality.

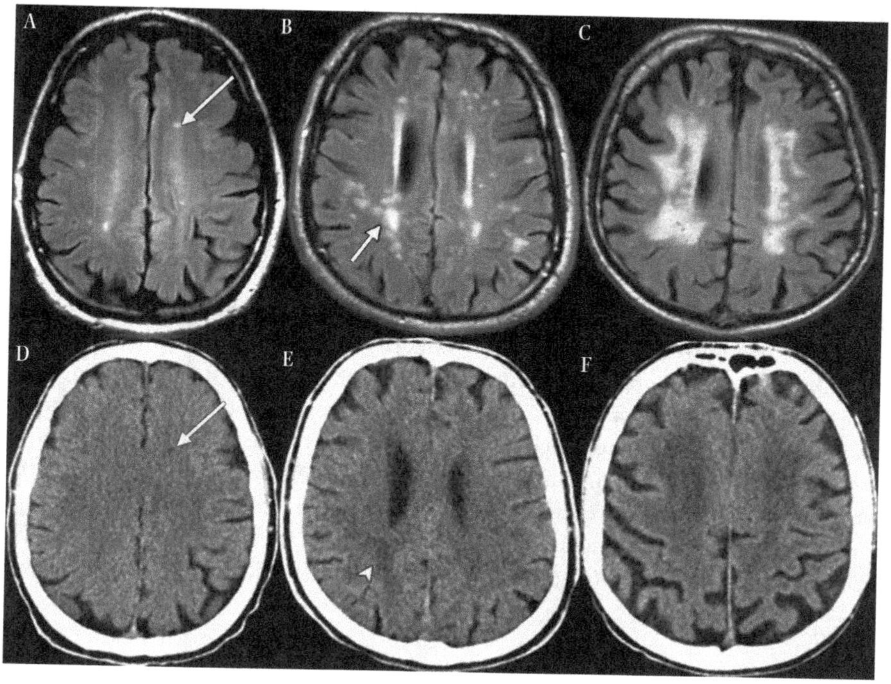

Figure 8.9 These axial images on the top row are from a FLAIR sequence and depict various levels of white matter hyperintense (WMH) foci compared to their CT counterpart below. As in Figures 8.3 and 8.4, the CT below is cut at the same level. Note the superiority of the FLAIR sequence over CT imaging for detecting white matter abnormalities. Since CT is based on an X-ray beam-density function, a darker image within what would be expected to be white matter parenchyma reflects less density and therefore less healthy white matter. Arrows in A and D point to the deep white matter of the left cerebral hemisphere just above the lateral ventricle. In the MRI, the arrow points to a punctate region of hyperintense signal; note the darker corresponding image on CT (arrow). Using the Fazekas et al. four-point scale (see Figure 8.5) where 0 reflects no identifiable WMHs, and 3, the highest rating, the image on the left was rated by Wattjes et al. (2009) as a "1." In B and E, the WMHs are beginning to become confluent (arrowhead in B and E), garnering a "2" rating, with the images to the right (C and F) showing confluent WMHs and a "3" rating.

Illustration used with permission from Wattjes et al. (2009) and the Radiological Society of North America. p.180.

Corpus Callosum

The corpus callosum (CC) is the largest of the brain commissures, easy to identify in the mid-sagittal MRI plane, with equally easy to identify normal appearance and landmarks (Georgy, Hesselink, & Jernigan, 1993; see Figure 8.10). Integrity of the CC represents a window into global white matter integrity where the CC is particularly vulnerable to change in morphology and MR signal intensity in disorders like MS and TBI (Bodini et al., 2013; Mesaros et al., 2009). There is a typical thinning of the CC with aging as well. Despite the fact that the CC thins with the aging process, excessive thinning of the CC occurs with degenerative disorders like Alzheimer's disease, probably reflective of not just white matter pathology but neuronal loss and secondary axonal degeneration, hence the loss of white matter (see Zhu, Gao, Wang, Shi, & Lin, 2012; Zhu et al., 2014). Meguro et al. (2003) showed that CC atrophy based on visual ratings in a mixed typical-aging and dementia group, including those with probable Alzheimer's disease, was associated with greater levels of executive deficits on neuropsychological testing.

There is a higher frequency of abnormal corpus callosum morphology in developmental disorders as well as in very low birthweight infants assessed later in life (Skranes et al., 2007), where the rating system by Spencer et al. (2005) as shown in Figure 8.10 was relatively effective in relating to cognitive impairment. Specifically, increased qualitative scores reflecting presence of an identifiable abnormality were associated with lower scores on intellectual assessment (Skranes et al., 2007). There may also be small size of the CC in schizophrenia, both qualitatively and quantitatively assessed (see Meisenzahl et al., 1999; Tibbo, Nopoulos, Arndt, & Andreasen, 1998) and associated with more negative symptoms. Anomalies in CC morphology have been associated with other neuropsychiatric disorders as well (Georgy et al., 1993). Additionally, in neuropsychiatric

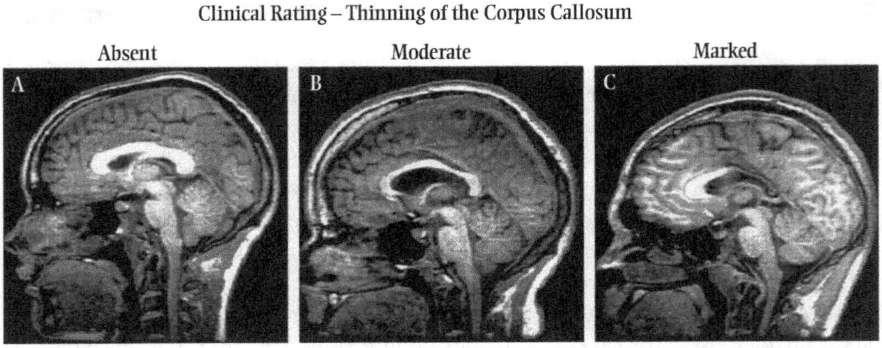

Figure 8.10 Corpus callosum (CC) clinical ratings according to Spencer et al. (2005) in cases of developmental disorder. See also Figure 8.11,which shows three cases with differing levels of CC thinning and how the Spencer et al. ratings could be performed.

Used with permission from the American Association of Neuroradiology and Williams and Wilkens, p. 2694.

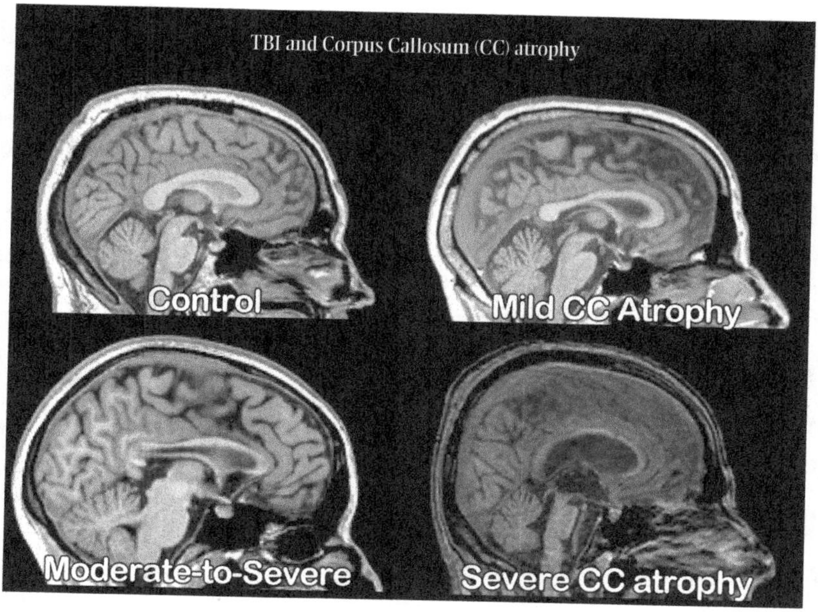

Figure 8.11 Midsagittal views of the corpus callosum depict the normal appearance of the corpus callosum in the upper left and three levels of CC atrophy, using the Spencer et al. ratings from Figure 8.10, in three cases of CC atrophy associated with traumatic brain injury (TBI). Reduced CC size often is associated with reduced processing speed on neuropsychological measures.

disorder associated CC anomalies, there may be other qualitative anomalies in other brain regions (Kennedy & Adolphs, 2012; Lawrie et al., 1997).

At the level of gross morphology, possibly the most studied qualitative as well as quantitative CC finding is in TBI, where severity is often associated with varying degrees of CC atrophy (Bigler & Maxwell, 2011; Gale, Johnson, Bigler, & Blatter, 1995), as depicted in Figure 8.11. It should be noted that an anatomical (T1-weighted) mid-sagittal MRI is the standard in clinical MRI and is often commented on by the neuroradiologist in the interpretive clinical report, although typically not in terms of a formal CC rating. The simple rating schema of Spencer et al. may be used regardless of the disorder.

Third (III) Ventricle

The third (III) ventricle sits at midline surround by the left and right sides of the thalamus as depicted in Figure 8.12 (white arrow in the Control subject). If there is volume loss anywhere in the cerebrum, the III ventricle has a tendency to widen. It will also widen in cases of hydrocephalus, but typically that is transient and potentially reversible if the reason for the hydrocephalus is some form of CSF obstruction. Reider-Groswasser and colleagues (1997) almost two decades ago showed how simple clinical ratings or linear measures, as shown in Figure

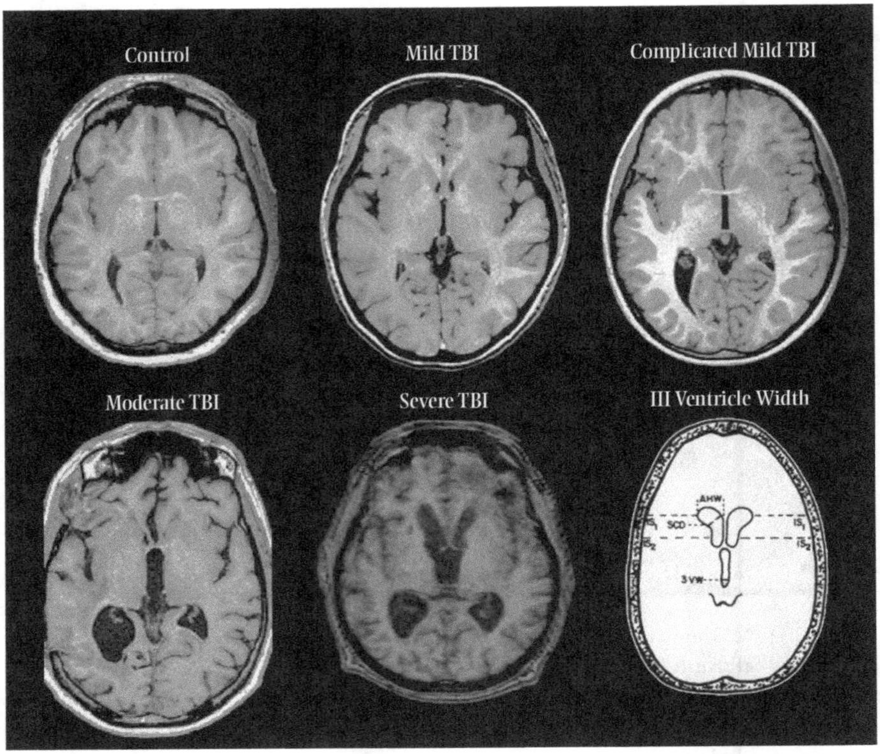

Figure 8.12 Third (III) ventricle ratings as observed in TBI. Note the illustration in the lower right corner that depicts where III ventricle width may be determined. The other measures involve linear distance and the width of the anterior horns of the lateral ventricle [from Reider-Groswasser et al. (1997) and the American Association for Neuroradiology, p. 149]. Note how thin the midline appearance is for the control subject (upper left). As TBI severity increases, accompanied by generalized cerebral atrophy and reduced brain volume, III ventricle width increases.

8.12, may be used to identify III ventricular dilatation and relate that to cognitive and behavioral outcome from acquired brain injury (see also Groswasser et al., 2002; Reider-Groswasser et al., 1997; Reider et al., 2002). Because of its midline location, pathology that results in parenchymal volume anywhere in the brain will typically result in III ventricle expansion.

Clinically, III ventricle width has also been examined in schizophrenia and age-mediated cognitive disorders (Cullberg & Nyback, 1992; Erkinjuntti et al., 1993; Johansson et al., 2012; Sandyk, 1993; Slansky et al., 1995; Soininen et al., 1993), even using coarse measures generated by ultrasonography (Wollenweber et al., 2011). Regardless of the imaging technique used, expansion of the III ventricle is a marker of brain pathology where greater expansion typically relates to worse neuropsychological outcome.

Hemosiderin Deposition Rating

Regardless of etiology, microhemorrhages, also referred to as "microbleeds," reflect vascular pathology of some sort that, as it increases, potentially relates to neuropsychological outcome. Figure 8.13 shows susceptibility weighted imaging (SWI)–identified regions of hemosiderin deposition. Hemosiderin is a blood byproduct from hemorrhage that has ferritin (iron), and is therefore sensitive to MR signal detection techniques. Ischemic vascular disease is associated with not only microhemorrhages but WMHs. Clinically, microbleeds are typically just counted, where in vascular disease microbleeds may be positively related to WMHs (Charidimou, Jager, & Werring, 2012; Goos et al., 2010; Noh et al., 2014), but this may not be the case in TBI (Riedy et al., 2015). In TBI, an increasing number of microbleeds has been related to worse neuropsychological outcome (Scheid & von Cramon, 2010), including pediatric TBI (Beauchamp et al., 2013;

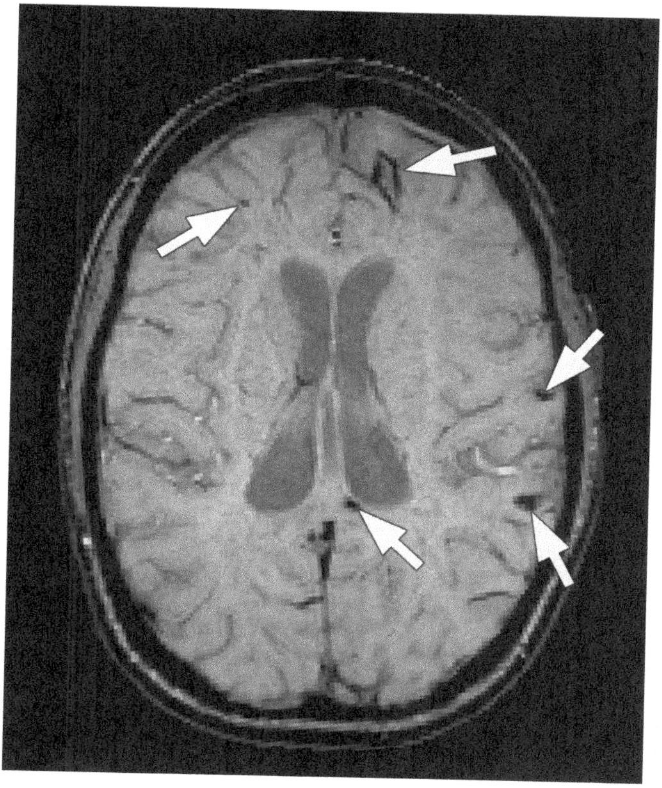

Figure 8.13 Axial view of susceptibility-weighted imaging (SWI) at the level of the body of the lateral ventricle in a patient who sustained a severe TBI. SWI is particularly sensitive in detecting hemosiderin deposition, reflecting prior hemorrhagic lesions. Although there are sophisticated methods for obtaining total hemosiderin burden, a simple frequency count is commonly done.

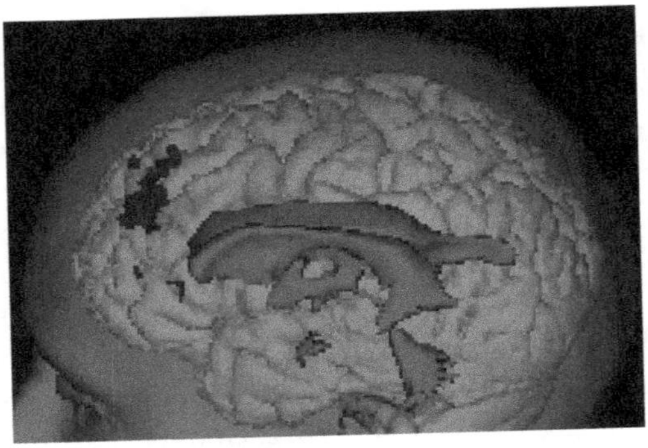

Figure 8.14 Three-dimensional (3-D) reconstruction of the brain, with the ventricular system depicted in the center of the image, to provide perspective. Darker areas represent individual areas where hemosiderin deposition could be detected, as shown in Figure 8.13. The one lesion in the posterior corpus callosum is obscured by the reconstruction of the ventricular system. Note the preponderance of hemorrhagic lesions within the frontal lobes, typical of TBI.

Bigler et al., 2013) and tends to occur more frequently within the frontal and temporal regions of the brain, as shown in Figure 8.14.

Changes in the Role of Neuropsychology with Advances in Neuroimaging

As implied in the introduction to this chapter, the role of neuropsychological assessment has changed as neuroimaging has improved, including the role that neuropsychological test findings play in the differential diagnosis of certain conditions. As an example, prior to contemporary neuroimaging, the workup of a patient with memory complaints and suspected early dementia would have largely relied on findings from neuropsychological assessments. Now, with automated quantitative neuroimage analysis techniques (Bigler, 2015), single-subject comparisons to a normative data set can be made, incorporating a wealth of neuroimaging information that, by itself yields diagnostic accuracy and classification that equals or surpasses just using neuropsychological findings alone—as high as 88% accurate in differentiating individuals with Alzheimer's disease from age-matched controls (see Moller et al., 2015; Schmand, Eikelenboom, van Gool, & Alzheimer's Disease Neuroimaging, 2012). Of course, neuroimaging alone does not provide any metrics that describe cognitive impairments that are essential in care, family planning, and treatment of the individuals with neurological conditions. Such a role will remain a robust and important contribution that clinical neuropsychology will play regardless of advances with neuroimaging. Likewise, given the broad spectrum of age-related cognitive complaints and the varieties of neurodegenerative diseases and neuropsychiatric disorders, the case can be made that neuropsychological assessment remains an important part of the workup of any individual with a cognitive complaint, especially in those younger than 65 (Finney, Minagar, & Heilman, 2016; Schmand, Eikelenboom, van Gool, & Alzheimer's Disease Neuroimaging, 2011; Sitek, Barczak, & Harciarek, 2015).

Another area in neuropsychology where neuroimaging has been particularly influential is in the field of epilepsy assessment. Prior to neuroimaging, neuropsychological assessment techniques were influential in the diagnostic decision process of determining lateralization, localization, and lesion detection, as reviewed by Loring (1991). Neuropsychological assessment remains an important part of the overall assessment of the patient with epilepsy (Hoppe & Helmstaedter, 2010), including pre-surgical assessment evaluations (Jones-Gotman et al., 2010; Loring, 2010). Just as with the neurodegenerative disorders, the neuropsychological examination in the patient with epilepsy remains the standard for assessing neurocognitive and neuroemotional functioning, but its role in lateralization of cognitive functioning and specification as to localization of function has changed with improved neuroimaging and electrophysiological methods (Baxendale & Thompson, 2010). With advances in functional MRI (fMRI), techniques are being standardized as neurocognitive probes to assess language, memory, and other cognitive functions in the patient with epilepsy, which have altered and will continue to influence the traditional role of neuropsychology in assessing that disorder (Sidhu et al., 2015).

Advanced Neuroimaging Techniques

Providing unique neuroanatomical information, one of the great neuroimaging discoveries at the end of the twentieth century was that MR water-diffusion metrics could be used to assess not only white matter integrity but connectivity using diffusion tensor imaging (DTI; Wilde, Hunter, & Bigler, 2012). DTI provides a wealth of metrics, including tractography that can be used to identify specific tracts and their physiological integrity within the brain (Chanraud, Zahr, Sullivan, & Pfefferbaum, 2010). The implications for neuropsychology using this technique are enormous (Sullivan & Bigler, 2015); however, the problem with DTI at this stage is that DTI metrics are in part dependent upon the machine environment generating the DTI sequence, and therefore a universally usable program like what has been developed for structural imaging (i.e., FreeSurfer [freesurfer.net]) has not yet been established. So, within a laboratory with an excellent and broad spectrum of normative scans, DTI permits exploring relationships of DTI metrics with specific neuropsychological measures—for example, motor performance on traditional neuropsychological tests like the finger-tapping test, and strength of grip-hand dynamometer measures with motor tracts (Travers et al., 2015), or language function involving the arcuate fasciculus (Paldino, Hedges, & Zhang, 2014). But how to clinically apply DTI findings and integrate them within neuropsychology and cognitive assessment of the individual patient, making the information clinically universal, is a work in progress, but with very significant positive gains being made (Strauss et al., 2015; Wilde et al., 2015).

Equally important neuroimaging discoveries generally contemporaneous with DTI were how to assess brain resting state and default mode network, established by a variety of functional neuroimaging techniques (Raichle et al., 2001). The "resting state" is inferred because the individual is merely lying in the scanner and does not have to be actively engaged in a cognitive task. The signal recording from MRI is the blood-oxygen-level–dependent (BOLD) signal—but there are resting state programs for positron emission tomography (PET) and electroencephalography (EEG) as well. These methods have tremendous clinical potential in terms of deriving networks and testing their integrity, but there is still no across-lab standardization, and how to handle within and between individual and lab variability has not been resolved (Chen et al., 2015).

Lastly, as already mentioned, fMRI neurocognitive probes are being specifically developed, which is likely to have a major impact on neuropsychology. This has been written about for over a decade (see Kozel & Trivedi, 2008), but it is rapidly moving toward greater clinical application (see Huettel, Song, & McCarthy, 2014) Also, a relatively new technology, functional near-infrared spectroscopy (fNIRS) has important implications for neuropsychology as well, because it provides a functional neuroimaging BOLD metric of cerebral cortex activation using localized infrared light beam technology. fNIRS does not have any of the restrictions of MR-based technologies, but at this stage it can only assess a limited amount of cerebral cortex (Stojanovic-Radic, Wylie, Voelbel, Chiaravalloti, & DeLuca, 2015). Nonetheless, this tool may become even more amenable to neuropsychological methods of assessment.

CONCLUSIONS

We are now well into the twenty-first century, with digitally sophisticated neuroimaging routinely being performed in most neurological and neuropsychiatric disorders. It is time for clinical neuropsychological assessment to begin to routinely utilize information from neuroimaging findings as part of the evaluation metric. This could begin with utilizing clinical rating methods, as outlined in this chapter. The incorporation of neuroimaging needs to be done with the highest degree of normative standards that have benefitted clinical neuropsychology as a discipline because, as Weinberger and Radulescu (2016) state, it is a disservice to all aspects of clinical neuroscience to be uncritically accepting of neuroimaging findings purportedly related as meaningful neurobehavioral correlates.

REFERENCES

Baxendale, S., & Thompson, P. (2010). Beyond localization: The role of traditional neuropsychological tests in an age of imaging. *Epilepsia, 51*(11), 2225–2230. doi:10.1111/j.1528-1167.2010.02710.x

Beauchamp, M. H., Beare, R., Ditchfield, M., Coleman, L., Babl, F. E., Kean, M., . . . Anderson, V. (2013). Susceptibility weighted imaging and its relationship to outcome after pediatric traumatic brain injury. *Cortex; A Journal Devoted to the Study of the Nervous System and Behavior, 49*(2), 591–598. doi:10.1016/j.cortex.2012.08.015

Bigler, E. D. (2015). Structural image analysis of the brain in neuropsychology using magnetic resonance imaging (MRI) techniques. *Neuropsychology Review, 25*(3), 224–249. doi:10.1007/s11065-015-9290-0

Bigler, E. D., Abildskov, T. J., Petrie, J., Farrer, T. J., Dennis, M., Simic, N., . . . Owen Yeates, K. (2013). Heterogeneity of brain lesions in pediatric traumatic brain injury. *Neuropsychology, 27*(4), 438–451. doi:10.1037/a0032837

Bigler, E. D., Kerr, B., Victoroff, J., Tate, D. F., & Breitner, J. C. (2002). White matter lesions, quantitative magnetic resonance imaging, and dementia. *Alzheimer Disease and Associated Disorders, 16*(3), 161–170.

Bigler, E. D., & Maxwell, W. L. (2011). Neuroimaging and neuropathology of TBI. *NeuroRehabilitation, 28*(2), 63–74. doi:10.3233/NRE-2011-0633

Bigler, E. D., Yeo, R. A., & Turkheimer, E. (1989). *Neuropsychological Function and Brain Imaging*. New York: Plenum Press.

Bilder, R. M. (2011). Neuropsychology 3.0: Evidence-based science and practice. *Journal of the International Neuropsychological Society: JINS, 17*(1), 7–13. doi:10.1017/S1355617710001396

Bodini, B., Cercignani, M., Khaleeli, Z., Miller, D. H., Ron, M., Penny, S., . . . Ciccarelli, O. (2013). Corpus callosum damage predicts disability progression and cognitive dysfunction in primary-progressive MS after five years. *Human Brain Mapping, 34*(5), 1163–1172. doi:10.1002/hbm.21499

Boone, K. B., Miller, B. L., Lesser, I. M., Mehringer, C. M., Hill-Gutierrez, E., Goldberg, M. A., & Berman, N. G. (1992). Neuropsychological correlates of white-matter lesions in healthy elderly subjects. A threshold effect. *Archives of Neurology, 49*(5), 549–554.

Chanraud, S., Zahr, N., Sullivan, E. V., & Pfefferbaum, A. (2010). MR diffusion tensor imaging: A window into white matter integrity of the working brain. *Neuropsychology Review, 20*(2), 209–225. doi:10.1007/s11065-010-9129-7

Charidimou, A., Jager, H. R., & Werring, D. J. (2012). Cerebral microbleed detection and mapping: Principles, methodological aspects and rationale in vascular dementia. *Experimental Gerontology, 47*(11), 843–852. doi:10.1016/j.exger.2012.06.008

Chen, B., Xu, T., Zhou, C., Wang, L., Yang, N., Wang, Z., . . . Weng, X. C. (2015). Individual variability and test-retest reliability revealed by ten repeated resting-state brain scans over one month. *PLoS One, 10*(12), e0144963. doi:10.1371/journal.pone.0144963

Chen, W., Song, X., Zhang, Y., Darvesh, S., Zhang, N., D'Arcy, R. C., . . . Rockwood, K. (2010). An MRI-based semiquantitative index for the evaluation of brain atrophy and lesions in Alzheimer's disease, mild cognitive impairment and normal aging. *Dementia and Geriatric Cognitive Disorders, 30*(2), 121–130. doi:10.1159/000319537

Cullberg, J., & Nyback, H. (1992). Persistent auditory hallucinations correlate with the size of the third ventricle in schizophrenic patients. *Acta Psychiatrica Scandinavica, 86*(6), 469–472.

DeCarli, C., Frisoni, G. B., Clark, C. M., Harvey, D., Grundman, M., Petersen, R. C., . . . Scheltens, P. (2007). Qualitative estimates of medial temporal atrophy as a predictor of progression from mild cognitive impairment to dementia. *Archives of Neurology, 64*(1), 108–115. doi:10.1001/archneur.64.1.108

Dennis, M., Spiegler, B. J., Simic, N., Sinopoli, K. J., Wilkinson, A., Yeates, K. O., . . . Fletcher, J. M. (2014). Functional plasticity in childhood brain disorders: When, what, how, and whom to assess. *Neuropsychology Review, 24*(4), 389–408. doi:10.1007/s11065-014-9261-x

Erkinjuntti, T., Lee, D. H., Gao, F., Steenhuis, R., Eliasziw, M., Fry, R., . . . Hachinski, V. C. (1993). Temporal lobe atrophy on magnetic resonance imaging in the diagnosis of early Alzheimer's disease. *Archives of Neurology, 50*(3), 305–310.

Fazekas, F., Chawluk, J. B., Alavi, A., Hurtig, H. I., & Zimmerman, R. A. (1987). MR signal abnormalities at 1.5 T in Alzheimer's dementia and normal aging. *AJR: American Journal of Roentgenology, 149*(2), 351–356. doi:10.2214/ajr.149.2.351

Filley, C. M., & Bigler, E. D. (Eds.). (2017). *Neuroanatomy for the Neuropsychologist.* In Morgan, J. E. & Ricker, J. H. (eds). Textbook of Clinical Neuropsychology. (2nd Edition). New York: Taylor & Francis.

Finney, G. R., Minagar, A., & Heilman, K. M. (2016). Assessment of mental status. *Neurologic Clinics, 34*(1), 1–16. doi:10.1016/j.ncl.2015.08.001

Gabrieli, J. D., Ghosh, S. S., & Whitfield-Gabrieli, S. (2015). Prediction as a humanitarian and pragmatic contribution from human cognitive neuroscience. *Neuron, 85*(1), 11–26. doi:10.1016/j.neuron.2014.10.047

Gale, S. D., Johnson, S. C., Bigler, E. D., & Blatter, D. D. (1995). Nonspecific white matter degeneration following traumatic brain injury. *Journal of the International Neuropsychological Society: JINS, 1*(1), 17–28.

Georgy, B. A., Hesselink, J. R., & Jernigan, T. L. (1993). MR imaging of the corpus callosum. *AJR: American Journal of Roentgenology, 160*(5), 949–955. doi:10.2214/ajr.160.5.8470609

Goos, J. D., Henneman, W. J., Sluimer, J. D., Vrenken, H., Sluimer, I. C., Barkhof, F., . . . van der Flier, W. M. (2010). Incidence of cerebral microbleeds: A longitudinal study in a memory clinic population. *Neurology, 74*(24), 1954–1960. doi:10.1212/WNL.0b013e3181e396ea

Groswasser, Z., Reider, G., II, Schwab, K., Ommaya, A. K., Pridgen, A., Brown, H. R., . . . Salazar, A. M. (2002). Quantitative imaging in late TBI. Part II: Cognition and work after closed and penetrating head injury: A report of the Vietnam head injury study. *Brain Injury, 16*(8), 681–690. doi:10.1080/02699050110119835

Guo, H., Song, X., Schmidt, M. H., Vandorpe, R., Yang, Z., LeBlanc, E., . . . Rockwood, K. (2014). Evaluation of whole brain health in aging and Alzheimer's disease: A standard procedure for scoring an MRI-based brain atrophy and lesion index. *Journal of Alzheimer's Disease: JAD, 42*(2), 691–703. doi:10.3233/JAD-140333

Hannay, H. J., Bieliauskas, L. A., Crosson, B., Hammeke, T., Hamsher, K. D., & Koffler, S. (1998). Proceedings of the Houston Conference on Specialty Education and Training in Clinical Neuropsychology. *Archives of Clinical Neuropsychology, 13*(Special Issue).

Heo, J. H., Lee, S. T., Kon, C., Park, H. J., Shim, J. Y., & Kim, M. (2009). White matter hyperintensities and cognitive dysfunction in Alzheimer disease. *Journal of Geriatric Psychiatry and Neurology, 22*(3), 207–212. doi:10.1177/0891988709335800

Hoppe, C., & Helmstaedter, C. (2010). Sensitive and specific neuropsychological assessments of the behavioral effects of epilepsy and its treatment are essential. *Epilepsia, 51*(11), 2365–2366.

Huettel, S. A., Song, A. W., & McCarthy, G. (2014). *Functional Magnetic Resonance Imaging* (3rd ed.). Sunderland, MA: Sinauer Associates.

Jang, J. W., Park, S. Y., Park, Y. H., Baek, M. J., Lim, J. S., Youn, Y. C., & Kim, S. (2015). A comprehensive visual rating scale of brain magnetic resonance imaging: Application in elderly subjects with Alzheimer's disease, mild cognitive impairment, and normal cognition. *Journal of Alzheimer's Disease: JAD, 44*(3), 1023–1034. doi:10.3233/JAD-142088

Johansson, L., Skoog, I., Gustafson, D. R., Olesen, P. J., Waern, M., Bengtsson, C., . . . Guo, X. (2012). Midlife psychological distress associated with late-life brain atrophy and white matter lesions: A 32-year population study of women. *Psychosomatic Medicine, 74*(2), 120–125. doi:10.1097/PSY.0b013e318246eb10

Jones-Gotman, M., Smith, M. L., Risse, G. L., Westerveld, M., Swanson, S. J., Giovagnoli, A. R., . . . Piazzini, A. (2010). The contribution of neuropsychology to diagnostic assessment in epilepsy. *Epilepsy and Behavior, 18*(1–2), 3–12. doi:10.1016/j.yebeh.2010.02.019

Kennedy, D. P., & Adolphs, R. (2012). The social brain in psychiatric and neurological disorders. *Trends in Cognitive Sciences, 16*(11), 559–572. doi:10.1016/j.tics.2012.09.006

Kertesz, A. (1983). *Localization in Neuropsychology*. San Diego: Academic Press.

Koedam, E. L., Lehmann, M., van der Flier, W. M., Scheltens, P., Pijnenburg, Y. A., Fox, N., . . . Wattjes, M. P. (2011). Visual assessment of posterior atrophy development of a MRI rating scale. *European Radiology, 21*(12), 2618–2625. doi:10.1007/s00330-011-2205-4

Kozel, F. A., & Trivedi, M. H. (2008). Developing a neuropsychiatric functional brain imaging test. *Neurocase, 14*(1), 54–58. doi:10.1080/13554790701881731

Lawrie, S. M., Abukmeil, S. S., Chiswick, A., Egan, V., Santosh, C. G., & Best, J. J. (1997). Qualitative cerebral morphology in schizophrenia: A magnetic resonance imaging study and systematic literature review. *Schizophrenia Research, 25*(2), 155–166. doi:10.1016/S0920-9964(97)00019-4

Leaper, S. A., Murray, A. D., Lemmon, H. A., Staff, R. T., Deary, I. J., Crawford, J. R., & Whalley, L. J. (2001). Neuropsychologic correlates of brain white matter lesions depicted on MR images: 1921 Aberdeen Birth Cohort. *Radiology, 221*(1), 51–55. doi:10.1148/radiol.2211010086

Lesser, I. M., Boone, K. B., Mehringer, C. M., Wohl, M. A., Miller, B. L., & Berman, N. G. (1996). Cognition and white matter hyperintensities in older depressed patients. *The American Journal of Psychiatry, 153*(10), 1280–1287.

Lezak, M. D. (1976). *Neuropsychological Assessment*. New York: Oxford University Press.

Lindeboom, J., & Weinstein, H. (2004). Neuropsychology of cognitive ageing, minimal cognitive impairment, Alzheimer's disease, and vascular cognitive impairment. *European Journal of Pharmacology, 490*(1–3), 83–86. doi:10.1016/j.ejphar.2004.02.046

Loring, D. W. (1991). A counterpoint to Reitan's note on the history of clinical neuropsychology. *Archives of Clinical Neuropsychology, 6*(3), 167–171.

Loring, D. W. (2010). History of neuropsychology through epilepsy eyes. *Archives of Clinical Neuropsychology, 25*(4), 259–273. doi:10.1093/arclin/acq024

Meguro, K., Constans, J. M., Shimada, M., Yamaguchi, S., Ishizaki, J., Ishii, H., . . . Sekita, Y. (2003). Corpus callosum atrophy, white matter lesions, and frontal executive dysfunction in normal aging and Alzheimer's disease. A community-based study: The Tajiri Project. *International Psychogeriatrics/IPA, 15*(1), 9–25.

Meisenzahl, E. M., Frodl, T., Greiner, J., Leinsinger, G., Maag, K. P., Heiss, D., . . . Moller, H. J. (1999). Corpus callosum size in schizophrenia—a magnetic resonance imaging analysis. *European Archives of Psychiatry and Clinical Neuroscience, 249*(6), 305–312.

Menendez-Gonzalez, M., Lopez-Muniz, A., Vega, J. A., Salas-Pacheco, J. M., & Arias-Carrion, O. (2014). MTA index: A simple 2D-method for assessing atrophy of the medial temporal lobe using clinically available neuroimaging. *Frontiers in Aging Neuroscience, 6*, 23. doi:10.3389/fnagi.2014.00023

Mesaros, S., Rocca, M. A., Riccitelli, G., Pagani, E., Rovaris, M., Caputo, D., . . . Filippi, M. (2009). Corpus callosum damage and cognitive dysfunction in benign MS. *Human Brain Mapping, 30*(8), 2656–2666. doi:10.1002/hbm.20692

Moller, C., Pijnenburg, Y. A., van der Flier, W. M., Versteeg, A., Tijms, B., de Munck, J. C., . . . Wink, A. M. (2015). Alzheimer disease and behavioral variant frontotemporal dementia: Automatic classification based on cortical atrophy for single-subject diagnosis. *Radiology, 279*(3), 838–848. doi:10.1148/radiol.2015150220

Noh, Y., Lee, Y., Seo, S. W., Jeong, J. H., Choi, S. H., Back, J. H., . . . Na, D. L. (2014). A new classification system for ischemia using a combination of deep and periventricular white matter hyperintensities. *Journal of Stroke and Cerebrovascular Diseases: The Official Journal of National Stroke Association, 23*(4), 636–642. doi:10.1016/j.jstrokecerebrovasdis.2013.06.002

Paldino, M. J., Hedges, K., & Zhang, W. (2014). Independent contribution of individual white matter pathways to language function in pediatric epilepsy patients. *NeuroImage. Clinical, 6*, 327–332. doi:10.1016/j.nicl.2014.09.017

Pasquier, F., Hamon, M., Lebert, F., Jacob, B., Pruvo, J. P., & Petit, H. (1997). Medial temporal lobe atrophy in memory disorders. *Journal of Neurology, 244*(3), 175–181.

Pasquier, F., Leys, D., Weerts, J. G., Mounier-Vehier, F., Barkhof, F., & Scheltens, P. (1996). Inter- and intraobserver reproducibility of cerebral atrophy assessment on MRI scans with hemispheric infarcts. *European Neurology, 36*(5), 268–272.

Prins, N. D., & Scheltens, P. (2015). White matter hyperintensities, cognitive impairment and dementia: An update. *Nature Reviews. Neurology, 11*(3), 157–165. doi:10.1038/nrneurol.2015.10

Raichle, M. E., MacLeod, A. M., Snyder, A. Z., Powers, W. J., Gusnard, D. A., & Shulman, G. L. (2001). A default mode of brain function. *Proceedings of the National Academy of Science U S A, 98*(2), 676–682. doi:10.1073/pnas.98.2.676

Reider-Groswasser, I., Costeff, H., Sazbon, L., & Groswasser, Z. (1997). CT findings in persistent vegetative state following blunt traumatic brain injury. *Brain Injury, 11*(12), 865–870.

Reider, G., II, Groswasser, Z., Ommaya, A. K., Schwab, K., Pridgen, A., Brown, H. R., . . . Salazar, A. M. (2002). Quantitive imaging in late traumatic brain injury. Part I: Late imaging parameters in closed and penetrating head injuries. *Brain Injury, 16*(6), 517–525. doi:10.1080/02699050110119141

Riedy, G., Senseney, J. S., Liu, W., Ollinger, J., Sham, E., Krapiva, P., . . . Oakes, T. R. (2015). Findings from structural MR imaging in military traumatic brain injury. *Radiology*, 150438. doi:10.1148/radiol.2015150438

Sandyk, R. (1993). The relationship of thought disorder to third ventricle width and calcification of the pineal gland in chronic schizophrenia. *The International Journal of Neuroscience, 68*(1–2), 53–59.

Scheid, R., & von Cramon, D. Y. (2010). Clinical findings in the chronic phase of traumatic brain injury: Data from 12 years' experience in the Cognitive Neurology Outpatient Clinic at the University of Leipzig. *Deutsches Arzteblatt International, 107*(12), 199–205. doi:10.3238/arztebl.2010.0199

Scheltens, P., Barkhof, F., Leys, D., Pruvo, J. P., Nauta, J. J., Vermersch, P., . . . Valk, J. (1993). A semiquantative rating scale for the assessment of signal hyperintensities on magnetic resonance imaging. *Journal of the Neurological Sciences, 114*(1), 7–12.

Scheltens, P., Barkhof, F., Valk, J., Algra, P. R., van der Hoop, R. G., Nauta, J., & Wolters, E. C. (1992). White matter lesions on magnetic resonance imaging in clinically diagnosed Alzheimer's disease. Evidence for heterogeneity. *Brain: A Journal of Neurology, 115(Pt 3)*, 735–748.

Scheltens, P., Launer, L. J., Barkhof, F., Weinstein, H. C., & van Gool, W. A. (1995). Visual assessment of medial temporal lobe atrophy on magnetic resonance imaging: Interobserver reliability. *Journal of Neurology, 242*(9), 557–560.

Scheltens, P., Leys, D., Barkhof, F., Huglo, D., Weinstein, H. C., Vermersch, P., . . . Valk, J. (1992). Atrophy of medial temporal lobes on MRI in "probable" Alzheimer's disease and normal ageing: Diagnostic value and neuropsychological correlates. *Journal of Neurology, Neurosurgery, and Psychiatry, 55*(10), 967–972.

Scheltens, P., Pasquier, F., Weerts, J. G., Barkhof, F., & Leys, D. (1997). Qualitative assessment of cerebral atrophy on MRI: Inter- and intra-observer reproducibility in dementia and normal aging. *European Neurology, 37*(2), 95–99.

Schmand, B., Eikelenboom, P., van Gool, W. A., & Alzheimer's Disease Neuroimaging, I. (2011). Value of neuropsychological tests, neuroimaging, and biomarkers for diagnosing Alzheimer's disease in younger and older age cohorts. *Journal of the American Geriatric Society, 59*(9), 1705–1710. doi:10.1111/j.1532-5415.2011.03539.x

Schmand, B., Eikelenboom, P., van Gool, W. A., & Alzheimer's Disease Neuroimaging, I. (2012). Value of diagnostic tests to predict conversion to Alzheimer's disease in young and old patients with amnestic mild cognitive impairment. *Journal of Alzheimer's Disease: JAD, 29*(3), 641–648. doi:10.3233/JAD-2012-111703

Schoenberg, M. R., Marsh, P. J., & Lerner, A. J. (2011). Neuroanatomy primer: Structure and function of the human nervous system. In M. R. Schoenberg & J. G. Scott (Eds.), *The Little Black Book of Neuropsychology: A Syndrome-Based Approach*. New York: Springer Science+Business Media LLC.

Sidhu, M. K., Stretton, J., Winston, G. P., Symms, M., Thompson, P. J., Koepp, M. J., & Duncan, J. S. (2015). Memory fMRI predicts verbal memory decline after anterior temporal lobe resection. *Neurology, 84*(15), 1512–1519. doi:10.1212/WNL.0000000000001461

Sitek, E. J., Barczak, A., & Harciarek, M. (2015). Neuropsychological assessment and differential diagnosis in young-onset dementias. *Psychiatric Clinics of North America, 38*(2), 265–279. doi:10.1016/j.psc.2015.01.003

Skranes, J., Vangberg, T. R., Kulseng, S., Indredavik, M. S., Evensen, K. A., Martinussen, M., . . . Brubakk, A. M. (2007). Clinical findings and white matter abnormalities seen on diffusion tensor imaging in adolescents with very low birth weight. *Brain: A Journal of Neurology, 130*(Pt 3), 654–666. doi:10.1093/brain/awm001

Slansky, I., Herholz, K., Pietrzyk, U., Kessler, J., Grond, M., Mielke, R., & Heiss, W. D. (1995). Cognitive impairment in Alzheimer's disease correlates with ventricular width and atrophy-corrected cortical glucose metabolism. *Neuroradiology, 37*(4), 270–277.

Soininen, H., Reinikainen, K. J., Puranen, M., Helkala, E. L., Paljarvi, L., & Riekkinen, P. J. (1993). Wide third ventricle correlates with low choline acetyltransferase activity of the neocortex in Alzheimer patients. *Alzheimer Disease and Associated Disorders, 7*(1), 39–47.

Song, X., Mitnitski, A., Zhang, N., Chen, W., & Rockwood, K. (2013). Dynamics of brain structure and cognitive function in the Alzheimer's disease neuroimaging initiative. *Journal of Neurology, Neurosurgery, and Psychiatry, 84*(1), 71–78. doi:10.1136/jnnp-2012-303579

Spencer, M. D., Gibson, R. J., Moorhead, T. W., Keston, P. M., Hoare, P., Best, J. J., . . . Johnstone, E. C. (2005). Qualitative assessment of brain anomalies in adolescents with mental retardation. *AJNR. American Journal of Neuroradiology, 26*(10), 2691–2697.

Stojanovic-Radic, J., Wylie, G., Voelbel, G., Chiaravalloti, N., & DeLuca, J. (2015). Neuroimaging and cognition using functional near infrared spectroscopy (fNIRS) in multiple sclerosis. *Brain Imaging and Behavior, 9*(2), 302–311. doi:10.1007/s11682-014-9307-y

Strauss, S., Hulkower, M., Gulko, E., Zampolin, R. L., Gutman, D., Chitkara, M., . . . Lipton, M. L. (2015). Current clinical applications and future potential of diffusion tensor imaging in traumatic brain injury. *Topics in Magnetic Resonance Imaging, 24*(6), 353–362. doi:10.1097/RMR.0000000000000071

Sullivan, E. V., & Bigler, E. D. (2015). Neuroimaging's role in neuropsychology: Introduction to the special issue of *Neuropsychology Review* on neuroimaging in neuropsychology. *Neuropsychology Review, 25*(3), 221–223. doi:10.1007/s11065-015-9296-7

Tibbo, P., Nopoulos, P., Arndt, S., & Andreasen, N. C. (1998). Corpus callosum shape and size in male patients with schizophrenia. *Biological Psychiatry, 44*(6), 405–412.

Toga, A. (2015). *Brain Mapping: An Encyclopedic Reference*. New York: Academic Press.

Travers, B. G., Bigler, E. D., Tromp do, P. M., Adluru, N., Destiche, D., Samsin, D., . . . Lainhart, J. E. (2015). Brainstem white matter predicts individual differences in manual motor difficulties and symptom severity in autism. *Journal of Autism and Developmental Disorders, 45*(9), 3030–3040. doi:10.1007/s10803-015-2467-9

Tschanz, J. T., Welsh-Bohmer, K. A., Plassman, B. L., Norton, M. C., Wyse, B. W., Breitner, J. C., & Cache County Study Investigators. (2002). An adaptation of the modified Mini-Mental State Examination: Analysis of demographic influences and normative data: The Cache County study. *Neuropsychiatry, Neuropsychology, and Behavioral Neurology, 15*(1), 28–38.

Tsui, Y. H., McDonnell, Z., Finuf, C., Hall, A., Gilmartin, M., Cummock, J., . . . Cache County Study Investigators. (2014). Scheltens et al. ratings for white matter hyperintensities in the Cache County study on memory health and aging. *Journal of International Neuropsychological Society, 20*(Suppl S1), 154–155.

Tuladhar, A. M., van Norden, A. G., de Laat, K. F., Zwiers, M. P., van Dijk, E. J., Norris, D. G., & de Leeuw, F. E. (2015). White matter integrity in small vessel disease is related to cognition. *NeuroImage. Clinical, 7*, 518–524. doi:10.1016/j.nicl.2015.02.003

van de Pol, L. A., Korf, E. S., van der Flier, W. M., Brashear, H. R., Fox, N. C., Barkhof, F., & Scheltens, P. (2007). Magnetic resonance imaging predictors of cognition in mild cognitive impairment. *Archives of Neurology, 64*(7), 1023–1028. doi:10.1001/archneur.64.7.1023

Wahlund, L. O., Barkhof, F., Fazekas, F., Bronge, L., Augustin, M., Sjogren, M., . . . Scheltens, P. (2001). A new rating scale for age-related white matter changes applicable to MRI and CT. *Stroke: A Journal of Cerebral Circulation, 32*(6), 1318–1322.

Wattjes, M. P., Henneman, W. J., van der Flier, W. M., de Vries, O., Traber, F., Geurts, J. J., . . . Barkhof, F. (2009). Diagnostic imaging of patients in a memory clinic: Comparison of MR imaging and 64-detector row CT. *Radiology, 253*(1), 174–183. doi:10.1148/radiol.2531082262

Weinberger, D. R., & Radulescu, E. (2016). Finding the elusive psychiatric "lesion" with 21st-century neuroanatomy: A note of caution. *The American Journal of Psychiatry, 173*(1), 27–33. doi:10.1176/appi.ajp.2015.15060753

Wilde, E. A., Bouix, S., Tate, D. F., Lin, A. P., Newsome, M. R., Taylor, B. A., . . . York, G. (2015). Advanced neuroimaging applied to veterans and service personnel with traumatic brain injury: State of the art and potential benefits. *Brain Imaging and Behavior, 9*(3), 367–402. doi:10.1007/s11682-015-9444-y

Wilde, E. A., Hunter, J. V., & Bigler, E. D. (2012). A primer of neuroimaging analysis in neurorehabilitation outcome research. *NeuroRehabilitation, 31*(3), 227–242. doi:10.3233/NRE-2012-0793

Wollenweber, F. A., Schomburg, R., Probst, M., Schneider, V., Hiry, T., Ochsenfeld, A., . . . Behnke, S. (2011). Width of the third ventricle assessed by transcranial sonography can monitor brain atrophy in a time- and cost-effective manner--results from a longitudinal study on 500 subjects. *Psychiatry Research, 191*(3), 212–216. doi:10.1016/j.pscychresns.2010.09.010

Zhu, M., Gao, W., Wang, X., Shi, C., & Lin, Z. (2012). Progression of corpus callosum atrophy in early stage of Alzheimer's disease: MRI based study. *Academic Radiology, 19*(5), 512–517. doi:10.1016/j.acra.2012.01.006

Zhu, M., Wang, X., Gao, W., Shi, C., Ge, H., Shen, H., & Lin, Z. (2014). Corpus callosum atrophy and cognitive decline in early Alzheimer's disease: Longitudinal MRI study. *Dementia and Geriatric Cognitive Disorders, 37*(3–4), 214–222. doi:10.1159/000350410

9

Use of Reporting Guidelines for Research in Clinical Neuropsychology: Expanding Evidence-Based Practice Through Enhanced Transparency

MIKE R. SCHOENBERG, KATIE E. OSBORN, AND JASON R. SOBLE

The advancement of evidence-based practice in clinical neuropsychology depends on the availability of transparent, peer-reviewed, readily accessible research to guide patient care decisions (Bilder, 2011; Chelune, 2010; Loring & Bowden, 2014; Miller, Schoenberg, & Bilder, 2014). Ideally, all published research should report four basic aspects: (1) What were the hypotheses tested and rationale for addressing them, (2) how were hypotheses tested, including materials and methods used, (3) what were the results, including direction, certainty, and size of effects, and (4) what are the implications of the results within the context of existing literature (Bradford-Hill, 1965). Statistical procedures should be described in sufficient detail to enable someone with access to the data to replicate and verify findings (International Committee of Medical Journal Editors, 1988, updated 2014).

Systematic evaluation of the quality of published research reports has unfortunately found lapses in published studies that did not meet basic needs for research reproducibility or application to clinical decision making (Altman, 2002; Altman & Dore, 1990; Schulz, Chalmers, Altman, Grimes, & Dore, 1995). A study comparing the quality of randomized control trials that were published in 2000 and 2006 found pervasive deficits in reporting fundamental aspects of research methodology in the 2000 trials, which did not substantially improve for studies published in 2006 (Hopewell, Dutton, Yu, Chan, & Altman, 2010). Indeed, key methodological factors such as randomization and blinding methods, sample-size calculations, and primary end-point determinants have been omitted from a majority of published trials (Altman, 2013). Even more concerning, data regarding harmful adverse events frequently have been omitted or misrepresented in published reports (Ioannidis, 2009). Accordingly, the biomedical sciences have widely adopted reporting guidelines in order to facilitate higher quality and transparency among published research manuscripts (Des Jarlais, Lyles, Crepaz, & Trend-Group, 2014; Moher, Schulz, Altman, & CONSORT-Group, 2001; von Elm et al., 2007).

Reporting guidelines specify aspects of research that should be included in published research reports. The particular details of research that need to be reported vary depending on the type of study, but common aspects include specifying the hypothesis, methods, primary and secondary outcome variables, statistical procedures, results, and discussion. Various checklists have been developed to help authors and editors assure adherence to publication guidelines such that the key elements of a particular study are communicated (Chan, Heinemann, & Roberts, 2014). Comprehensive information about many widely accepted reporting guidelines are available through the EQUATOR (Enhancing the Quality and Transparency of Health Research) Network website at http://www.equator-network.org/reporting-guidelines/.

In this chapter, several reporting guidelines relevant to the field of clinical neuropsychology will be described, including the Consolidated Standards of Reporting Trials (CONSORT), the Standards for Reporting of Diagnostic Accuracy (STARD, Bossuyt et al., 2003), the Strengthening the Reporting of Observational Studies in Epidemiology (STROBE), the Preferred Reporting Items for Systematic Reviews and Meta-Analyses (PRISMA), and the Patient Reported Outcome Measurement Information System (PROMIS). Following an overview of the guidelines, the benefits of using the guidelines to identify and rank quality evidence will be highlighted. These guidelines include the minimum criteria needed for studies to be included in systemic reviews or meta-analyses. Furthermore, evidence-based practice requires the published study to include the elements identified by a publication guideline to allow clinicians to judge for themselves how the implications may be applicable to a particular patient. This chapter will dovetail with Chapters 11 and 12, where techniques for the rapid interpretation and application of the quality clinical evidence will be described and will include one or more examples of critical appraisal of systematic reviews.

OVERVIEW OF FIVE WIDELY ADOPTED REPORTING GUIDELINES: CONSORT, STROBE, STARD, PRISMA, AND PROMIS

This section provides brief synopses of several commonly accepted reporting guidelines for publishing research and psychometric instrument development. For more comprehensive information regarding any of the guidelines, please refer to the online resources listed in Table 9.1.

Table 9.1 REPORTING GUIDELINES OF RELEVANCE TO NEUROPSYCHOLOGY

Guideline	Methodological Purview	Overview	Online Resources
CONSORT	Randomized clinical trials	25-item checklist and flow diagram displaying participants' progression through the trial	www.consort-statement.org www.equator-network.org
STROBE	Observational studies in epidemiology	6 available checklists; vary based on reporting context and study type (i.e., cohort vs. case-control vs. cross-sectional)	www.strobe-statement.org www.equator-network.org
STARD	Diagnostic accuracy studies	25-item checklist and flow diagram displaying study design and patient flow	www.stard-statement.org www.equator-network.org
PRISMA	Systematic reviews and meta-analyses	27-item checklist and a four-phase flow diagram	www.prisma-statement.org www.equator-network.org
PROMIS	Instrument development and validation	List of 9 overriding standards, each with corresponding checklists	www.nihpromis.org

Consolidated Standards of Reporting Trials (CONSORT) Statement

The CONSORT Statement is a set of evidence-based reporting recommendations to facilitate complete and transparent communication of key aspects of randomized trials (Schulz, Altman, & Moher, 2010). It was originally published in 1996 and then updated in 2001, and again in 2010 (Moher et al., 2010). Although the CONSORT checklist and flow diagram were primarily developed as tools for authors, its guidelines can serve as helpful resources for anyone involved in the evaluation of randomized trials, including editors, peer reviewers, and consumers of clinical research (Altman, 2013).

The CONSORT Statement recommends that information be included that covers all aspects of reporting for randomized trials, with particular emphasis on transparency regarding methodology and key study methods, procedures, and statistical analyses. The guidelines require authors to report crucial details often omitted from clinical trials, such as details of randomization, information pertaining to participant dropouts, unanticipated harms, and aspects of trial implementation that differed from planned methodology (Altman, 2013). Indeed, by establishing a minimum set of reporting requirements, the

CONSORT recommendations minimize bias within the scientific literature and provide necessary safeguards against the publication of misleading or outright skewed findings. The current version of the CONSORT Statement, including the full 25-item checklist and recommended flow diagram, is available online at www.consort-statement.org. The CONSORT reporting guidelines have been endorsed by over 50% of the core medical journals in the *Abridged Index Medicus* on PubMed and have been formally endorsed by *Neuropsychology* and *Neuropsychology Review* (Schulz et al., 2010). Furthermore, the CONSORT reporting guideline requirements are generally included in the American Psychological Association Journal Article Reporting Standards (APA JARS; APA Publications and Communications Board Working Group on Journal Article Reporting Standards, 2008).

Strengthening the Reporting of Observational Studies in Epidemiology (STROBE)

Much research within the field of clinical neuropsychology does not typically lend itself well to randomized controlled-trial designs. Accordingly, hypotheses must often be tested using quasi-experimental and observational approaches, making the STROBE criteria particularly relevant to any discussion concerning research reporting guidelines within clinical neuropsychology (Loring & Bowden, 2014). The STROBE Statement, published in 2007, was designed to enhance transparency of published research in which the etiology or clinical condition of a study population is predetermined (i.e., not manipulated or controlled by the investigator as part of the study: Loring & Bowden, 2014; Vandenbroucke, 2009; von Elm et al., 2007). Given the propensity of confounding variables to influence the relationships between etiological or clinical factors of interest and outcome variables, complete and transparent reporting of participant and methodological details is essential for accurate interpretation of findings in observational studies. The STROBE Statement includes a 22-item checklist covering key elements with respect to the design and reporting of observational research (Vandenbroucke et al., 2007; von Elm et al., 2007). The elements composing the checklist were designed to systematically address minimum guidelines for complete and transparent reporting, while maintaining enough flexibility so as not to require overly rigid reporting templates (Loring & Bowden, 2014). Readers are referred to the STROBE Statement website (www.strobe-statement.org) for access to the complete STROBE checklist. Beyond the guidelines, the STROBE initiative provides a comprehensive review of the rationale for development and application of the STROBE guidelines that is freely available (e.g., www.STROBE-checklist.org or www.EQUATOR-network.org). The STROBE statement, as reporting guidelines, has been endorsed by the International Committee of Biomedical Journal Editors as part of their Uniform Requirements for submitting manuscripts to biomedical journals (Alfonso, Bermejo, & Segovia, 2004). Similarly, the APA JARS include the content identified by the STROBE publication guidelines.

Standards for the Reporting of Diagnostic Accuracy Studies (STARD)

The goal of the STARD Initiative is to promote complete, transparent, and accurate reporting of diagnostic accuracy studies in order to identify potential threats to internal validity and better assess the generalizability of results (Bossuyt et al., 2003). The STARD Initiative uses a 25-item checklist that addresses the critical elements related to diagnostic accuracy, study design, and reporting. The checklist can be obtained from the STARD website (www.stard-statement.org). A flow diagram is also available and provides additional information regarding subject inclusion orexclusion, test execution order, and the number of patients undergoing the test under evaluation (index test) and subsequent reference tests (Bossuyt et al., 2003). The original 2003 STARD guidelines and checklist were updated in 2014, and the revised 2015 STARD guideline (Bossuyt, Cohen, Gatsonis, & Korevaar, 2016) and checklist are available as open-access article and checklist (see www.stard-statement.org or www.equator-network.org/reporting-guideines/stard/). An extension specific for diagnostic studies in dementia has been developed that is termed the "STARDdem Guideline" (Noel-Storr et al., 2014) and is likely to be applicable to diagnostic studies in neuropsychology research more generally.

Preferred Reporting Items for Systematic Reviews and Meta-Analyses (PRISMA)

The PRISMA statement provides a set of guidelines related to developing and reporting protocols for systematic reviews and meta-analyses and is an update of the now-outdated Quality Of Reporting Of Meta-Analyses (QUOROM) guidelines (Moher, Liberati, Tetzlaff, Altman, & Group, 2009). A 27-item checklist that includes the critical items for transparent reporting is available on the PRISMA statement website (http://www.prisma-statement.org/statement.htm). The reader is also referred to Moher and colleagues (Moher et al., 2009) for further explanation of the meaning and rationale for each of the 27 items. A four-step flowchart also is included on the PRISMA website in order to clarify the flow of information through the different phases of a systematic review (i.e., the number of initial records identified, eligibility/inclusion, and exclusion with rationale for exclusion). More recently, the PRISMA guidelines have been adapted for use with journal and conference abstracts (Beller et al., 2013), as well as for systematic reviews that specifically focus on health equity (Welch et al., 2012). The PRISMA website (www.PRISMA-statement.org) provides researchers and authors with extensive resources and tools to assist in designing and conducting systematic reviews and meta-analyses. The PRISMA guidelines for publication have been endorsed by over 200 journals and are supported by major biomedical journal editor organizations, including: Centre for Reviews and Dissemination, Cochrane Collaboration, Council of Science Editors, National Evidence-Based Healthcare Collaborating Agency (NECA), and Word Association of Medical Editors (PRISMA-statement.org).

Patient-Reported Outcome Measurement Information System (PROMIS)

Although they are not part of the formal EQUATOR Network system of published reporting guidelines, we think it is essential to discuss the PROMIS guidelines, given the prominent role of test development and validation within clinical neuropsychology. PROMIS is funded by the National Institutes of Health (NIH) and promotes instrument development and validation through rigorous empirical methodology with the goal of providing clinicians with precise and valid measures (PROMIS website, retrieved 25 January 2015). The following nine standards have been developed by PROMIS as the scientific foundation for instrument development:

1. Definition of Target Concept and Conceptual Model,
2. Composition of Individual Items,
3. Item Pool Construction,
4. Determination of Item Bank Properties,
5. Testing and Instrument Formats,
6. Validity,
7. Reliability,
8. Interpretability, and
9. Language Translation and Cultural Adaptation.

A detailed description of each standard can be found on the PROMIS website: http://www.nihpromis.org/Documents/PROMISStandards_Vers2.0_Final.pdf. The PROMIS guidelines include what have been identified as essential elements of psychology and neuropsychology test development (Plake & Wise, 2014), but they include specific aspects in the development and measurement of health outcomes.

BENEFITS AND POTENTIAL PITFALLS OF ADOPTING REPORTING GUIDELINES FOR PUBLISHED RESEARCH IN CLINICAL NEUROPSYCHOLOGY

The initial impetus for the establishment of formal reporting guidelines occurred decades ago, following several reviews that revealed pervasive omissions and misrepresentations of crucial methodological elements in clinical research published by major medical journals (Altman & Dore, 1990; Pocock, Hughes, & Lee, 1987; Schulz et al., 1995). Since adopting reporting guidelines, many journals have seen marked improvements in the quality and transparency of published research (Alvarez, Meyer, Gourraud, & Paul, 2009; Moher, Jones, & Lepage, 2001; Plint et al., 2006). Nonetheless, a review of studies evaluating psychological and social work interventions revealed that clinical psychology and related behavioral sciences fields are lagging behind the biomedical sciences with regard to reporting guideline adherence (Grant, Mayo-Wilson, Melendez-Torres, &

Montgomery, 2013). *Neuropsychology* (published by the American Psychological Association) and *Neuropsychology Review* are the only neuropsychology-specific journals to have formally adopted the CONSORT Statement for its published clinical trials, although *Archives of Clinical Neuropsychology* and *The Clinical Neuropsychologist* also recently expressed an intention to begin adhering to the reporting guidelines adopted by most major biomedical journals (Lee, 2016; Schoenberg, 2014). Other journals published by the American Psychological Association that publish neuropsychology work, such as *Psychological Assessment*, adhere to the APA JARS criteria, which include aspects of CONSORT, STOBE, STARD, and PRISMA publication guidelines. Further widespread adoption of reporting guidelines by neuropsychology journals is a logical next step toward enhancing the evidence base of the field through the facilitation of high-quality, transparent research.

The potential benefits of implementing formal reporting standards for neuropsychology-related research publications are far-reaching. Authors are obvious beneficiaries of uniform reporting guidelines, given the decreased ambiguity such guidelines would facilitate with respect to methodological inclusion criteria needed to withstand the peer-review process. One of the authors of the STROBE guidelines suggested novice researchers and authors such as doctoral students stand the most to gain from uniform reporting standards, as the guidelines exemplify how and why certain key elements must be included in scientific writing (Vandenbroucke, 2009). However, we argue that previous reviews on reporting practices suggest that even seasoned researchers and authors stand to benefit from such added guidance (Altman & Dore, 1990; Pocock et al., 1987; Schulz et al., 1995).

Journal editors and peer reviewers would benefit from wider adoption of uniform reporting guidelines for neuropsychology journals. In many respects, reporting guidelines have been met with an outpouring of support by leadership within major scientific journals. For example, 585 journals have endorsed the CONSORT Statement to date, constituting over half of the medical journals indexed on PubMed *Abridged Index Medicus* (CONSORT Statement website, retrieved 24 January 2015) as well as *Neuropsychology*. The STROBE Statement has been similarly met with support by the scientific community, with the International Committee of Medical Journal Editors including it in its uniform requirements for biomedical journal manuscript submissions (International Committee of Medical Journal Editors, 1988, updated 2014). Likewise, the PRISMA has been endorsed by over 170 journals (PRISMA Statement website, retrieved 24 January 2015) and has been cited over 13,000 times to date.

Despite this overwhelming display of support, some researchers and authors still debate who should shoulder the responsibility for ensuring reporting guideline adherence, with research suggesting best adherence happens when editors require authors to adhere to publication guidelines (Altman & Simera, 2010; Fuller, Pearson, Peters, & Anderson, 2015; Hopewell et al., 2010; Scott-Lichter & Editorial Policy Committee of Council of Science Editors, 2012; Vandenbroucke, 2009). Journal editors have raised concerns regarding the practical burden associated with checking manuscripts for consistency with guideline recommendations, and questions have been raised as to whether peer reviewers can realistically be tasked with this duty (Vandenbroucke, 2009). Journals have adapted to these demands in varying ways. For instance, the *British Medical Journal* requires its authors to include completed checklists along with manuscript submissions in order to ensure reporting guideline adherence without unduly taxing its editors or reviewers (*British Medical Journal* article submission requirements webpage, retrieved 19 January 2015). The *Journal of Clinical Epidemiology* expressed a more flexible approach, endorsing the utility of reporting guidelines as a tool to assist authors, but emphasizing that such guidelines should not be used as a strict template nor as a method for journals to judge manuscript quality (Knottnerus & Tugwell, 2003, 2008). In a special issue of *The Clinical Neuropsychologist*, the process that submitting authors followed to adhere to publication guidelines, which included the STROBE checklists, were published to highlight the ease with which authors could adhere to publication standards across several study designs (Benitez, Hassenstab, & Bangen, 2014; Marcopulos et al., 2014; Soble et al., 2014).

Last, but certainly not least, clinicians and other healthcare consumers certainly have much to gain as a result of wider adoption of reporting guidelines, particularly with regard to the continued development of clinical neuropsychology as an evidence-based practice. Evidence-based medicine depends on the conduct and judicious use of sound scientific discovery to inform clinical decision making (Sackett, Rosenberg, Gray, Haynes, & Richardson, 1996). By enhancing the completeness and transparency of published research, reporting guidelines will help the clinician determine the applicability and generalizability of findings to their patient populations and clinical contexts. Furthermore, such added transparency will promote independent replication of studies, as well as enable better syntheses of reported findings through systematic reviews and meta-analyses (Ioannidis, 2005; Miller et al., 2014). In order to promote the integration of neuropsychological factors and outcomes within broader areas of biomedical science and clinical practice, neuropsychology researchers must join the ranks of other medical and healthcare researchers in adapting to meet the needs for more transparent and complete reporting practices (Miller et al., 2014; Schoenberg, 2014).

REFERENCES

Alfonso, F., Bermejo, J., & Segovia, J. (2004). [New recommendations of the International Committee of Medical Journal Editors. Shifting focus: from uniformity in technical requirements to bioethical considerations]. *Revista Española de Cardiología, 57*(6), 592–593.

Altman, D. G. (2002). Poor-quality medical research: What can journals do? *Journal of the American Medical Association, 287*, 2765–2767.

Altman, D. G. (2013). Transparent reporting of trials is essential. *The American Journal of Gastroenterology, 108*, 1231–1235. doi:10.1038/ajg.2012.457

Altman, D. G., & Dore, C. J. (1990). Randomisation and baseline comparisons in clinical trials. *Lancet, 335*, 149–153.

Altman, D. G., & Simera, I. (2010). Responsible reporting of health research studies: Transparent, complete, accurate and timely. *Journal of Antimicrobial Chemotherapy, 65*(1), 1–3. doi:10.1093/jac/dkp410

Alvarez, F., Meyer, N., Gourraud, P. A., & Paul, C. (2009). CONSORT adoption and quality of reporting of randomized controlled trials: A systematic analysis in two dermatology journals. *British Journal of Dermatology, 161*(5), 1159–1165. doi:10.1111/j.1365-2133.2009.09382.x

APA Publications and Communications Board Working Group on Journal Article Reporting Standards. (2008). Reporting standards for research in psychology: Why do we need them? What might they be? (2008). *The American Psychologist, 63*(9), 839–851. doi:10.1037/0003-066x.63.9.839

Beller, E. M., Glasziou, P. P., Altman, D. G., Hopewell, S., Bastian, H., Chalmers, I., Gotzsche, P. C., Lasserson, T., Tovey, D., for the PRISMA for Abstracts Group. (2013). PRISMA for abstracts: Reporting systematic reviews in journal and conference abstracts. *PLOS Medicine, 10*(4), e1001419. doi:10.1371/journal.pmed.1001419

Benitez, A., Hassenstab, J., & Bangen, K. J. (2014). Neuroimaging training among neuropsychologists: A survey of the state of current training and recommendations for trainees. *Clinical Neuropsychology, 28*(4), 600–613. doi:10.1080/13854046.2013.854836

Bilder, R. M. (2011). Neuropsychology 3.0: Evidence-based science and practice. *Journal of the International Neuropsychological Society, 17*, 383–384.

Bossuyt, P. M., Cohen, J. F., Gatsonis, C. A., & Korevaar, D. A. (2016). STARD 2015: Updated reporting guidelines for all diagnostic accuracy studies. *Annals of Translational Medicine, 4*(4), 85. doi:10.3978/j.issn.2305-5839.2016.02.06

Bossuyt, P. M., Reitsma, J. B., Bruns, D. E., Gatsonis, C. A., Glasziou, P. P., Irwig, L. M., . . . de Vet, H. C. (2003). Towards complete and accurate reporting of studies of diagnostic accuracy: The STARD initiative. *British Medical Journal, 326*(7379), 41–44.

Bradford-Hill, A. (1965). Reasons for writing. *British Medical Journal, 2*, 870.

Chan, L., Heinemann, A. W., & Roberts, J. (2014). Elevating the quality of disability and rehabilitation research: Mandatory use of the reporting guidelines. *Canadian Journal of Occupational Therapy, 81*(2), 72–77. doi:10.1177/0008417414533077

Chelune, G. L. (2010). Evidence-based research and practice in clinical neuropsychology. *The Clinical Neuropsychologist, 24*, 454–467.

Des Jarlais, D. C., Lyles, C., Crepaz, N., & Trend-Group. (2014). Improving the reporting quality of nonrandomized evaluations of behavioral and public health interventions: The TREND statement. *American Journal of Public Health, 94*, 361–366.

Fuller, T., Pearson, M., Peters, J., & Anderson, R. (2015). What affects authors' and editors' use of reporting guidelines? Findings from an online survey and qualitative interviews. *PLoS One, 10*(4), e0121585. doi:10.1371/journal.pone.0121585

Grant, S. P., Mayo-Wilson, E., Melendez-Torres, G. J., & Montgomery, P. (2013). Reporting quality of social and psychological intervention trials: A systematic review of reporting guidelines and trial publications. *PLoS One, 8*(5), e65442. doi:10.1371/journal.pone.0065442

Hopewell, S., Dutton, S., Yu, L. M., Chan, A. W., & Altman, D. G. (2010). The quality of reports of randomised trials in 2000 and 2006: Comparative study of articles indexed in PubMed. *British Medical Journal Open, 340*, c723.

International Committee of Medical Journal Editors [homepage on the Internet]. Recommendations for the Conduct, Reporting, Editing and Publication of Scholarly Work in Medical Journals [accessed 30Aug2016] Available from: http://www.ICMJE.org.

Ioannidis, J. P. (2005). Why most published research findings are false. *PLOS Medicine, 2*(8), e124. doi:10.1371/journal.pmed.0020124

Ioannidis, J. P. (2009). Adverse events in randomized trials: Neglected, restricted, distorted, and silenced. *Archives of Internal Medicine, 169*, 1737–1739.

Knottnerus, A., & Tugwell, P. (2003). The standards for reporting of diagnostic accuracy. *Journal of Clinical Epidemiology, 56*, 1118–1127.

Knottnerus, A., & Tugwell, P. (2008). STROBE—A checklist to strengthen the reporting of observational studies in epidemiology. *Journal of Clinical Epidemiology, 61*, 323.

Lee, G. P. (2016). New Editor-in-Chief introductory comments. *Archives of Clinical Neuropsychology, 31*(3), 195–196. doi:10.1093/arclin/acw008

Loring, D. W., & Bowden, S. C. (2014). The STROBE Statement and neuropsychology: Lighting the way toward evidence-based practice. *The Clinical Neuropsychologist, 28*(4), 556–574. doi:10.1080/13854046.2012.762552

Marcopulos, B. A., Caillouet, B. A., Bailey, C. M., Tussey, C., Kent, J. A., & Frederick, R. (2014). Clinical decision making in response to performance validity test failure in a psychiatric setting. *Clinical Neuropsychology, 28*(4), 633–652. doi:10.1080/13854046.2014.896416

Miller, J. B., Schoenberg, M. R., & Bilder, R. M. (2014). Consolidated Standards Of Reporting Trials (CONSORT): Considerations for neuropsychological research. *The Clinical Neuropsychologist, 28*(4), 575–599. doi:10.1080/13854046.2014.907445

Moher, D., Hopewell, S., Schulz, K. F., Montori, V., Gotzsche, P. C., Devereaux, P. J., . . . Altman, D. G. (2010). CONSORT 2010 explanation and elaboration: Updated guidelines for reporting parallel group randomised trials. *British Medical Journal Open, 340*, c869. doi:10.1136/bmj.c869

Moher, D., Jones, A., & Lepage, L. (2001). Use of the CONSORT statement and quality of reports of randomized trials: A comparative before-and-after evaluation. *Journal of the American Medical Association, 285*(15), 1992–1995.

Moher, D., Liberati, A., Tetzlaff, J., Altman, D. G., & PRISMA Group. (2009). Preferred reporting items for systematic reviews and meta-analyses: The PRISMA statement. *PLOS Medicine, 6*(7), e1000097. doi:10.1371/journal.pmed.1000097

Moher, D., Schulz, K. F., Altman, D. G., & CONSORT-Group. (2001). The CONSORT statement: Revised recommendations for improving the quality of reports of parallel-group randomized trials. *Journal of the American Medical Association, 285*(15), 1987–1991.

Noel-Storr, A. H., McCleery, J. M., Richard, E., Ritchie, C. W., Flicker, L., Cullum, S. J., . . . McShane, R. (2014). Reporting standards for studies of diagnostic test accuracy in dementia: The STARDdem Initiative. *Neurology, 83*(4), 364–373. doi:10.1212/wnl.0000000000000621

Plake, B. S., & Wise, L. L. (2014). What is the role and importance of the revised AERA, APA, NCME standards for educational and psychological testing? *Educational Measurement: Issues and Practice, 33*(4), 4–12. doi:10.1111/emip.12045

Plint, A. C., Moher, D., Morrison, A., Schulz, K. F., Altman, D. G., Hill, C., & Gaboury, I. (2006). Does the CONSORT checklist improve the quality of reports of randomised controlled trials? A systemic review. *Medical Journal of Australia, 185*(5), 263–267.

Pocock, S. J., Hughes, M. D., & Lee, R. J. (1987). Statistical problems in the reporting of clinical trials. A survey of three medical journals. *New England Journal of Medicine, 317*(7), 426–432. doi:10.1056/nejm198708133170706

Sackett, D. L., Rosenberg, W. M., Gray, J. A., Haynes, R. B., & Richardson, W. S. (1996). Evidence based medicine: What it is and what it isn't. *British Medical Journal, 312*(7023), 71–72.

Schoenberg, M. R. (2014). Introduction to the special issue on improving neuropsychological research through use of reporting guidelines. *The Clinical Neuropsychologist, 28*(4), 549–555. doi:10.1080/13854046.2014.934020

Schulz, K. F., Altman, D. G., & Moher, D. (2010). CONSORT 2010 statement: Updated guidelines for reporting parallel group randomised trials. *PLOS Medicine, 7*, e1000251. doi:10.1371/journal.pmed.1000251

Schulz, K. F., Chalmers, I., Altman, D. G., Grimes, D. A., & Dore, C. J. (1995). The methodological quality of randomization as assessed from reports of trials in specialist and general medical journals. *The Online Journal of Current Clinical Trial, Doc. No. 197* (81 paragraphs).

Scott-Lichter, D., & Editorial Policy Committee of Council of Science Editors. (2012). *CSE's White Paper on Promoting Integrity in Scientific Journal Publications, 2012 Update* (3rd revised ed.). Council of Science Editors, Wheat Ridge, CO.

Soble, J. R., Silva, M. A., Vanderploeg, R. D., Curtiss, G., Belanger, H. G., Donnell, A. J., & Scott, S. G. (2014). Normative data for the Neurobehavioral Symptom Inventory (NSI) and post-concussion symptom profiles among TBI, PTSD, and nonclinical samples. *Clinical Neuropsychology, 28*(4), 614–632. doi:10.1080/13854046.2014.894576

Vandenbroucke, J. P. (2009). STREGA, STROBE, STARD, SQUIRE, MOOSE, PRISMA, GNOSIS, TREND, ORION, COREQ, QUOROM, REMARK ... and CONSORT: For whom does the guideline toll? *Journal of Clinical Epidemiology, 62*, 594–596. doi:10.1016/j.jclinepi.2008.12.003

Vandenbroucke, J. P., von Elm, E., Altman, D. G., Gotzsche, P. C., Mulrow, C. D., Pocock, S. J., ... Egger, M. (2007). Strengthening the Reporting of Observational Studies in Epidemiology (STROBE): Explanation and elaboration. *Epidemiology, 18*, 805–835. doi:10.1097/EDE.1090b1013e3181577511

von Elm, E., Altman, D. G., Egger, M., Pocock, S. J., Gotzsche, P. C., Vandenbroucke, J. P., & STROBE-Initiative. (2007). The Strengthening of Reporting of Observational Studies in Epidemiology (STROBE) statement: Guidelines for reporting of observational studies. *Lancet, 370*, 1453–1457.

Welch, V., Petticrew, M., Tugwell, P., Moher, D., O'Neill, J., Waters, E., White, H., the PRISMA-Equity Bellagio Group. (2012). PRISMA-Equity 2012 extension: Reporting guidelines for systematic reviews with a focus on health equity. *PLOS Medicine, 9*(10), e1001333. doi:10.1371/journal.pmed.1001333

10

How Do I Know When a Diagnostic Test Works?

MARTIN BUNNAGE

Diagnostic validity is a crucial component of effective practice in clinical neuropsychology. Healthcare practitioners are in the privileged position of being able to help members of society with some of their health concerns. To be able to do this as efficiently and effectively as possible, it is necessary to have valid procedures by which to make decisions. Decision-making in healthcare is often imperfect, but some approaches are more overtly scientific than others (Ruscio, 2007; Straus et al., 2011).

In the pursuit of evidence-based practice, it is appropriate to acknowledge the weaknesses and biases human decision-makers display and instead combine clinical skills and observations with assessment tools and decision-making methods that maximize expertise and diagnostic validity (Haynes et al., 2002). Diagnostic validity is a special application of criterion-related validity, which has long been discussed within applied psychology as the most direct method by which to validate tests (e.g., see Strauss and Smith, 2009; Faust, 2003).

Within the practice of clinical neuropsychology, diagnostic decision-making occurs at many levels. Sometimes the focus is on diagnosis when it relates to deciding upon the likely presence or absence of a disease. At other times, the focus is on making prognostic statements that rely on the diagnosis of specific signs or symptoms. In each scenario, efforts are made to bring some order to the wealth of information available during a clinical encounter. Clinicians formulate meaningful questions and then try to answer them in a valid way that allows for inferences of interest to be made that benefit the patient (Schoenberg & Scott, 2011). The questions may be very varied, for example, whether the person has suffered from a traumatic brain injury, whether the person has a dyspraxia or a memory disorder, which may then be used to infer damage within the cerebrum, or whether from a neuropsychological perspective the person being assessed is safe to return to their former work role as a skilled professional.

When trying to understand the scientific basis of diagnostic decision-making, practitioners are often discomfited by the apparent mechanistic and mathematical presentation of the relevant principles, even though research suggests that careful, objective techniques are likely to increase judgement accuracy (Grove & Meehl, 1996). In the current chapter, mathematical formulae have been kept to an absolute minimum, and wherever possible, ideas and principles are illustrated using scenarios and tests common to clinical neuropsychologists.

Consider the following example. A clinician has a test of memory and wants to know whether or not someone has a memory problem sufficient to meet the suggested diagnostic criteria of mild cognitive impairment (MCI; see Albert et al., 2011). The diagnostic question being asked is whether or not someone has a memory problem. The presence or absence of a memory problem is something that is not known in direct or absolute terms, if it were there would be no need to test for it. Instead, the clinician has a conceptual understanding of what memory is and there are some operational definitions of how a problem with memory manifests compared to what healthy memory function displays.

Specifically, "memory" can be defined as the ability to learn, retain, and recall new information. Healthy memory function might be defined statistically as a score on a test of this ability that falls within the range of scores observed in the relevant reference group, in this case, members of the community without known deficit (Wechsler, 2010). The clinician could then adopt, for example, the criteria suggested by Albert et al. (2011) to define abnormal memory within the context of possible MCI, that is, a score on the memory test of 1–1.5 standard deviations below the mean for a patient's age- and education-matched peers.

In practice, when considering this question, the clinician might conceptualize memory as the ability to learn, retain, and recall stimulus material via prose recall or verbal paired-associate learning. Defined in this way normal memory would be indicated by a score on these tests above the 7th percentile (that is, 1.5 standard deviations below the mean) when compared with age- and education-matched peers and consider a memory deficit to be indicated by a score below the 7th percentile.

If the clinician applied these tests to patients, some of whom had a memory disorder and some of whom did not, the clinician would get a range of performance on the memory tests that had some degree of relationship with the presence or absence of the underlying memory disorder. Strauss and Smith (2009) provide detailed discussion of the more general research strategy of criterion-related validity. Many of the patients who perform below the 7th percentile on the test will demonstrate evidence of a memory disorder in their everyday life. These people can be described in the terminology of criterion-related validity as "true positives." The test scores says these people have a "memory disorder," and they appear to demonstrate problems with memory in day-to-day life.

A second category includes the people who perform below the 7th percentile on the test but nonetheless do not demonstrate any memory problems in their everyday life. These people may be described as "false positives."

Table 10.1 CATEGORICAL DESCRIPTIONS REFLECTING THE ASSOCIATION BETWEEN THE RESULTS OF A TEST FOR IMPAIRMENT IN A COGNITIVE ABILITY USED TO DETECT THE "CONDITION OF INTEREST" (COI) SHOWN IN THE ROWS, AND THE REAL-LIFE PRESENCE OF THE "CONDITION OF INTEREST" SHOWN IN THE COLUMNS. ALSO SHOWN ARE THE METRICS OF SENSITIVITY AND SPECIFICITY.

	COI Is Present	**COI Is Not Present**
Test says "yes" to COI	True Positives A	False Positives B
Test says "no" to COI	False Negatives C	True Negatives D
	Sensitivity = A/A + C	**Specificity = D/D + B**

A third category of patients will be those who perform above the 7th percentile on the test and do not demonstrate any problem behavior in their everyday life that would suggest the presence of a memory disorder. These people are our "true negatives." The test says "no memory disorder," and the persons so identified appear to have no memory disorder.

Finally, a fourth category of patients will be those who perform above the 7th percentile on the test but nonetheless demonstrate behavior in their everyday life that would suggest the presence of a memory disorder. These people are "false negatives." The test says "no memory disorder" but they appear to have a memory disorder. The association between the results of a test for the "condition of interest" and the real-life presence of the condition of interest are represented in Table 10.1.

While it would be excellent for the practice of clinical neuropsychology to rest firmly on the basis of tests without any false negative or false positive results, this is unfortunately not the case, nor is it the case for most diagnostic tests (Straus et al., 2011). All tests are imperfect to some extent, and as a consequence, classification accuracy of every test can be quantified in terms of the four cells shown in Table 10.1, that is, true positives, false positives, false negatives and true negatives (Straus et al., 2011).

SENSITIVITY AND SPECIFICITY

The relationship between the true positive, true negative, false positive, and false negative results on a test can be expressed as the test sensitivity and specificity in relation to a specific criterion. The comparison criterion is usually termed the "external validity criterion" or "gold standard" for a criterion with the best available validity (Straus & Smith, 2009). For example, the sensitivity and specificity of a memory test for detecting memory impairment in everyday life could be compared to an external validity criterion defined by an informant's objective ratings of a person's performance in their everyday life. Another example of an external validity criterion would be expert clinician-panel consensus ratings of the presence of a diagnosis.

To continue the MCI example, sensitivity reflects how many people with a memory disorder in their everyday life have a positive test result. In this case, the number of people with a memory disorder in everyday life who have a memory test score below the 7th percentile. Usually there is an imperfect relationship between these two sources of classification. Consequently, whilst, with a good test, most of the people with a memory disorder in everyday life will score below the 7th percentile on this memory test (i.e., the test is sensitive to the presence of a memory disorder), there will be some people who have a memory disorder in everyday life but who score better on the test. This scenario reflects a false negative (i.e., the test says there is no memory disorder when in fact there is). Also there will be some people who score below the 7th percentile on the test who have no apparent memory disorder in everyday life. This scenario reflects a false positive (i.e., the test says there is a memory disorder when in fact there is not). These further metrics are shown in Table 10.1.

"Sensitivity" is calculated from the number of true positives as a percentage of the total number of "positives" in the population. In Table 10.1, this value would be reflected by the equation **A/A + C.**

"Specificity" reflects how many people without a memory disorder in real life have a negative test result, in this case, defined as a memory score above the 7th percentile. As before, whilst most people without a memory disorder will score above the 7th percentile on this memory test, there will also be some people who do not have a memory disorder but who score poorly on the test. The latter scenario reflects a false positive error. Specificity is calculated from the number of true negatives as a percentage of the total number of "negatives" in the population. In Table 10.1, this would be reflected by the equation **D/D + B.**

Sensitivity and specificity are often expressed as percentages or decimal proportions reflecting the outcomes of the two equations above. Tools for calculating these values and other values described below are readily available on the Internet, for example, see http://ktclearinghouse.ca/cebm/practise/ca/calculators/statscalc or http://www.cebm.net.

There is usually a tradeoff between sensitivity and specificity for any given test. No diagnostic test is perfect, consequently, as sensitivity increases, it is usually at the expense of specificity and vice versa, as shown in Figure 10.1. If a clinician is trying to capture all the people with the condition of interest, represented by the darker distribution in Figure 10.1, then the ability of the test to do so increases as the cut-score used moves from the left to the right in Figure 10.1. That is, from "A" to "B" and finally to "C". Using the cut-score of "C," almost all those in the darker distribution are below the cut-score and so would be correctly identified by the test. In this circumstance, the sensitivity of the test is high. However, as the cut-score changes from "A" to "B" and finally to "C," it can also be seen that the number of people within the lighter distribution (which represents people without the condition) who are correctly classified decreases because more of their scores fall below the cut-score as it moved to "C." That is, as the sensitivity of the test increases, the number of false positive test results also increases, which means the specificity of the test decreases.

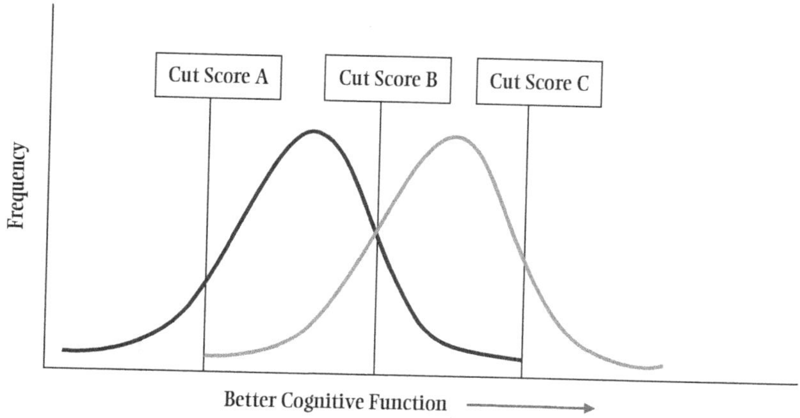

Figure 10.1 The trade-off between sensitivity and specificity when using three different cut-scores to distinguish between scores within the condition of interest distribution (darker curve on the left) versus those within the control group distribution (lighter curve on the right).

The opposite is also true: as the cut-score changes from "C" to "B" to "A," the number of false positives decreases, but so does the number of true positives identified by the test. In this latter circumstance, where the cutoff score moves from right to left in Figure 10.1, the specificity of the test increases, but at the expense of the sensitivity of the test.

Invariably, in clinical practice, the distribution of scores on tests between those who have, and those who do not have, the condition of interest overlaps. It is also the case in clinical practice that the cut-scores used to help guide the interpretation of test results need not be absolute or fixed. Consequently, the relationship between the sensitivity and specificity of a test result and the condition of interest will vary, depending upon the cut-score that is used. The choice of cut-off can also be used to help favor either sensitivity or specificity, depending upon the clinical question that is being asked. Sometimes, particularly when screening, it is usually more helpful to emphasize sensitivity over specificity (Straus et al., 2011). The reason for weighting sensitivity is that the goal of screening is usually to identify all the people who may have the condition of interest. It is more important not to miss people with the condition of interest (false negative errors) than it is to minimize potential false positive errors. Subsequently, the people whose scores are classified as positive at the first screening assessment can be reassessed with a test with a high specificity. This strategy is known as the "two-step diagnostic process" (Straus et al., 2011).

Alternatively, in some scenarios, it would be more important to emphasize specificity rather than sensitivity, that is, for decisions where the costs of false-positive errors might be high. Such a circumstance might apply with tests used to help identify people who are potentially feigning their cognitive problems. In this scenario, given the cost of wrongly diagnosing malingering, test cut-scores are often weighted to emphasize high specificity, sometimes at the expense of sensitivity (Gervais et al., 2004).

POSITIVE AND NEGATIVE LIKELIHOOD RATIOS

A likelihood ratio is a way of estimating how much a test result should shift a clinician's index of suspicion in the direction of the "condition of interest" being present or absent. Strictly defined, likelihood ratios reflect the change in the likelihood of a diagnosis, after obtaining a positive or negative test result. In the memory disorder example above, the likelihood ratios are a direct way of indicating the change in the likelihood of a person having a memory disorder in everyday life, depending on whether that person obtained a positive or negative test result. In essence, the positive likelihood ratio shows how much more likely it is that the person tested has a memory disorder in everyday life when they obtain a positive score, namely, a score below the 7th percentile on the memory test. In the case of a negative test result, a negative likelihood ratio shows how much less likely it is that the person has a memory disorder in everyday life when they score above the 7th percentile on the memory test.

These likelihoods can be calculated by the following equations (see Grimes & Shultz, 2002):

$$\text{Positive Likelihood Ratio } (\text{LR}+) = \frac{\text{Probability that a person with the condition has a positive test result}}{\text{probability than an individual without the condition has a positive test result}}.$$

$$\text{Negative Likelihood Ratio } (\text{LR}-) = \frac{\text{Probability that a person with the condition has a negative test result}}{\text{probability that an individual without the condition has a negative test result}}.$$

In terms of the values in Table 10.1, these formulae can be written as:

$$\text{LR+} = (\text{A/A+C}) \;/\; (\text{B/B+D})$$
$$\text{LR−} = (\text{C/A+C}) \;/\; (\text{D/B+D})$$

These equations can also be written in terms of sensitivity and specificity, namely:

$$\text{LR+} = \text{sensitivity} \;/\; (1 - \text{specificity})$$
$$\text{LR−} = (1 - \text{sensitivity}) \;/\; \text{specificity}$$

As likelihood ratios for a positive test result increase significantly above 1, there is an increased probability of the condition of interest being present after a positive test result is obtained. Conversely, as the likelihood ratio for a negative test result decreases significantly below 1, there is a decreased probability of the condition being present after a negative test result is obtained. As positive likelihood ratios increase above 10, for example, the probability of the condition being present is greatly increased when a positive test result is obtained. Conversely, as a negative likelihood ratio decreases below 0.1, for example, the probability of the condition being present is greatly reduced when the test result is negative.

The positive likelihood ratio is a way of thinking about a positive test result affecting the base-rate estimate to increase the likelihood of the diagnosis. Conversely, a negative likelihood ratio is a way of thinking about a negative test result affecting the base-rate estimate to reduce the likelihood of the diagnosis. In this way, the pre-test odds (base rate) are changed by the likelihood ratio, resulting in the post-test odds. Likelihood ratios are interpreted with reference to an estimated or known pre-test probability (also referred to as the "clinical prevalence" or "base rate"). A nomogram for interpreting diagnostic test results is shown in Figure 10.2. In the nomogram, a line is drawn from the pre-test probability through the likelihood ratio to estimate the post-test probability (see Fagan, 1975).

An online calculator is also available to estimate post-test probability using likelihood ratios, see http://araw.mede.uic.edu/cgi-bin/testcalc.pl

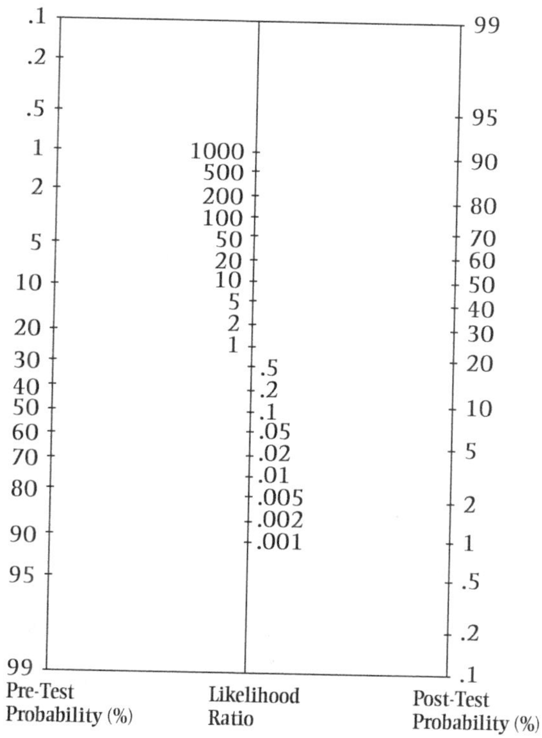

Figure 10.2 Nomogram for interpreting diagnostic test results.

Table 10.2 Examples showing how the likelihood ratio changes selected pre-test probability (base-rate) values, to re-estimate the probability of the diagnosis after obtaining the test result, termed the "post-test probability."

Pre-Test Probability (Base Rate)	Likelihood Ratio	Post-Test Probability
1%	.1	<0.1%
1%	.5	1%
1%	2	2%
1%	5	5%
1%	10	9%
10%	.1	1%
10%	.5	5%
10%	2	18%
10%	5	36%
10%	10	53%
25%	.1	3%
25%	.5	14%
25%	2	40%
25%	5	62%
25%	10	77%

To assist in the appreciation of the relationship between selected pre-test probability values, likelihood ratio values, and post-test probability, examples of the calculation are presented in Table 10.2. The interested reader could also plot the numbers presented in Table 10.2 on the nomogram presented at Figure 10.2 to see how the nomogram reduces the need for calculations to obtain an estimate of post-test probability. As can be seen from Table 10.2, the likelihood ratio allows re-estimation of the probability of the condition of interest after obtaining a positive or negative test result. In other words, the likelihood ratio acts on the base rate of the condition of interest within the population tested. This latter relationship is explored further in the following section.

POSITIVE AND NEGATIVE PREDICTIVE VALUE AND THE PREVALENCE OF THE CONDITION OF INTEREST (BASE RATE)

In clinical practice, a diagnostic test is applied to a population of interest. A clinician uses the test to help answer a question about the group membership of the person tested. For example, a memory test is used to help answer the question of whether or not the person tested is a member of the impaired-memory group or the unimpaired-memory group. Frederick and Bowden (2009) noted that, unlike the true positive and false positive classification rate of a test, the positive predictive power and negative predictive power of a test is affected by the base rate of the condition of interest within the population tested. The definition and calculation of the positive and negative predictive values of a test are reported in relation to the four quantities in Table 10.1.

The "positive predictive value" refers to the number of people with a positive test result who actually have the condition of interest. In the memory example above, we would be asking how many people who obtain a memory test score below the 7th percentile when tested have a memory disorder in everyday life. This can be represented mathematically as **A/A + B** for the values in Table 10.1. The "negative predictive value" refers to the number of people with a negative test result who do not actually have the condition of interest. In the memory example, this would be the number of people with a memory test score above the 7th percentile who do not have a memory disorder in everyday life. This can be represented mathematically as **D/C + D** in Table 10.1.

The performance of a test in relation to a diagnostic decision is further affected by a property of the population being tested rather than of the test itself. This property is the "prevalence" (or base-rate or pre-test probability) of the condition of interest in the population being tested. In terms of the memory disorder example, this would be the number of people who actually have a memory disorder in everyday life, out of all the people being tested. This percentage is referred to as the base-rate or prevalence or pre-test probability of the condition of interest in the population.

If we considered a community-based example, the proportion of people with a memory disorder in everyday life among all those being tested would be much lower than if we considered a population of people attending a tertiary-referral dementia diagnosis clinic. In the latter setting, it would be reasonable to assume the number of people attending with a memory disorder in everyday life would be higher.

A specific example of the impact of the prevalence of the condition of interest on the diagnostic performance of a test can be seen in the study of Mioshi et al. (2006) of the diagnostic validity of the Addenbrooke Cognitive Examination–Revised. These researchers noted the sensitivity, specificity, likelihood ratios, and positive and negative predictive values of the test when making a dementia diagnosis using cut-scores of 82 and 88 on the Addenbrooke test at different levels of prevalence.

Consider the results of Mioshi et al. (2006) in relation to their cut-score of 88. At an estimated prevalence of 40% the positive predictive value of the test was 0.85, meaning that there was a .85 probability that a person with a score at 88 or below had dementia. This positive predictive value changed dramatically, however, when the presumed prevalence was 5%. At this level of prevalence, the positive predictive value of the test became 0.31, meaning that there was only a .31 probability that a person with a score at 88 or below had dementia. In other words, as the prevalence of the condition of interest, in this case dementia, lessened in the population tested, the validity of a positive test result indicating the presence of dementia also declined. At 5% prevalence, a positive test score was diagnostically accurate only 31% of the time. That is, at this 5% prevalence, a positive test score was a false positive 69% of the time. A positive test result is, therefore, at this low level of prevalence, much more likely to be incorrect than it is correct at detecting dementia.

These ideas are further expanded below using hypothetical data applied to our previously discussed memory disorder example. In that example, the diagnosis being made was whether or not someone had a memory disorder in everyday life, and the cut-score on the memory test used was the 7th percentile.

Lets assume we started from an estimated prevalence of 50%, that is, the original research study used to derive the cut-score was made up of two equal-sized groups that were matched in terms of their demographic and clinical characteristics other than the presence of memory disorder. If a valid memory test is used, it might be expected to have a sensitivity of, say, 0.78 and a specificity of 0.82, to choose two arbitrary hypothetical values. Further suppose that the cut-score is derived from research to classify people into either the "memory disorder in everyday life group" (disorder present) or the "no memory disorder in everyday life group" (disorder not present). Suppose also, in this hypothetical example, that there are 125 people in each of these two groups. These properties of the test are represented in Table 10.3. The numbers of people in each cell (A to D) in Table 10.3 are determined by our hypothetical sensitivity and specificity values.

The sensitivity of the test shown in Table 10.3 is given by A/A + C, which in this example is 97/125 = 0.78 (rounded to two decimal places). The specificity of the test is given by D/D + B which in this example is 103/125 = 0.82. In this example, the base rate of the condition of interest was set to 50%, that is, the disorder is present in 125 people (A + C) and is not present in 125 people (B + D), so the base rate is 125/250.

The positive predictive value of the test is given by A/A + B, which in this example is 97/119 = 82%. This value indicates that there is a probability of .82 that a positive test result comes from a person with the condition of interest, in this example, memory disorder. The negative predictive value of the test is represented by D/C + D, which in this example is 103/131 = 79%. This value indicates that there is a probability of .79 that a negative test result comes from a person without memory disorder.

Table 10.3 NUMBER OF PEOPLE CLASSIFIED INTO THE DIAGNOSTIC CATEGORIES REFLECTED BY CELLS A TO D FOR THE HYPOTHETICAL MEMORY DISORDER EXAMPLE, WITH A STUDY PREVALENCE OR BASE RATE OF 50%.

	Disorder Is Present	**Disorder Is Not Present**	**Total**
Test says "yes"	True Positives A 97	False Positives B 22	119
Test says "no"	False Negatives C 28	True Negatives D 103	131
Total	125	125	

The interpretation of the usefulness of the test changes, however, if the base rate of the condition changes, especially if the base rate falls to a lower level than was represented in the research study. Base rates will change if the population tested is different from the research study population, for example, if all the people from a community-based population are tested. When compared with the research study population, the community-based population would have a lower base rate of the condition of interest. The base rate is lower because the prevalence of the condition of interest will be diluted across many more people than in the research study, where the condition of interest was deliberately identified and concentrated into one of the groups tested.

If the same test and cut-off from the original research study are applied to the community-based population, the interpretation of the test results will be different. This is because, in the community-based population, the base rate of the condition of interest is lower. Let us suppose, in this example, that a base rate of 9% reflects the frequency of memory disorder in the community-based population. A reworking of the preceding calculations, but with the lower base rate, is shown in Table 10.4.

For the example in Table 10.4, the sensitivity of the test is given by A/A + C and stays the same as in the previous example, that is, it is 97/125 = 0.78. The specificity of the test is represented by D/D + B and stays the same as in the previous example, that is, it is 1030/1250 = 0.82. However, in Table 10.4, the base rate of the condition is now 9%, the disorder is present in 125 people and is not present in 1,250 people, that is, 125/(125 + 1250).

Therefore, the positive predictive value of the test, which is represented by A/A + B, is now in this example 97/317 = 31%. That is, the probability of a positive test result coming from a person with memory disorder is now only .31. To put it another way, out of all the positive test results obtained, 31% are true positives and reflect the presence of the condition of interest and 69% are false positives. The negative predictive value of the test is represented by D/C + D, which in this example is now 1030/1058 = 97%, that is, out of all the negative test results

Table 10.4 NUMBER OF PEOPLE CLASSIFIED INTO THE DIAGNOSTIC CATEGORIES REFLECTED BY CELLS A TO D FOR THE HYPOTHETICAL MEMORY DISORDER EXAMPLE, WITH A BASE RATE OF 9%.

	Disorder Is Present	Disorder Is Not Present	Total
Test says "yes"	True Positives A 97	False Positives B 220	317
Test says "no"	False Negatives C 28	True Negatives D 1030	1058
Total	125	1250	

obtained, 97% are true negatives and reflect the absence of the condition of interest and 3% are false negatives.

These calculations and the numbers in Table 10.4 show that, when the base rate of the condition of interest tends towards zero, we can become more confident in negative test results but less confident in positive test results. The negative predictive value increased from 79% to 97% as the base rate decreased in these two examples. A negative test result was more likely to be accurate and the number of false-negatives less as the base rate of the condition of interest decreased. However, the positive predictive value decreased from 81% to 31% as the base rate decreased from 50% to 9%. That is, a positive test result was less likely to be accurate and the number of false positives increased in proportion to the true positives as the base rate of the condition of interest decreased.

So, in general, when the base rate of the condition of interest is low, a test that appears to have good diagnostic properties (when calculated under the high base-rate conditions often found in published research studies) can actually perform so poorly that a positive test result is more likely to be wrong than it is right, that is, a positive test result is more likely to be a false positive than a true positive. The impact of prevalence upon the predictive power of diagnostic tests is discussed in detail in Baldessarini et al. (1983).

The implication of these calculations is that, when applying these principles to diagnostic decision-making in clinical practice, it is necessary to have some idea of the base rate of the condition of interest within the clinical setting in which the test is being used. This information allows for the calculations necessary to estimate how the test will perform when taken from the research setting to a clinical setting with a different base rate. Returning to the Mioshi et al. (2006) example, while sensitivity and specificity were high using the cut-score of 88, the positive predictive value of the test was shown to be poor at low base rates, it was 0.31 at a 5% base rate. In other words, at this low base rate, a positive test result was much more likely to be a false positive than a true positive. At the higher base rate of 40%, the positive predictive value was much higher, at 0.85, indicating a much reduced likelihood of false positive test results. Before using this test at the prescribed cut-offs to make diagnostic decisions, any clinician would be wise to estimate the base rate of the condition of interest in the population being tested to avoid the error of interpreting a false positive as a true positive.

Putting these ideas together allows for the calculation of the post-test probability at any specified base rate.

The post-test probability is calculated as follows:

$$\text{Post-Test Probability} = \text{Prevalence} / (1 - \text{Prevalence}) \times \text{Likelihood Ratio} / \\ \left[\text{Prevalence} / \left((1 - \text{Prevalence}) \times \text{Likelihood Ratio}\right) + 1\right]$$

In the example described here, with a prevalence of 9%, the post-test probability of the person with a memory test score below the 7th percentile having a memory problem in everyday life is calculated as follows, when using the data presented in Table 10.4. LR+ = 4.41, Prevalence = 0.09, Post-Test Probability = 30% probability of a memory disorder in everyday life. When the prevalence is assumed to be 50%, the post-test probability becomes: LR+ = 4.41, Prevalence = 0.5, Post-Test Probability = 82% probability of a memory disorder in everyday life. See http://araw.mede.uic.edu/cgi-bin/testcalc.pl for an online calculator.

RELIABILITY OF MEASUREMENT

When considering the likely diagnostic validity of a test procedure, it is also crucial to consider the reliability of the test result. When thinking about diagnostic decision-making, we are essentially attempting to arrive at a decision, namely, is the condition of interest present or not? The reliability of our test result has a crucial bearing on the confidence we have in the decision we are making. Put simply, nothing can be more valid than it is reliable. On average, a test result cannot correlate better with some diagnostic outcome than it can correlate with itself. If a test score is not relatively reliable, it cannot have high validity and therefore cannot be of high diagnostic utility (Schmidt & Hunter, 1996).

When thinking about diagnostic validity as described above, it is necessary to turn the score on a test into a decision. This is usually achieved by considering whether the obtained test score falls above or below a cut-score that has been empirically derived to maximize the accuracy of classification. For example, when considering performance validity during cognitive testing, Schroeder et al. (2012) highlighted cut-scores of less than or equal to 6 or 7 on the Reliable Digit Span measure as being optimal, depending upon the population being tested. Any decision about whether or not a score falls above or below a specific cut-off needs to consider the reliability of the score itself. The reliability of the Digit Span subtest is high, which encourages confidence in the obtained result but if, for example, the test score were very unreliable, one could only have limited confidence that the score obtained at one assessment would reflect the person's true score. If the test score is unreliable and a patient is tested again, their score might vary, and thus the patient could be classified as being above or below the cut-off at different points in time merely as a consequence of poor measurement reliability. Such measurement unreliability fundamentally undermines the diagnostic validity possible with any test of lower reliability. Reliability of test scores is examined in detail in Chapter 5 of the current volume.

CRITICALLY APPRAISED TOPIC

With the Critically Appraised Topic (CAT) procedure, evidence for the validity of a diagnostic test, including the evidence noted above, is critically appraised to help a clinician answer a specific question (see Bowden et al., 2013; and Chapters 11 and 12 of this volume). Critical appraisal supports clinicians in translating the research evidence available to them into practical guidance regarding how to interpret a particular test score in a particular circumstance.

In summary, the CAT procedure is a systematic way of collating, appraising, and making use of the available research evidence to guide clinical practice.

The CAT procedure encourages clinicians to critically evaluate the quality of the scientific evidence available to them and use the calculations herein to help them determine the most appropriate way to interpret the results of testing undertaken with their patient. For further discussion, the reader is referred to Chapter 11 of this volume where a CAT of a performance validity test is presented.

REFERENCES

Albert, M. S., DeKosky, S. T., Dickson, D., Dubois, B., Feldman, H. H., Fox, N. C., ... Phelps, C. H. (2011). The diagnosis of mild cognitive impairment due to Alzheimer's disease: Recommendations from the National Institute of Aging–Alzheimer's Association workgroups on diagnostic guidelines for Alzheimer's disease. *Alzheimer's Dementia, 7*(3), 270–279.

Baldessarini, R. J., Finklestein, S., & Arana, G. W. (1983). The predictive power of diagnostic tests and the effect of prevalence of illness. *Archives of General Psychiatry, 40*, 569–573.

Bowden, S. C., Harrison, E. J., & Loring, D. W. (2013). Evaluating research for clinical significance: Using critically appraised topics to enhance evidence-based neuropsychology. *The Clinical Neuropsychologist, 28*(4), 653–668.

Faust, D. (2003). Alternatives to four clinical and research traditions in malingering detection. In P. W. Halligan, C. Bass, & D. A. Oakley (Eds.), *Malingering and Illness Deception* (pages 107–121). Oxford: Oxford University Press.

Fagan, T. J. (1975). Nomogram for Bayes's theorem. *New England Journal of Medicine, 293*(5), 257.

Frederick, R. I., & Bowden, S. C. (2009). The test validation summary. *Assessment, 16*(3), 215–236.

Gervais, R. O., Rohling, M. L., Green, P., & Ford, W. (2004). A comparison of WMT, CARB, and TOMM failure rates in non-head injury disability claimants. *Archives of Clinical Neuropsychology, 19*, 475–487.

Grimes, D. A., & Schulz, K. F. (2002). An overview of clinical research: The lay of the land. *Lancet, 359*(9300), 57–61.

Grove, W. M., & Meehl, P. E. (1996). Comparative efficiency of informal (subjective, impressionistic) and formal (mechanical, algorithmic) prediction procedures: The clinical-statistical controversy. *Psychology, Public Policy and Law, 2*(2), 293–323.

Haynes, R. B., Devereaux, P. J., & Guyatt, G. H. (2002). Clinical expertise in the era of evidence-based medicine and patient choice. *Evidence Based Medicine, 7*, 36–38.

Mioshi, E., Dawson, K., Mitchell, J., Arnold, R., & Hodges, J. R. (2006). The Addenbrooke's Cognitive Examination–Revised (ACE-R): A brief cognitive test battery for dementia screening. *International Journal of Geriatric Psychiatry, 21*, 1078–1085.

Ruscio, J. (2007). The clinician as subject. Practitioners are prone to the same judgment errors as everyone else. In S. O. Lilenfield & W. T. O'Donohue (Eds.), *The Great Ideas of Clinical Science: 17 Principles That Every Mental Health Professional Should Understand* (pages 29–48). New York: Routledge.

Schoenberg, M. R., & Scott, J. G. (Eds.). (2011). *The Little Black Book of Neuropsychology: A Syndrome-Based Approach*. New York: Springer.
Schroeder, R. W., Twumasi-Ankrah, P., Baade, L. E., & Marshall, P. S. (2012). Reliable digit span: A systematic review and cross-validation study. *Assessment, 19*(1), 21–30.
Schmidt, F. L., & Hunter, J. E. (1996). Measurement error in psychological research: Lessons from 26 research scenarios. *Psychological Methods, 1*(2), 199–223.
Strauss, M. E., & Smith, G. T. (2009). Construct validity: Advances in theory and methodology. *Annual Review of Clinical Psychology, 5*, 1–25.
Straus, S. E., Glasziou, P., Richardson, W. S., & Haynes, R. B. (2011). *Evidence-Based Medicine. How to Practice and Teach It* (4th ed.). Churchill Livingstone Elsevier.
Wechsler, D. (2010). *Wechsler Memory Scale–Fourth UK Edition. Administration and Scoring Manual.* London: Pearson Education, Pearson Assessment.

FURTHER READING

Straus, S. E., Glasziou, P., Richardson, W. S., & Haynes, R. B. (2011). *Evidence-Based Medicine. How to Practice and Teach It* (4th ed.). Churchill Livingstone Elsevier.

11

Applying Diagnostic Standards to Performance Validity Tests and the Individual Case

DAVID T. R. BERRY, JORDAN P. HARP, LISA MASON KOEHL, AND HANNAH L. COMBS

In a meta-analysis based on research sponsored by the American Psychological Association Board of Professional Affairs, Meyer and colleagues (Meyer et al., 2001) reviewed evidence on the effect sizes (a quantitative measure of the strength of a phenomenon) characterizing psychological and medical diagnostic tests and procedures. They concluded that the validity of the two domains was comparable. This approach held that the quality of medical diagnostic procedures is a benchmark against which to judge that of psychological tests. This suggests that psychologists should be aware of and responsive to improvements in methodologies used to evaluate medical tests.

In fact, since the Meyer et al. (2001) publication, there have been major initiatives in medicine to improve the quality of published evaluations of diagnostic accuracy as well as the usefulness of systematic reviews of these protocols. One driving force has been the development of standardized protocols to evaluate individual publications and summary reviews in the field by the Cochrane Collaboration (http://www.cochrane.org/cochrane-reviews). Although the Cochrane organization initially focused primarily on treatments, more recently it has also begun to address the accuracy of diagnostic procedures, and by late 2014, it was preparing a manual to guide these reviews (http://srdta.cochrane.org/handbook-dta-reviews).

A second major impetus to improving the quality of studies of medical diagnostic techniques was a systematic review of the effect of various technical flaws on the reported accuracy of the procedures. Lijmer et al. (1999) concluded, "These data provide empirical evidence that diagnostic studies with methodological shortcomings may overestimate the accuracy of a diagnostic test, particularly those including unrepresentative patients or applying different reference standards" (p. 1061). They further emphasized the importance of adequate methodology, complete and reliable reporting of results, and comprehensive clarity on methods employed in the study.

Developments aimed at standardizing and improving the quality of medical treatments and diagnostic evaluations have proliferated over the past decade (e.g., Developing and Evaluating Communication strategies to support Informed Decisions and practice based on Evidence [DECIDE], Treweek et al., 2013; GRADEpro Guideline Development Toolkit [GRADE], Hsu et al., 2011; Quality Assessment tool for Diagnostic Accuracy Studies—2 [QUADAS-2], Whiting et al., 2011). An influential framework for evaluating the diagnostic accuracy of medical tests is STARD (Standards for Reporting of Diagnostic Accuracy: Bossuyt et al., 2003). The STARD criteria cover 25 issues that should be addressed by both primary source and review papers evaluating diagnostic test accuracy. The tremendous impact these guidelines have had on medicine may be readily documented by a Science Citation Index search on the number of times the original STARD publication (and nearly identical papers in other journals) has been referenced. As of October 10, 2014, these guidelines had been cited over 2,000 times. In sharp contrast, a contemporaneous search using EBSCO Information Services (EBSCO) host and the PsychINFO database revealed nine publications mentioning STARD in the title or abstract, with only three in outlets that appeared to be primarily psychological or neuropsychological in focus (*Brain Impairment, Journal of Personality Assessment,* and *Psychological Trauma: Theory, Research, and Practice*). Thus, as of late 2014, the STARD criteria appeared to be rather less influential in the psychological than in the medical literature. This disparity should concern clinical psychologists and neuropsychologists wishing to maximize quality in their investigations of the diagnostic accuracy of psychological instruments and procedures.

One area where the field of clinical neuropsychology has witnessed strong interest over the past two decades is detection of "malingering" (the deliberate fabrication or exaggeration of physical or psychological symptoms or deficits in pursuit of external goals), as demonstrated in the publication of hundreds of papers on the topic as well as several edited volumes (Boone, 2007; Larrabee, 2007; Rogers, 2012). The present chapter will explore application of the STARD criteria to performance validity tests (PVTs; Larrabee, 2012), which are intended to "diagnose" or identify invalid performances in neuropsychological evaluations.

METHODOLOGICAL QUALITY INDICATORS FOR PERFORMANCE VALIDITY TESTS AND MEDICAL DIAGNOSTIC PROCEDURES

In the medical literature, quantitative evaluations of treatments as well as diagnostic procedures are commonly referred to as "systematic reviews." In contrast, although the intended goals are usually quite similar, this type of evaluation is typically known as a "meta-analytic review" in the psychological and neuropsychological literature. There have been several such reviews of tests and scales intended to detect false reports of psychopathology (Berry, Baer, & Harris, 1991;

Rogers, Sewell, Martin, & Vitacco, 2003) as well as invalid approaches to neuropsychological test performance by those taking the tests (Sollman & Berry, 2011; Vickery, Berry, Inman, Harris, & Orey, 2001). These studies focused on summarizing effect sizes and basic diagnostic statistics. However, many of them coded methodological characteristics and explored the relationship of these with the summary statistics. For example, Table 11.1 lists the methodological variables extracted in a meta-analysis of the accuracy of selected PVTs (Sollman & Berry, 2011).

These methodological indicators were initially derived from recommendations by a pioneer in the area of detection of malingered psychological deficits, Richard Rogers (1988). These guidelines were intended to improve research quality in the area and were updated in Rogers (2012), and adapted in reviews such as the previously noted Sollman and Berry (2011). Given this provenance, it is not surprising that they are much less clinically than research-oriented. Although there is typically a degree of arbitrariness in devising scoring criteria used for quality evaluations, it is striking how little attention to clinical generalizability of results appears in the criteria listed in Table 11.1. An additional issue of note is the amount of coverage given to simulator malingering designs (i.e., normal subjects asked to feign deficits on testing), an approach that would seem uncommon in the medical diagnostic literature. However, malingering is a psychological construct, and analog production of psychological phenomena is viewed as a legitimate procedure for understanding the construct validity of psychological tests (Anastasi & Urbina, 1997). For example, administration of a putative test of anxiety before and after experimental induction of the emotion should document a predictable difference in scores on the two occasions. Similarly, instructing participants to feign psychological or neuropsychological deficits during administration of test batteries has been useful in investigating the sensitivity of malingering-detection instruments, although of course an appropriate clinical control group is required to determine specificity (Rogers et al., 2003; Sollman & Berry, 2011).

Column 2 of Table 11.2 provides a summary of the STARD criteria. In considering these entries, it is important to note that the "index test" is the procedure undergoing evaluation, whereas the "reference test" is the procedure used as the "gold standard" or "external validity criterion" (Anastasi & Urbina, 1997). It can be seen that there is remarkably little overlap between the STARD criteria and the methodological variables evaluated in Table 11.1, with the former covering many important technical aspects of the procedures employed in diagnostic studies. This suggests that extant meta-analyses of PVTs are probably not of the quality recommended for contemporary evaluations of medical diagnostic tests, a conclusion that is likely to be of concern to clinicians who utilize these procedures. This issue may also hold for standard neuropsychological tests.

A point that seems important to emphasize is that the STARD criteria do not function simply as "quality control" standards for diagnostic studies (although this is a useful application). In addition, they allow a reader to understand the nature of the clinical population to which the respective study results may be

Table 11.1 Methodological Characteristic Scoring System from a Meta-Analysis of Performance Validity Tests

	Response Options and Points			Score
For All Study Types:				
Were enough participants evaluated?	*N* total	1 group	Neither = 0	
	>20 = 2	>10 = 1		
Did groups match on age, gender, education, and race/ethnicity?	3–4 of these = 2	1–2 of these = 1	0/Don't know [K] = 0	
		Both Designs: Total		/ 4
For Simulation Evaluations:				
Was feigning group clinically relevant? that is:				
From a neurological, psychiatric, or other clinical sample?	Yes = 2		No = 0	
(If no to above), from a non-student sample?	Yes = 1		No = 0	
Were preexisting internal validity weaknesses ruled out by ensuring:				
Honest [HON] group not compensation-seeking or in litigation?	Yes = 1		No = 0	
No other indicators of decreased motivation to fulfill role?	Yes = 1		No = 0	
Was clinical practice approximated, through:				
Administration of >1 psychological or neuropsychological test?	Yes = 1		No = 0	
Administration of more than 1 feigning index? (for comparison)	Yes = 1		No = 0	
Test-administrator blinding?	Yes = 1		No = 0	
Were simulators prepared for their role by being given:				
A scenario to relate to?	Yes = 1		No = 0	
Preparation time before testing?	Yes = 1		No = 0	
Provision of or access to outside resources?	Yes = 1		No = 0	
Coaching on disorder symptoms?	Yes = 1		No = 0	
Coaching on how to evade detection by feigning tests?	Yes = 1		No = 0	
Was feigners' motivation to fulfill role improved by giving:				
Admonition to work hard to avoid detection?	Yes = 1		No = 0	
An explanation of why they should try to evade detection?	Yes = 1		No = 0	

Adequate financial incentive for successful feigning?	>$10 = 2	<$10 = 1	$0 = 0	
Was internal validity checked by post-test questioning of Subjects [S]'s:				
Self-reported effort at compliance?		Yes = 1	No = 0	
Self-reported comprehension of instructions?		Yes = 1	No = 0	
Perceived success at fulfilling role?		Yes = 1	No = 0	
		Enhanced Simulation Total		/ 19
For Known-Groups Evaluations:				
Was validity of criterion classification maximized by:				
Using multiple feigning measures to classify honest and feigners?	>2 = 2	1 = 1	None = 0	
Using the highest level of certainty in classifying feigners?	Significantly < chance = 2	Below cut score = 1	Non-objective = 0	
Excluding "indeterminate" participants' data?		Yes = 1	No = 0	
Was potential for classification contamination examined by:				
Evaluating group differences on compensation-seeking status?		Yes = 1	No = 0	
Evaluating group differences on neuropsychological tests?		Yes = 1	No = 0	
Shows that significant differences (effects) on the above exist?		Yes = 1	No = 0	
		Known-Groups Total		/ 12
	GRAND TOTAL for applicable design questions from above			

Source: Unpublished appendix from Sollman & Berry (2011).

Table 11.2 STARD DIAGNOSTIC QUALITY CONTROL CHECKLIST

STARD Item #	STARD Criteria	Application of STARD to Schipper et al. (2008)
1a	Clearly identified as a diagnostic accuracy study?	Not explicitly stated. Determination of "Operating Characteristics" of the manual LMT noted in Abstract (p. 345). Sensitivity, Specificity, and Area Under the Curve (AUC) data presented on p. 347, 4th paragraph.
1b	Are keywords *sensitivity* & *specificity* used?	Not included as keywords but appear in text (p. 347, 4th & 5th paragraphs).
2	Does research question include diagnostic accuracy of the index test?	Not explicitly, although text states goal is to compare the computerized and manual forms of the test (p. 346, 1st paragraph) with Sensitivity, Specificity, and AUC compared on p. 347, last paragraph.
3	Does study population have appropriate: • Inclusion/exclusion criteria? • Setting? • Location? • Spectrum of disease?	Inclusion criteria appear on p. 346, 2nd & 3rd paragraphs. Exclusion criteria appear in 3rd paragraph of this page. Setting and location not specified. Spectrum of disease not specified except in terms of means & standard deviations for Glasgow Coma Scale scores and duration of loss of consciousness (p. 346, 2nd paragraph).
4	Was subject recruitment accomplished by: • Presenting symptoms? • Results from previous tests? • Fact that patients had already received index test or reference standard? • Obtaining appropriate spectrum of disease? • Excluding other conditions in controls?	Archival study (p. 346, 2nd paragraph). Participants selected because they had received both index and reference tests. Spectrum of TBI not entirely clear, but wide range implied by GCS and duration of loss of consciousness (p. 346, paragraph 2). Estimated base rate of malingering (20%, p. 347, 1st paragraph) toward the lower end of published prevalence rates. No statement regarding exclusion on the basis of comorbid conditions present.
5	Was sampling: • Consecutive? • Or were additional criteria used?	Archival study. Requirements were: Administered full neuropsychological battery, received all 3 PVTs, failed none or >2 of them (p. 346, 2nd and 3rd paragraphs).
6	Was data collection: • Prospective or retrospective?	Archival study; retrospective data collection (p. 346, 2nd paragraph).
7	Were reference standard and rationale described?	Reference standards described on p. 346, 3rd paragraph, but no rationale provided. Rationale and description provided for index test (p. 346, first paragraph, and p. 345, first paragraph).
8	Were technical specifications for index & reference tests described, including: • Materials? • Methods? • Timing? • Citations?	PVT citations on p. 346, 1st and 2nd paragraphs. Methods and timing of administration not specified.

STARD Item #	STARD Criteria	Application of STARD to Schipper et al. (2008)
9	Were definition & rationale given for index & reference tests': • Units? • Cutoffs? • Categories of result? • Above predetermined?	Units implied (percentage correct) for index test (LMT, p. 347, 4th paragraph). Units for Reference tests not explicitly described. Cutoff for LMT given on p. 347, 4th paragraph. Categories of results described on p. 346, 3rd paragraph. Cutoffs were described as recommended cutting scores for TOMM, DMT (p. 346, 3rd paragraph) and LMT (p. 347, 4th paragraph).
10	Were index & reference test administrators & readers described, including: • Number? • Training? • Expertise?	Not described.
11	For index & reference tests, were: • Readers blind? • Any other data known to readers?	Not described.
12	• How was diagnostic accuracy calculated? • How was uncertainty quantified?	Sensitivity, specificity, and AUC calculated and presented on p. 347, paragraph 4. Only AUC included 95% confidence intervals.
13	Was test reproducibility (reliability) reported?	Not provided.
14	Were start & stop dates of recruitment provided?	Not provided.
15	Were participant characteristics described, including: • Clinical? • Demographic?	Demographic, TBI, and compensation-seeking characteristics for entire sample described on p. 346, 2nd paragraph. Probable Feigners and Honest characteristics were compared on p. 347, 2nd paragraph.
16	Was flow diagram with number included and excluded, along with reasons, provided?	Flow diagram not provided. However, p. 346, 3rd paragraph, tracks assignments of all participants.
17	Were the following details provided: • Time between Index and Reference tests? • Any interventions in interval?	Time between tests not explicitly addressed, but likely that index test and tests contributing to reference standard were completed during same evaluation. Possible interventions not addressed, but seem unlikely.

(*Continued*)

STARD Item #	STARD Criteria	Application of STARD to Schipper et al. (2008)
18	Were the following details addressed: • Severity/spectrum of disease appropriate in target patients with criteria? • Other diagnoses in controls? • Specify how above 2 defined?	Not explicitly stated, but likely severity and spectrum of TBI comparable to that found in outpatient neuropsychological assessment practice. As noted earlier, base rate of 20% feigning in this sample was lower than reported in many other compensation-seeking samples. Comorbid conditions not detailed. Criteria for TBI not explicitly addressed. Criteria for feigning and honest group assignments addressed on p. 346, 3rd paragraph.
19	Is there a: • Table with cross-tabulation of results from Index and Reference tests? • Are indeterminate and technical failures included in table?	Not present. Indeterminate classification described on p. 346, 3rd paragraph, but not included in a table.
20	Any adverse results from testing described?	Not discussed, but unlikely.
21	Are there estimates of diagnostic accuracy with confidence intervals?	Estimated sensitivity, specificity, and AUC presented on p. 347, 4th paragraph. Only AUC provided standard error value.
22	Was handling of index test results in terms of following described: • Indeterminate? • Missing responses? • Outliers?	Indeterminate subjects were excluded from diagnostic accuracy calculations. Missing responses and outliers not mentioned.
23	Was variability of accuracy across following variables addressed: • Sites? • Subgroups? • Readers?	Not addressed.
24	Was test reproducibility addressed in terms of stability and rater agreement?	Not addressed.
25	Was clinical applicability of findings discussed?	Only briefly discussed on p. 347, last paragraph.

Note: STARD = Standards for Reporting of Diagnostic Accuracy; Bossuyt et al. (2003). Index test is procedure being evaluated. Reference test is "gold standard."

generalized. Thus, a publication that shows that a given diagnostic procedure performs well in an inpatient setting may not necessarily provide data that are applicable to an outpatient setting. This might be due to variations in the severity of the disease in the different settings, differing pathways to testing, etc. Reviewing a study using the STARD criteria directs the reader to issues bearing on the generalizability of results.

To facilitate progress in this area, subsequent sections of this chapter will explore the nature of PVTs, issues relatively specific to studying these instruments, application of STARD criteria to a representative study of a PVT, description of a relevant clinical case scenario, as well as introduction and completion of a clinician-friendly worksheet to determine if the target study provides appropriate information for an individual case question.

PERFORMANCE VALIDITY TESTS

Prior to applying the STARD criteria to a PVT, it may be helpful to consider briefly the development, nature, and application of PVTs in clinical neuropsychology. It has long been known that, as tests of ability, neuropsychological procedures require the active cooperation of test-takers in order to obtain valid data that may be used to appreciate the nature and extent of any brain dysfunction (Boone, 2007). Furthermore, research with normal individuals asked to feign brain damage on neuropsychological tests has indicated that many simulators are successful in producing plausible deficits on these procedures (Larrabee, 2007). Beginning in the 1980s, more sophisticated tests for identification of invalid approaches to neuropsychological testing were validated and published. Methodological issues were recognized as important very early in this research area (Rogers, 1988).

The most popular current PVTs involve questions or items with a forced choice between two alternative answers. This method allows calculation of the expected number of correct answers, given complete absence of the ability in question. For example, in a recognition memory task with two choices possible on each of 50 trials, completely random responding should produce about 50% correct choices, and a level statistically significantly below this may also be calculated. Performances that are statistically significantly below chance suggest an active avoidance of the correct answer in favor of the incorrect option. This "statistically significantly below chance" level was initially the benchmark for identifying malingered neuropsychological deficits. However, later work in groups instructed to fake deficits suggested that this criterion was too conservative in identifying feigners. Subsequently, cutting scores based on performance of non–compensation-seeking patients with the disorder in question were widely adopted and proved to be more effective overall than the statistically significantly below chance criterion (Vickery et al., 2001).

The primary designs for validation studies of PVTs have been simulation and known-groups methodologies. In simulation designs (which are thought to maximize internal validity, or the extent to which changes in the dependent variable are attributable to manipulation of the independent variable), a group is instructed to feign deficits on test batteries that include PVTs, and results are compared to those from a group with a known pathology, such as traumatic brain injury (TBI), that is tested in a context with no external motivation for faking deficits. The Known-Groups design (which is thought to maximize external validity, or the extent to which results are generalizable to other settings, populations, etc., and is much closer to typical studies of medical diagnostic tests) usually involves administering previously validated PVTs (reference tests) as well as a new PVT (index test) to a series of patients with a target disorder, such as TBI. The previously validated PVTs, and sometimes other criteria (e.g., Slick, Sherman, & Iverson, 1999) are then used to classify each patient as honest or feigning. Results from the new PVT are compared in the two groups classified on the basis of their performances on previously validated PVTs. Both these designs allow determination of effect sizes as well as estimated sensitivity (percent of those known to have a target condition who have a positive test sign) and specificity (percent of those known not to have a target condition who have a negative test sign). Together with known or estimated base rates of the condition in question, these two statistics can be used to estimate Positive Predictive Power (percentage of those with a positive test sign who actually have the target condition) and Negative Predictive Power (percentage of those with a negative test sign who do not have the target condition).

Vickery et al. (2001) meta-analyzed results from published studies of the accuracy of the most well-studied PVTs and reported an average effect size (Cohen's *d*) of 1.1, as well as average sensitivity of .56 and specificity of .96. Sollman and Berry (2011) reported on a similar review of the most commonly studied PVTs published since the previous meta-analysis and found a mean effect size of 1.5, sensitivity of .69, and specificity of .90. Along with many other publications in the area, these results supported routine clinical use of PVTs, especially in cases where compensation-seeking, such as litigation or the pursuit of disability awards, was present.

In 2005, the National Academy of Neuropsychology published a policy statement on PVTs (Bush et al., 2005), indicating that "the assessment of symptom validity is an essential part of a neuropsychological evaluation. The clinician should be prepared to justify a decision not to assess symptom validity as part of a neuropsychological evaluation" (p. 421). Along with similar statements by other professional organizations (Heilbronner et al., 2009), it is clear that PVTs are a well-established part of the fabric of neuropsychological assessment.

APPLICATION OF STARD CRITERIA TO A PERFORMANCE VALIDITY TEST

One of the PVTs evaluated in the meta-analysis by Sollman and Berry (2011) was the Letter Memory Test (LMT: Inman et al., 1998). The original LMT was a computer-administered recognition memory test with 45 items. Each item included a stimulus of consonant letters (e.g., VXW), a delay period, and then a recognition trial that included the original stimulus as well as one or more foils. Across nine blocks of trials, face difficulty was manipulated by increasing the number of consonant letters in the stimulus varying from 3 to 4 to 5, and by increasing the number of choices on the recognition trial from 2 to 3 to 4. Orey, Cragar, and Berry (2000) described a manual form of the test with stimulus and recognition materials printed on 3″ X 5″ index cards. Schipper, Berry, Coen, and Clark (2008) published a cross-validation of the manual form of the test, which will be the target article for application of the STARD criteria here.

The third column of Table 11.2 summarizes application of the STARD criteria to the manuscript by Schipper et al. (2008). It may be seen that a large number of the STARD criteria were not addressed, or only briefly covered, in this paper. Thus, if these criteria were followed in evaluating the paper for publication, it might not have been accepted in a journal that required adherence to STARD guidelines for reports on diagnostic tests. More substantively, several of the omitted STARD criteria in the paper raise the possibility that various types of bias that might have affected results were not addressed, and these will be covered next. Parenthetically, it should be noted that several other publications support the validity of the LMT (Alwes, Clark, Berry, & Granacher, 2008; Dearth et al., 2005; Inman & Berry, 2002; Inman et al., 1998; Vagnini et al., 2006; Vickery et al., 2004).

For reviewing evidence on the accuracy of diagnostic test procedures, "bias" has been defined as "systematic error or deviation from the truth, either in results or in their inferences" (Reitsma et al., 2009, p. 4). The information missing from the report by Schipper et al. (2008) raises the possibility of the presence of several types of bias, including, but not limited to, the following: The minimal description of selection criteria for participants means that the spectrum of patients for whom the results are generalizable is unclear, and thus it is uncertain to which groups the findings may apply. In terms of the reference standard, the description of the accuracy of the combination of the Test of Memory Malingering (TOMM) and the Digit Memory Test (DMT) on pp. 346–347 is helpful, but it does not entirely rule out bias due to the criterion variables. In other words, the extent to which application of these reference tests may have resulted in inaccurate classifications is ambiguous. The brief description of injury severity for TBI patients on p. 346 is insufficient to understand completely their standing on disease progression and recovery variables, which again obscures the appropriate population to which results might generalize. Although the selection of participants' data is described as an "archival" approach, the lack of description of the process by which participants were referred for neuropsychological evaluations, as well as failure to specify the criteria for choice of PVTs administered in a given examination, raise the possibility of partial verification as well as differential verification biases. These biases arise in cases in which the group used to determine sensitivity undergoes different procedures from the group used to determine specificity values, which may affect generalizability of results. Failure to specify whether index test administrators and interpreters were blind to reference test results raises the possibility of diagnostic review bias, commonly termed "criterion contamination" in the psychometric literature. Criterion contamination, in which findings from the criterion variables may affect interpretation of predictor variables, typically results in an overestimation of validity. The number of indeterminate outcomes (only one PVT failed) was described on p. 346. As results from these participants were excluded from the calculations of sensitivity and specificity values, it is likely that one or both of these parameters is overestimated in the present study. The issue of withdrawals from neuropsychological evaluations is not addressed in the report, which also may affect the accuracy of test parameters. Together, these potential sources of bias suggest that results from this study should be applied only cautiously to new patient groups. This exercise illustrates how systematic application of the STARD criteria to review of an article directs our attention to important issues that may limit the applicability of reported results. Of course, similar issues may arise in published studies of other PVTs as well as standard neuropsychological tests.

The data presented in Table 11.2 suggest that STARD criteria may be readily applied to a published study of a PVT. Although STARD provides a meticulous assessment of the quality and generalizability in an evaluation of the diagnostic validity of a PVT, this application may be too time-consuming for a busy clinician confronted with a novel clinical problem. Therefore, it may be helpful to illustrate the application of a briefer, but still acceptable, set of criteria to a common clinical concern. This will be addressed by setting out a hypothetical assessment scenario and working through the application of these criteria to the problem.

CLINICAL PROBLEM

A 40-year-old man presents to a psychological provider with memory complaints approximately a year following a motor vehicle accident with a reported mild concussion. The patient relates that he was rear-ended while stopped at an intersection. He reports problems with attention and prospective memory, stating that he must rely on lists to function at work and in his personal life since the accident. In passing, the patient mentions that he is considering pressing charges and possibly pursuing civil litigation against the other driver involved in the accident.

The relevant question, then, is whether or not, in the case of 40-year-old male with a mild TBI and subjective memory symptoms, there is a PVT that provides reliable diagnostic information beyond clinical impression to determine if a compensation-seeking evaluee is putting forth his best effort.

APPLYING THE CRITICALLY APPRAISED TOPIC WORKSHEET

Although limitations of the Schipper et al. study (2008) were noted, for the sake of consistency, this article will also be used as the target for a briefer worksheet. Straus and colleagues (Straus, Richardson, Glasziou, & Hayes, 2011) illustrate the use of templates to assist clinicians in evaluating research articles for methodological quality, practical importance, and clinical generalizability. It is important to appreciate that the entries in the Critically Appraised Topic (CAT) worksheets are a condensed subset of the STARD criteria. Thus, these worksheets allow the relatively rapid implementation of major STARD criteria. There are CAT worksheets designed to allow clinicians to analytically evaluate available evidence on diagnosis, prognosis, harm, and therapy. For most psychologists and neuropsychologists, the diagnostic CAT worksheet provides the most utility as it provides a systematic way to evaluate research evidence on measures relevant to clinical practice in this area. Furthermore, the CAT approach allows clinicians to relate this evidence to individual patients in specific diagnostic settings. Although these methods may not be necessary for clinical questions that fall under a clinician's expertise, the framework can be used to find and interpret evidence for novel clinical questions or to update an area of knowledge.

The subsequent diagnostic CAT example is based on the worksheet accessible online at http://ktclearinghouse.ca/cebm/practise/ca and is used to illustrate the clinical utility of the CAT method for PVTs. Although CAT worksheets are most valuable when dealing with novel clinical questions, the TBI problem is used

Table 11.3.1 CAT Worksheet Example, Part 1

Are the results of this diagnostic study valid?	
1. Was there an independent, blind comparison with a reference ("gold") standard of diagnosis?	LMT results were checked against results from two other PVTs, the Test of Memory Malingering (TOMM) and the Digit Memory Test (DMT), using recommended cutting scores for all. An objective algorithm using results from TOMM and DMT classified each participant into Honest, Probable Feigning, and Indeterminate groups. While not carried out under "blind" conditions, use of the algorithm should decrease subjective factors, although not eliminate them.
2. Was the diagnostic test evaluated in an appropriate spectrum of patients (like those in whom it would be used in practice)?	Results may be applicable to those from outpatient neuropsychological evaluations. However, details of rationale for choosing PVTs, presence of comorbid disorders, referral pathway, and other potentially relevant issues were not described.
3. Was the reference standard applied regardless of the diagnostic test result?	Unclear, as this was an archival study.
4. Was the test (or cluster of tests) validated in a second, independent group of patients?	This was a cross-validation of the manual LMT, with results reported to be similar to those from the computerized version of the test.
Conclusion—yes, the results of this diagnostic study are probably valid, as described above.	

Source: Schipper, L. J., Berry, D. T. R., Coen, E. M., & Clark, J. A. (2008). Cross-validation of a manual form of the Letter Memory Test using a known-groups methodology. *The Clinical Neuropsychologist, 22*, 345–349.

Table 11.3.2 CAT Worksheet Example, Part 2 Are the Valid Results of This Diagnostic Study Important?

EXAMPLE CALCULATIONS		Target Disorder (Probable Cognitive Feigning)		
		Present	**Absent**	**Totals**
1.Diagnostic test result (LMT)	Positive (<93% on LMT)	8 a	1 b	9 a + b
	Negative (≥93% on LMT)	2 c	38 d	40 c + d
Totals		10 a + c	39 b + d	49 a + b + c + d
Test-Based Operating Characteristics				
2. Sensitivity = a/(a + c) = 8/10 = 80%				
3. Specificity = d/(b + d) = 38/39 = 97.5%				
4. Likelihood ratio for a positive test result = LR+ = sensitivity/(1 - specificity) = 80%/2.5% = 32				
5. Likelihood ratio for a negative test result = LR– = (1 - sensitivity)/ specificity = 20%/97.5% = 0.21				
Sample-Based Operating Characteristics				
6. Sample positive predictive value = a/(a + b) = 8/9 = 88.9%				
7. Sample negative predictive value = d/(c + d) = 38/40 = 95%				

8. Sample base rate = (a + c)/(a + b + c + d) = 10/49 = 0.20
Population-Based Operating Characteristics (Revised Estimates)
9. Pre-test probability (estimated population base rate) = 0.35 (mid-range compensation-seeking mild TBI base rate; Greve, Bianchini, & Doane, 2006)
10. Pre-test odds = prevalence/(1 - prevalence) = 35%/65% = 0.54
11. Post-test odds for a positive test result = pre-test odds x LR+ = 0.54 x 32.0 = 17.3
12. Post-test odds for a negative test result = pre-test odds x LR− = 0.54 x 0.21 = .11
13. Post-test probability if test sign is positive = 17.3/18.3 = .95
14. Post-test probability if test sign is negative = 0.11/1.11 = .10
Conclusion—Yes, the LMT has moderately strong sensitivity and strong specificity, suggesting that it would be potentially useful.

Note—data in above table and statistics appearing below based on p. 347, paragraph 4, Schipper et al. (2008).

Table 11.3.3 CAT WORKSHEET EXAMPLE, PART 3 CAN YOU APPLY THIS VALID, IMPORTANT EVIDENCE ABOUT A DIAGNOSTIC TEST IN CARING FOR YOUR PATIENT?

1. Is the diagnostic test available, affordable, accurate, and precise in your setting?	Yes, the LMT is available for purchase from its author, has been cross-validated, and appears comparable in operating characteristics to other PVTs. Training as a neuropsychologist or psychometrist entails accuracy and precision in administering neuropsychological tests.
2. Can you generate a clinically sensible estimate of your patient's pre-test probability (from personal experience, prevalence statistics, practice databases, or primary studies)? • Are the study patients similar to your own? • Is it unlikely that the disease possibilities or probabilities have changed since the evidence was gathered?	Yes, and the literature on assessment of mild traumatic brain injury suggests a base rate of about 30–40% for malingered neurocognitive dysfunction when the evaluation includes a forensic component. For current purposes, a pre-test feigning base rate of 35% was assumed, based on reports in the literature. The compensation-seeking subjects in the study are comparable to the current patient. There does not appear to be any reason to believe that the base rate of malingered neurocognitive dysfunction in this population has changed over time.
3. Will the resulting post-test probabilities affect your management and help your patient? • Could it move you across a test-treatment threshold? • Would your patient be a willing partner in carrying it out?	Yes. Failing the LMT provides a positive predictive power value of .89, making it likely that Malingered Neurocognitive Dysfunction (MNCD) is present. Passing the LMT provides a negative predictive power of .95 at the specified base rate of 35%. The LMT is no more uncomfortable to take than most other neuropsychological tests.
4. Would the consequences of the test help your patient?	Failing the LMT provides moderately strong evidence of feigned cognitive deficits. While not necessarily likely to be viewed as helpful by the compensation-seeking patient, such a result could result in early termination of testing. Passing the LMT provides strong evidence of valid test results.

Conclusion—Yes, failing the LMT raises the probability of feigned deficits from about .35 to .89 at the estimated base rate of 35%. Passing the LMT reduces the probability of feigned deficits from .35 to .05 at the estimated base rate of 35%.

to illustrate this approach in a hypothetical patient in need of effort screening. The diagnostic worksheet is made up of three parts, with multiple additional sub-questions: (1) Are the results of this study valid? (2) Are the valid results of this study important? (3) Can you apply this valid, important study about a diagnostic test to your patient? Once a clinician is experienced in using the CAT method, a worksheet can be completed reasonably quickly. Table 11.3.1–11.3.3 provides data and answers to these questions, with more comments and elaborate answers provided than are necessarily required for most issues. Once again, it is emphasized the issues probed in the CAT worksheet and Table 11.3.1–11.3.3 are a subset of the STARD criteria.

Results from Table 11.3.2 suggest that the LMT is probably a valid PVT that may be applied, albeit with caution, to addressing the possibility of feigned neuropsychological deficits. As noted, failing the LMT greatly raises the probability of faking (from an estimated representative, fixed pre-test probability of .35 to a post-test probability of .95; see Table 11.3.2, footnotes 9 and 13). Passing the LMT lowers the likelihood of feigning (from an estimated representative, fixed pre-test probability of .35 to a post-test probability of .10; see Table 11.3.2, footnotes 9 and 14). Of course, these predictive powers would be altered in different base-rate environments, a fact that completion of the CAT forces the clinician to take in to account. So an alternative representation of the diagnostic value of the LMT is communicated by the likelihood ratio (LR)+ of 32 (Table 11.3.2), which indicates that a positive result on the LMT greatly increases the likelihood of faking on the part of this test-taker.

Thus, the CAT results support careful use of the LMT in an evaluation of a potentially compensation-seeking patient, such as the one described in the clinical vignette described (see Table 11.3.3). CAT worksheets provide a reasonably rapid framework for addressing major STARD issues when considering a PVT. Psychologists and neuropsychologists could potentially improve both their clinical and research activities through application of STARD criteria to diagnostic tests.

REFERENCES

Alwes, Y. R., Clark, J. A., Berry, D. T. R., & Granacher, R. P. (2008). Screening for feigning in a civil forensic setting. *The Journal of Clinical and Experimental Neuropsychology, 30*, 1–8.

Anastasi, A., & Urbina, S. (1997). *Psychological Testing* (7th ed.). Upper Saddle River, NJ: Simon & Schuster.

Berry, D. T. R., Baer, R. A., & Harris, M. J. (1991). Detection of malingering on the MMPI: A meta-analysis. *Clinical Psychology Review, 11*, 585–598.

Boone, K. B. (2007). *Assessment of Feigned Cognitive Impairment: A Neuropsychologic al Perspective*. New York: Guilford Press.

Bossuyt, P. M., Reitsma, J. B., Bruns, D. E., Gatsoni, C. A., Glasziou, P. P., Irwig, L. M., . . . de Vet, H. C. W. (2003). Towards complete and accurate reporting of studies of diagnostic accuracy: The STARD initiative. *British Medical Journal, 326*, 41–44.

Bush, S. S., Ruff, R. M., Troster, A. I., Barth, J. T., Koffler, S. P., Pliskin, N. H., . . . Silver, C. H. (2005). Symptom validity assessment: Practice issues and medical necessity: NAN Policy & Planning Committee. *Archives of Clinical Neuropsychology, 20*, 419–426.

Dearth, C. D., Berry, D. T. R., Vickery, C. D., Vagnini, V. L., Baser, R. E., Orey, S. A., & Cragar, D. E. (2005). Detection of feigned head injury symptoms on the MMPI-2 in head injured patients and community controls. *Archives of Clinical Neuropsychology, 20*, 95–110.

Greve, K. W., Bianchini, K. J., & Doane, B. M. (2006). Classification accuracy of the test of memory malingering in traumatic brain injury: Results of a known-groups analysis. *Journal of Clinical and Experimental Neuropsychology, 28*, 1176–1190.

Heilbronner, R. L., Sweet, J. J., Morgan, J. E., Larrabee, G. J., Millis, S. R., & Conference Participants. (2009). American Academy of Clinical Neuropsychology Consensus Conference statement on the neuropsychological assessment of effort, response bias, and malingering. *The Clinical Neuropsychologist, 23*, 1093–1129.

Hsu, J., Brozek, J. L., Terracciano, L., Kries, J., Compalati, E., Stein, A. T., . . . Schünemann, H. J. (2011). Application of GRADE: Making evidence-based recommendations about diagnostic tests in clinical practice guidelines. *Implementing Science, 6*, 62.

Inman, T. H., & Berry, D. T. R. (2002). Cross-validation of indicators of malingering: A comparison of nine neuropsychological tests, four tests of malingering, and behavioral observations. *Archives of Clinical Neuropsychology, 17*, 1–23.

Inman, T. H., Vickery, C. D., Berry, D. T. R., Lamb, D., Edwards, C., & Smith, G. T. (1998). Development and initial validation of a new procedure for evaluating adequacy of effort given during neuropsychological testing: The Letter Memory Test. *Psychological Assessment, 10*, 128–139.

Larrabee, G. J. (2007). *Assessment of Malingered Neuropsychological Deficits*. New York: Oxford University Press.

Larrabee, G. J. (2012). Performance validity and symptom validity in neuropsychological assessment. *Journal of the International Neuropsychological Society, 18*, 625–631.

Lijmer, J. G., Mol, B. W., Heisterkamp, S., Bonsel, G. J., Prinz, M. H., van der Meulen, J. H. P., & Bossuyt, P. M. M. (1999). Empirical evidence of design-related bias in studies of diagnostic tests. *Journal of the American Medical Association, 282*, 1061–1066.

Meyer, G. J., Finn, S. E., Eyde, L. D., Kay, G. G., Moreland, K. L., Dies, R. R., . . . Reed, G. M. (2001). Psychological testing and psychological assessment: A review of evidence and issues. *American Psychologist, 56*, 128–165.

Orey, S. A., Cragar, D. E., & Berry, D. T. R. (2000). The effects of two motivational manipulations on the neuropsychological performance of mildly head-injured college students. *Archives of Clinical Neuropsychology, 15*, 335–348.

Reitsma, J. B., Rutjes, A. W. S., Whiting, P., Vlassov, V. V., Leeflang, M. M. G., Deeks, J. J. (2009). Chapter 9: Assessing methodological quality. In J. J. Deeks, P. M. Bossuyt, & C. Gatsonis (Eds.), *Cochrane Handbook for Systematic Reviews of Diagnostic Test Accuracy Version 1.0.0*. The Cochrane Collaboration, 2009. Available from: http://srdta.cochrane.org/.

Rogers, R. (1988). *Clinical Assessment of Malingering and Deception* (1st ed.). New York: Guilford Press.

Rogers, R. (2012). *Clinical Assessment of Malingering and Deception* (3rd ed.). New York: Oxford Press.

Rogers, R., Sewell, K. W., Martin, M. A., & Vitacco, M. J. (2003). Detection of feigned mental disorders: A meta-analysis of the MMPI-2 and malingering. *Assessment, 10*, 160–177.

Schipper, L. J., Berry, D. T. R., Coen, E., & Clark, J. A. (2008). Cross-validation of a manual form of the Letter Memory Test using a Known-Groups methodology. *The Clinical Neuropsychologist, 22*, 345–349.

Slick, D. J., Sherman, E. M., & Iverson, G. L. (1999). Diagnostic criteria for malingered neurocognitive dysfunction: Proposed standards for clinical practice and research. *The Clinical Neuropsychologist, 13*, 545–561.

Sollman, M. J., & Berry, D. T. R. (2011). Detection of inadequate effort on neuropsychological testing: A meta-analytic update and extension. *Archives of Clinical Neuropsychology, 26*, 774–789.

Straus, S., Richardson, W. S., Glasziou, P., & Haynes, R. B. (2011). *Evidence-Based Medicine: How to Practice and Teach EBM* (4th ed.). Edinburgh: Churchill Livingstone.

Treweek, S., Oxman, A. D., Alderson, P., Bossuyt, P. M., Brandt, L., Brozek, J., . . . DECIDE Consortium. (2013). Developing and evaluating communication strategies to support informed decisions and practice based on evidence (DECIDE): Protocol and preliminary results. *Implementing Science, 8*, 6.

Vagnini, V. L., Sollman, M. J., Berry, D. T. R., Granacher, R. P., Clark, J. A., Burton, R., . . . Saier, J. (2006). Known-groups cross-validation of the Letter Memory Test in a compensation-seeking mixed neurologic sample. *The Clinical Neuropsychologist, 20*, 289–305.

Vickery, C. D., Berry, D. T. R., Dearth, C. S., Vagnini, V. L., Baser, R. E., Cragar, D. E., & Orey, S. A. (2004). Head injury and the ability to feign neuropsychological deficits. *Archives of Clinical Neuropsychology, 19*, 37–48.

Vickery, C. D., Berry, D. T. R., Inman, T. H., Harris, M. J., & Orey, S. A. (2001). Detection of inadequate effort on neuropsychological testing: A meta-analytic review of selected procedures. *Archives of Clinical Neuropsychology, 16*, 45–73.

Whiting, P. F., Rutjes. A. W., Westwood, M. E., Mallett, S., Deeks, J. J., Reitsma, J. B., . . . the QUADAS-2 Group. (2011). QUADAS-2: A revised tool for the quality assessment of diagnostic studies. *Annals of Internal Medicine, 155*, 529–536.

12

Critically Appraised Topics for Intervention Studies: Practical Implementation Methods for the Clinician-Scientist

JUSTIN B. MILLER

INTRODUCTION TO CRITICAL APPRAISAL

Evidence-based practice (EBP) is a well-established standard in medicine, integrating the best available research evidence, individual patient characteristics, and clinical expertise (Sackett, Rosenberg, Gray, Haynes, & Richardson, 1996), and it has become increasingly common throughout the behavioral health sciences over the past decade. As defined by the American Psychological Association Presidential Task Force, evidence-based psychology "promotes effective psychological practice and enhances public health by applying empirically supported principles of psychological assessment, case formulation, therapeutic relationships, and intervention" (p. 271; APA Presidential Task Force, 2006). There are multiple components of this definition that are of central relevance for clinical neuropsychology. Certainly psychological assessment should be firmly rooted in clinical practice, and there are critical appraisal methods available to aid development of a test battery with appropriate sensitivity and specificity to answer a specific referral question (see Chapters 7 and 10 in this volume). Although not the emphasis of the current chapter, a clinical case formulation can, and should, be scientifically grounded using evidence-based methods to facilitate diagnostic decisions. It is the point of intervention and, more specifically, making treatment decisions and recommendations, where the methods reviewed in this chapter take center stage.

The role of the neuropsychologist is multifaceted and has been defined to include "assessment, intervention, consultation, supervision, research and inquiry, consumer protection, and professional development" (National Academy of Neuropsychology Definition of a Clinical Neuropsychologist, 2001).

In each of these capacities, linking observable behaviors with brain functioning via objective methods is a fundamental component of professional practice that is inextricably tied to scientific evidence. In conjunction with clinician expertise, and patient characteristics, culture, and preferences, the act of linking science to practice lies at the core of evidence-based psychology (APA Presidential Task Force, 2006). For both diagnosticians and treatment providers, a major component of clinical practice is to make specific treatment recommendations that are custom-tailored to individual patients, identifying the interventions that are most likely to be beneficial. EBP guidelines emphasize the importance of integrating empirical evidence into clinical practice. However, guidelines may contain little in the way of specific guidance about how to integrate evidence with practice, leaving the individual practitioner responsible for identification of evidence and implementation of quality evidence in clinical practice. Despite robust scientific training in psychology, methods for assisting clinicians to integrate quality evidence in their practice are not included in most training programs and are relatively new in the training of professionals of all types. For most practicing clinicians, finding and applying quality evidence is easier said than done. Simply being able to read and comprehend information presented in scientific publications does not necessarily facilitate application of findings to real-world, individualized, clinical practice. And although empirically supported treatments (EST; Chambless & Hollon, 1998) have become increasingly common and provide systematic methods for determining the efficacy of treatments, simply being established as "empirically supported" is an insufficient basis for making specific treatment recommendations for individual patients.

In the absence of an evidence-based method, treatment recommendations are likely to be rooted in a combination of clinical experience and expertise. For many professionals, particularly those still in training and early-career practitioners, it would certainly not be uncommon to make recommendations based on prior training experiences, emulating the practices of former mentors. The further one gets from training, drawing on past experiences would similarly be expected to have an influence on treating current patients, especially those presenting with a clinical problem comparable to a former patient's. While this approach integrates clinical expertise, which is one of the core tenets of evidence-based medicine and practice, it fails to account for individual patient preferences. More importantly, these recommendations may or may not be rooted in *current* empirical evidence, the third primary tenet of EBP. Attention is drawn to the word *current*. Particularly for recommendations that are passed down from training generation to training generation, even if originally rooted in scientific evidence, research evidence continually evolves, and if a treatment method was applicable at one point in time, this does not necessarily mean it has stood the test of time. In addition, in parallel with developments in EBP, the understanding of "expertise" has evolved to focus on knowledge held by skilled practitioners that is reflective of the best available scientific practice (Haynes, 2002). By systematically reappraising the literature on a regular basis, evidence-based methods can address each of these shortcomings.

The primary aim of the present chapter is to review the methods designed to help with integrating evidence into clinical practice, namely, the methods of *critical appraisal* (critically appraised topics; CAT) for systematically evaluating the clinical relevance of empirical evidence, with particular emphasis in this chapter on neuropsychological intervention studies. Beginning with the development of a focused clinical question, the process of evaluating an intervention study with CAT analysis—including methods for assessing study quality, calculating patient-relevant statistics, and moving from group-level data to individual patient recommendations—will be reviewed in detail, with worked examples throughout. A secondary aim is to demonstrate the utility, and perhaps more important, the simplicity of making empirically based recommendations for patients, and how these data might be utilized and integrated into an EBP. Ultimately, the goal is to improve patient outcomes and facilitate the merging of science with clinical practice via a simple systematic method.

What Is a Critically Appraised Topic?

Developed as a clinical and educational tool to teach EBP and facilitate transfer of evidence to bedside care (Sauve et al., 1995; Wyer, 1997), critical appraisal is a systematic method for evaluating empirical research and translating quantitative findings from the scientific literature into meaningful, accessible metrics that facilitate real-time decision-making in clinical practice. CAT methods are particularly geared towards working with individual patients. Any topic that has been subjected to critical appraisal methods is therefore a "critically appraised topic (CAT)." There are multiple variants of critical appraisal techniques, including emphasis on diagnosis (see Chapters 7 and 11 of this volume), as well as prognosis, risk assessment, and intervention. Systematic reviews can also be subjected to CAT analysis, which is essentially a method of aggregating findings from several individual CAT analyses into one concise summary. Example summary sheets for CAT analyses are readily available online (e.g., http://www.cebm.net/critical-appraisal or http://ktclearinghouse.ca/cebm/toolbox/worksheets), and some programs automate CAT generation based on entered input (e.g., Center for Evidence-Based Medicine [CEBM] CATmaker). In order to conduct a CAT analysis with a systematic review, facility with conducting individual CATs is essential, and is hence an initial starting point for learning and the focus of this chapter.

While each of the main CAT variants is relevant for clinical practice, for the purpose of making treatment recommendations, methods for critically appraising intervention studies are of direct relevance for all clinicians. Although there are subtle variations among methods of CAT analysis, depending on the type of study being appraised, the core components of the effective critical appraisal that intervention CATs seek to establish are: (1) addressing a clearly focused clinical question, (2) evaluating the methodological rigor of retrieved evidence to determine the validity of the study methods, (3) assessing whether or not the results generated from the appraised study are both valid *and* important, and

Box 12.1 CLINICAL SCENARIO

Mr. G is a 72-year-old man with 16 years of education (former software engineer) who has become concerned about increasing forgetfulness despite continued maintenance of an active lifestyle. His mother and sister both developed dementia and he is worried about his future. A recent neuropsychological evaluation revealed normal cognitive functioning without evidence of emotional difficulty. During feedback, Mr. G was informed of results that suggest his experiences are consistent with normal aging. He has asked whether or not starting a computer-based cognitive training program would help prevent cognitive and memory decline.

(4) determining whether these valid and important results are applicable to a particular patient. From these determinations, quantifiable metrics are derived that are then used to provide tailored recommendations as to whether or not the reviewed intervention is likely to be beneficial. In addition to making informed treatment recommendations, a further benefit of CAT analysis is that it creates a condensed summary of the best available evidence, with practice recommendations that can be stored for later reference. These recommendations can then be used as an evidence-foundation for development of clinical policies and practice guidelines. As each step of the CAT methodology is reviewed, the specific procedures will be demonstrated and applied using a realistic hypothetical clinical scenario, presented in Box 12.1.

GENERATING A SPECIFIC CLINICAL QUESTION

The initial step in a CAT analysis is to identify a narrowly focused and clearly defined clinical question. On the surface, this may seem like a straightforward and simple task. In our case example, the question the patient has asked is whether or not cognitive training will help prevent cognitive decline. This could succinctly be summarized by asking: "Will *therapy X* help my patient?" Or, more broadly: "What type of therapy should be recommended?" While both are certainly viable clinical questions, they lack sufficient specificity for CAT analysis. In either question, there is no indication of for whom the therapy is being recommended. Neither is there specification of the type of problem to be addressed by this therapy, nor the desired outcome. This question could potentially be specified by asking: "Should this patient receive cognitive-behavioral therapy?" For even greater specificity: "Should this patient receive cognitive-behavioral therapy for treating his depression?" These latter questions certainly address for whom and for what purpose, but still neglect to identify a comparison treatment.

To facilitate the formulation of a clinically focused, answerable question for use in EBP, a framework has been established that identifies the individual components to consider. The *PICO* method emphasizes explicit identification of the

*P*atient (or *P*roblem), the *I*ntervention, the *C*omparison, and the *O*utcome, and can be applied to a multitude of clinical questions. Appropriate formulation of PICO-based questions can also assist with identifying relevant search terms and keywords to be used in the literature reviews. Although it is not entirely necessary to specify each component, the more information and detail are provided, the more refined the obtained results will be. In most instances, identifying the patient or problem is straightforward and obvious. In our scenario, for example, the patient is a 72-year-old college-educated man. Alternatively, identifying the patient's concern about increasing forgetfulness would frame the question using a problem-focused perspective. Either approach would be appropriate, though focusing on the patient's problem of interest may aid in establishing search terms. For even greater depth, describing both the patient and the problem of interest is feasible.

In the example provided, the patient himself has specified a particular intervention (i.e., computer-based cognitive training) that is of interest to him, though this is not always the case. This is where good clinical skill and expertise are needed to help identify potential interventions. Though some patients may be particularly well informed and come with interest in an identified intervention, more often the clinician is relied upon as the expert to suggest a treatment. Identifying a comparison condition may also be obvious in some instances where the patient's concerns are of a type familiar to the clinician, in others, the comparison may be implied, but in still others, it may need to be specified. When comparing medications, for example, a patient may want to know if one particular drug may be more effective than another, or whether or not a current medication has more side-effects than an alternative. In behavioral health and therapy, similar questions can be asked about the relative benefits of one type of intervention compared to another (e.g., prolonged exposure therapy vs. cognitive-processing therapy, mindfulness-based stress reduction vs. anxiolytic medication). In such instances, the alternative or comparison should be specified whenever possible. Oftentimes, however, the comparison may be no treatment or intervention at all (i.e., maintain status quo), which is the case in our example.

The fourth major component of a clinically focused question is to identify the outcome of interest. Even though this often serves as the starting point in formulating a question (e.g., What's the goal?), it is important to ensure that an articulated, operationalized, and realistic goal has been clearly specified. Doing so not only clarifies the goal, but also helps frame the scope and trajectory of intervention. For example, the outcome of interest in one study may be delay of cognitive decline or prevention of dementia, whereas in another study, the outcome of interest may be restoration of cognitive functioning or increasing functional independence. Each of these goals may be applicable to similar patient populations and comparable interventions, but reflect inversely related outcomes (i.e., reducing odds of adverse outcome vs. increasing odds of beneficial outcome). As will be shown later, this has particular relevance for the metrics derived from CAT analysis.

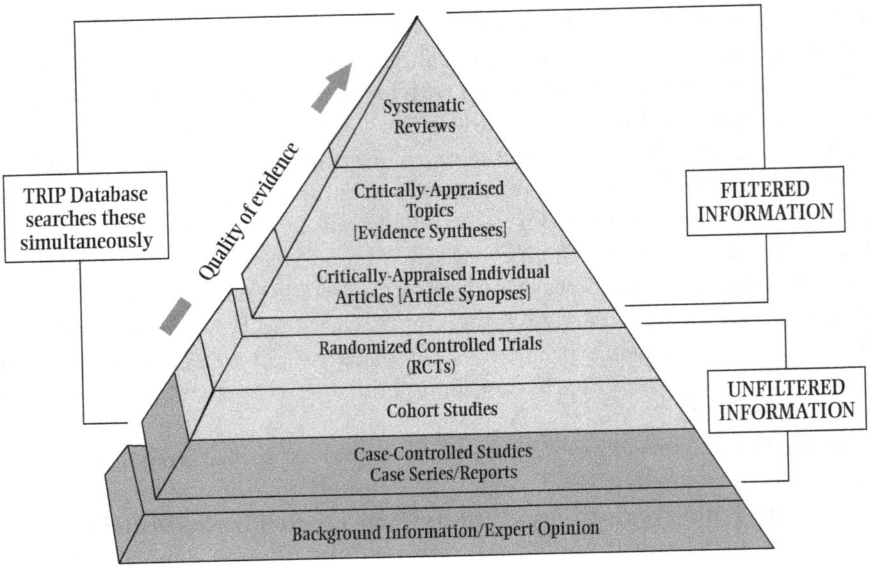

Figure 12.1 Levels of empirical evidence. EBM Pyramid and EBM Page Generator, (c) 2006 Trustees of Dartmouth College and Yale University. All rights reserved. Produced by Jan Glover, David Izzo, Karen Odato, and Lei Wang.

Depending on the nature of the question, an additional component of the PICO method is added that focuses on the study design (PICOS). For evaluating an individual intervention, a randomized controlled trial (RCT) is the highest level of evidence and should be used whenever possible. In the event that an RCT is not available, every effort should be made to find the next-best level of evidence and subsequently note the limited nature of available evidence (see Figure 12.1).

To tie all of this together, the PICO-based question derived from our clinical scenario would read: "A 72-year-old college-educated man with memory difficulty (patient and problem) is interested to know whether engaging in a computer-based cognitive training program (intervention) will help maintain cognitive and memory functioning over time (outcome) better than simple maintenance of an active lifestyle (comparison)." As can be seen in this example, the order of PICO components matters not, as long as each of the main elements are there. The increased level of specificity in this question should be readily apparent, and from this focused question, search terms and keywords can easily be derived to guide subsequent literature searches (e.g., "memory," "computer," and "cognitive training").

SYSTEMATICALLY RETRIEVING BEST AVAILABLE EVIDENCE

Once a question has been established, and potential search terms are identified, the next step is to identify the best available evidence that not only will address the clinical question of interest, but is also amenable to CAT analysis. Given the constantly expanding body of empirical literature, finding a relevant intervention study may not prove to be very challenging with utilization of available literature resources, particularly for more common clinical questions. Finding a study that provides the necessary data points for CAT analysis, however, can prove to be much more difficult. Published studies vary considerably in quality and completeness of reporting, and although reporting guidelines (e.g., Consolidated Standards of Reporting Trials: CONSORT) help promote comprehensive reporting, adherence to reporting guidelines is not consistent across publications. The difficulty in finding a high-quality well-reported study that contains the necessary data for CAT analysis should not be misconstrued as a shortcoming of the CAT method, however. Rather, it highlights the importance of proper reporting and the value in adherence to reporting guidelines in manuscript preparation.

One of the core tenets of EBP is that clinical decisions should be informed by the best available scientific evidence. Within the empirical literature, there are varying levels of scientific evidence, which can be arranged hierarchically (see Figure 12.1; also http://www.dartmouth.edu/~biomed/resources.htmld/guides/ebm_psych_resources.html or http://guides.library.harvard.edu/hms/ebm). Broadly defined, studies and empirical evidence can be classified as either "filtered" or "unfiltered" information. Filtered information is evidence that has been systematically screened and reviewed according to a prescribed methodology that seeks to assess the quality of the study. Because these sources have already been evaluated for quality, and often aggregated (e.g., meta-analysis), filtered evidence is often regarded as a higher level of evidence (http://www.cebm.net/ocebm-levels-of-evidence/). When available, filtered evidence should be used in CAT analysis. Examples include systematic review, with or without meta-analysis, as well as individual and aggregated critically appraised topics.

Unfiltered evidence is derived from original, peer-reviewed research papers such as those composing the primary literature, and it is generally considered a lower tier of evidence than filtered studies. RCTs, cohort and cross-sectional studies, archival studies, and case reports are all examples of unfiltered evidence, as the quality of these reports has not been vetted beyond the initial peer-review process. This is not to say that the quality of the evidence obtained from unfiltered evidence is poor. Rather, because the information reflects a primary analysis of the original data without additional scrutiny, it is generally considered less stringent. Primary studies such as these typically serve as the foundation from which the filtered evidence-base is derived.

With the availability of digital repositories, gone are the days of clinicians buried in the library stacks, manually searching through tables of contents, journal-by-journal, issue-by-issue. The increased accessibility of such vast collections of empirical evidence has been a tremendous boon for EBP. Perhaps the most well-known portal is PubMed, which is a free, online, searchable database that includes the MEDLINE database and is maintained by the National Center for Biotechnology Information (NCBI) at the United States National Library of Medicine (NLM; National Library of Medicine, 2014b). PubMed made its debut in 1996 (Canese, 2006), which coincides with one of the earliest published definitions of evidence-based medicine (i.e., Sackett et al., 1996). Articles within PubMed are indexed using Medical Subject Headings (MeSH) terms, which is a standardized language that utilizes a hierarchical organization of terms with increasing specificity that is intended to facilitate literature searches (National Library of Medicine, 2014a). PubMed contains both filtered and unfiltered data, and while the individual articles indexed in PubMed are not reviewed, the publishing journals indexed in PubMed must meet minimum criteria as set forth by the Literature Selection Technical Review Committee of the NLM. Therefore, the quality of individual articles retrieved directly through PubMed must be evaluated directly by the clinician.

The Cochrane Library is another online repository, published by the Cochrane Collaboration, an independent, multidisciplinary agency with a primary mission of "promot[ing] evidence-informed health decision-making by producing high-quality, relevant, accessible systematic reviews and other synthesized research evidence" (Cochrane Collaboration, 2014b). The systematic reviews in the Cochrane Library each address a clearly focused question targeted at health care interventions, and are regarded as some of the highest-quality filtered evidence available (Masic, Miokovic, & Muhamedagic, 2008). For CAT analysis of an intervention study, the Cochrane Library should be one of the earliest starting points, if not the first, in the literature search. As of early 2014, there were over 5,000 reviews published in the Cochrane Library (Cochrane Collaboration, 2014a), and the Library is updated on a regular basis as new reviews are added.

Yet another online tool for identifying research evidence is the Turning Research into Practice (TRIP) database. Although not a repository of evidence in and of itself, the TRIP database provides a search engine specifically designed to allow clinicians to easily search a multitude of evidence repositories using a single interface (www.tripdatabase.com). The TRIP site provides results from both filtered and unfiltered evidence, with the type of evidence clearly identified (e.g., systematic review, clinical trial, primary research) in the search results list. An added benefit of the TRIP database is the integration of a PICO-based search interface, which readily facilitates identification of high-quality evidence for CAT analysis. Between these and other search resources, employment of an appropriate and efficient search strategy is likely to yield evidence addressing the clinical question of interest, should such evidence exist. Although this is beyond the scope of this chapter, developing sound practices for reviewing the available literature, including a familiarity with the MeSH terminology, can certainly be helpful in conducting a targeted and efficient search (www.nlm.nih.gov/mesh/MBrowser.html). Utilizing Boolean operators (i.e., AND, OR, and NOT) to combine search terms is also beneficial and will aid in generating refined search results.

As previously mentioned, however, while it may be possible to find evidence that answers the specific clinical question, it may not be sufficient or amenable to CAT analysis. Specific data points are required to establish the relevant event rates in both treatment and comparison conditions, and while these are not unusual values to include in a paper, the quality of reporting varies tremendously among published studies, and these data can oftentimes prove elusive. For this reason, several specific sets of reporting guidelines have been developed, each of which targets a specific type of publication. Perhaps most relevant to neuropsychological interventions is the Consolidated Standards of Reporting Trials (CONSORT) statement, which includes a participant flowchart (Schulz, Altman, & Moher, 2010) and has been reviewed for neuropsychological studies (Miller, Schoenberg, & Bilder, 2014). Also of interest, the Preferred Reporting Items for Systematic Reviews and Meta-Analysis (PRISMA) statement (Moher, Liberati, Tetzlaff, & Altman, 2009) includes relevant points for inclusion in systematic reviews and meta-analysis. These checklists contain the minimum necessary criteria for transparent reporting of research findings, and are more and more becoming required components for publication. In order to complete a CAT analysis, for example, categorical outcome data must be readily available or able to be determined, as these data provide the basis for calculation of risk-reduction (RR), number-needed-to-treat (NNT), and related critical appraisal metrics. Adherence to the CONSORT statement will ensure that these data are readily reported, as a participant flowchart is required. In some studies, these data will be readily available and explicitly reported. In others, these values may need to be calculated (e.g., when the outcome is reported as a percentage of participants). Hence, when identifying evidence, seeking out studies that adhere to reporting guidelines can facilitate CAT analysis. Additional information on reporting guidelines is available through the Equator Network (www.equator-network.org), and readers are strongly encouraged to familiarize themselves with this information.

As has been previously mentioned, a core component of EBP is that the best available evidence is used. Figure 12.1 provides a general hierarchical framework, and several grading systems have been developed to further facilitate rapid assessment of evidence quality. Perhaps one of the most well-known is that from the Oxford Centre for Evidence-Based Medicine (CEBM), which provides a five-step model for various clinical questions (Howick et al., 2011). For all but prevalence studies, a systematic review is considered Level 1 evidence (http://www.cebm.net/ocebm-levels-of-evidence/). For an intervention study, a single RCT is considered Level 2 data, and a non-randomized trial is considered Level 3. The Grading of Recommendations Assessment, Development and Evaluation (GRADE) Working Group is another example of an international collaboration that has led to the development of a well-established method for grading the quality of evidence (www.gradeworkinggroup.org/index.htm). It is important to use the highest level of evidence available when conducting a CAT analysis, as the quality of output from critical appraisal is directly tied to the quality of input. However, as an aside, a common misunderstanding of the CAT process is that a successful CAT is only one that finds relevant, high-quality evidence. In fact, this is not the only purpose of a CAT. A successful CAT finds and evaluates the best available evidence, whether that evidence is derived from a high-quality study or a poor-quality study, or even no study at all. The outcome of the CAT is then to provide the clinician undertaking the CAT with an informed evaluation of the best available evidence, which may include the conclusion that there is no good evidence bearing on a particular question. Alternatively, it may be concluded that the best available evidence is derived form a poor-quality study that should not be relied upon to guide clinical practice.

To continue with our example, an initial search of the Cochrane Library returned no results (searched: June 20, 2015). Turning to PubMed to find a high-quality, well-reported systematic review of computerized cognitive training returned several results, though none were sufficiently reported to allow CAT analysis. Working down the evidence ladder, a single RCT was sought next. Search terms included: *cognitive training AND older adults* (note the use of the Boolean operator "and" to refine the search to results including both terms). Search filters applied were: *clinical trial, published in the last 5 years, studying humans*, and *published in English*. These search criteria returned 291 results. Titles and abstracts were initially reviewed, and promising articles were reviewed in detail (exemplifying the importance of a good title!). The 10-year update of the Advanced Cognitive Training for Independent and Vital Elderly (ACTIVE) cognitive training trial by Rebok et al. (2014) was identified as a relevant study and was selected for further CAT analysis. It is considered Level 2 evidence per the Oxford CEBM system, which, given the lack of a systematic review, was the highest level of evidence available at the time of the search (http://www.cebm.net/ocebm-levels-of-evidence/). The ACTIVE trial was one of the largest RCTs to date of cognitive training in older adults (n = 2,832; ages 65–94). Targeted cognitive domains included in the intervention were memory, processing speed, and reasoning and the comparison group was a no-contact control group (Ball et al., 2002). Further review of the paper found that categorical outcomes could be calculated from the data presented, thereby making this study useful for full CAT analysis.

CRITICALLY APPRAISE THE EVIDENCE: ARE THE RESULTS OF THIS STUDY VALID?

Once a relevant study has been identified, which is useful for CAT analysis, the process of critical appraisal begins. The initial step is to determine whether or not the study was executed with sufficient methodological rigor such that that the obtained findings and conclusions can be considered valid and reliable. Several checklists have been developed towards this end, which are designed to systematically evaluate whether or not the core components of a well-designed trial are present. Examples of checklists are available from several online resources, and each varies slightly in format and finer content points, though the primary components are similar and based on the most important elements of CONSORT criteria. Regardless of the checklist used, including an objective methodological review in the final CAT summary is strongly recommended for later reference.

When appraising an intervention trial, an initial point of determination is to establish whether or not participants were assigned to treatment groups at random. True randomization, when carried out effectively, methodologically minimizes potential biases relating to the risk of systematic differences between groups prior to the intervention that may threaten the internal validity of a study (see Cook & Campbell, 1979). Randomization also facilitates effective blinding of group membership (i.e., treatment vs. control) to study participants and experimenters, which further increases the internal validity of a trial. When reviewing an RCT, particularly those in which blinding was carried out, it should also be noted whether or not group membership was effectively concealed for the duration of the study. For many psychological and neuropsychological trials, however, blinding and concealment are not feasible, and in some instances, neither is true randomization, although blinding of outcome assessors is often feasible. These real-world compromises increase the importance of independent replication and careful control of treatment variables.

Of equal importance to the internal validity of a study, group characteristics of independent and non-experimental variables (e.g., demographic factors, health status, etc.) must be comparable at the start of the trial, before intervention. With proper randomization and sufficiently large samples, differences at baseline are less likely, but they may not be completely eliminated. In the event that differences exist prior to the intervention, they must be accounted for in subsequent analyses and clearly documented. An important point of note, only if a truly randomized study is not available or not feasible should a non-randomized trial be used for CAT analysis (Straus, Glasziou, Richardson, & Haynes, 2011). Whether or not randomization was used, and what kind (e.g., simple, blocked, matched), should be reported within the Methods section of a publication (if not the title or abstract), especially those adhering to CONSORT guidelines (Schulz, Altman, & Moher, 2010).

When developing an intervention trial, an important part of the experimental design is to find a balance between retaining study participants and allowing enough time to let any effects of treatment manifest. For example, a behavioral intervention targeting development of academic-study skills for adult college students with traumatic brain injury may take a semester, if not an entire year or longer, to demonstrate an effect. If the initial follow-up assessment is too soon, treatment effects may not be apparent or relevant, leading to a false-negative error. Thus, when reviewing papers, it is important to consider whether or not the length of time between intervention and follow-up assessments was long enough.

Subject attrition is also a critical component. While follow-up intervals need to be sufficient to allow treatment effects to manifest, it is also important to consider the amount of subject attrition over the course of a trial. Properly reported trials adhering to reporting guidelines will include these data, usually in a flowchart, which is a required component of CONSORT guidelines. If there has been a considerable degree of subject attrition over the course of a trial, it should raise concerns about possible biases complicating interpretation of the intervention, and additional analyses should have been conducted in order to explore any systematic differences between those who completed the intervention as designed (i.e., completers) and those who did not (i.e., non-completers). An added point of consideration is to discern whether or not the subjects were analyzed using an intention-to-treat (ITT) analysis (i.e., Were subjects analyzed according to the original randomization schedule and sample numbers, regardless of attrition?), or was a per-protocol analysis used (i.e., Were only subjects completing the entire trial retained in the final analysis?). Both approaches have their strengths and weakness, the discussion of which is beyond the scope of the present chapter, however, ITT analyses generally are preferred for superiority trials (i.e., those demonstrating the superiority of an intervention over another control condition: Gupta, 2011), and therefore are preferable for most CAT analyses.

If a per-protocol (completers) analysis was used, then ensuring that participants who completed the trial were analyzed according to the groups in which they were assigned and not just the group in which they finished the trial is also critical, as significant breaks in randomization assignment have the risk of introducing systematic group differences that were minimized via the original randomization. Although it would be unusual in a well-designed and carefully executed study, ITT analysis is important in trials where subjects were inadvertently randomized to the wrong group, or if participants crossed from one group to another. Making sure that, aside from the intervention itself, each of the study groups was treated comparably throughout the trial (e.g., same assessment time points and measures, similar interaction with study team members) is also important, as any systematic differences introduce bias, threatening the internal validity.

Continuing with the example, the study by Rebok et al. (2014) is clearly a randomized trial, and the comparison of baseline factors finds that the groups were, indeed, comparable at the outset of the trial after randomization. A small number of patients were incorrectly randomized and thus excluded from final analyses, however, the substantial majority of participants completed the trial as randomized. Given the adherence to CONSORT guidelines, a flowchart is provided within the published manuscript that clearly documents subject attrition, which appears minimal over the course of the trial (Rebok et al., 2014, Figure 1, p. 19). The treatment follow-up period of ten years is also most certainly an adequate time-frame to establish any effects. Participants were compared according to the groups they were assigned to, and groups were treated equally across the trial. Thus, although there was a small break in randomization at the outset of the intervention (1% of eligible sample), these individuals were excluded from analysis, and the remainder of the methodology is sound and of sufficient rigor that the obtained findings are considered valid. CAT analysis can proceed with confidence that the retrieved article is of high methods quality.

ARE THESE VALID RESULTS IMPORTANT?

Once the validity of the methodology has been established, quantitative data need to be extracted in order to critically evaluate the reported study outcomes. In order to do so, a 2 x 2 matrix of categorical outcomes needs to be created, which will allow the calculation of the relevant event rates. A sample matrix is presented in Table 12.1, which shows the required information for each of the

Table 12.1 Sample 2 x 2 Outcomes Matrix

	Outcome of Interest	**Did Not Meet Outcome**	**Group Total**
Treatment Group	A	B	(A + B) = Treatment *n*
Control Group	C	D	(C + D) = Control *n*

four cells. Note that each cell represents a unique group of participants, there should be no overlap in membership between cells. As previously mentioned, this can be far easier said than done, as these data are not always explicitly presented. Even for studies with high-quality methods, should these data not be available in the report, this would be a valid stopping point for further CAT analysis. Thus, without proper and thorough reporting, studies rated highly for methods quality can still produce less interpretable data.

Although these data may be directly reported in some papers, in others they may be more elusive. For examples, in the paper reviewed here, the research participants meeting outcome criteria are reported in terms of a percentage (found in Rebok et al., 2014, their Table 2, p. 21), thereby requiring working backwards to calculate the exact number of participants who met outcome criteria (note that, for this particular purpose, however, reporting percentages in this manner can facilitate CAT analysis, discussed later). When determining these values, it is very important to keep in mind the specific outcome of interest, and whether or not it is beneficial or harmful. In the Rebok et al. paper, the reported values relate to the categorical outcome variable of the number of people who remained "at or above baseline" (i.e., remained stable) over the course of the 10-year interval, which would be considered a benefit. If, however, the outcome of interest was cognitive decline (as is the case in the presently worked example), a further calculation would be necessary to establish the risk of harm, defined as cognitive decline. This highlights the importance of remaining mindful of the outcome of interest.

For both the treatment group and the control group, event rates need to be calculated for the outcome of interest. These are simply the proportion of individuals demonstrating the outcome of interest out of the total number of participants in the respective group, expressed as a percentage (this is why the use of percentages in the Rebok et al., 2014, paper is beneficial; see their Table 2, p. 21) or decimal proportion. In the case of an ITT analysis, the event rates are the proportion of people showing the outcome out of the total number of people randomized to that treatment condition. Referencing Table 12.1, the value in cell C represents the percentage of individuals in the control group who satisfy outcome criteria. Dividing this value by the total number of individuals in the control group renders the Control Event Rate (CER). An analogous value is calculated for the treatment, or experimental, group, referred to as the Experimental Event Rate (EER). The corresponding value in Table 12.1 would be the value of cell A divided by the total number of individuals in the experimental group (A/A + B). The CER and EER serve as the foundation of CAT analysis for a treatment study and are utilized to derive the remaining statistics. In any given intervention study, there will be an event rate associated with each of the treatment conditions, as well as for each control condition. The Rebok et al. (2014) paper, for example, would yield three EERs and three CERs (one experimental event rate and control event rate for each of the memory training, reasoning training, and processing-speed training conditions).

Using the calculated event rates, the extent of reduction in risk of the outcome can then be calculated in both absolute and relative terms, which is then used to determine the number of individuals to treat before an outcome is expected (for details of formula, see Straus et al., 2011). The Absolute Risk Reduction (ARR) is simply the extent to which an individual's risk of the outcome is reduced from receiving the treatment. ARR is the absolute value of the difference between the EER and the CER, that is, (|CER − EER|) (Straus et al., 2011). The Relative Risk Reduction (RRR) is an extension of the ARR, calculated as a function of the overall prevalence of the outcome in the specific control group studied. RRR is calculated by dividing the ARR by the CER and represents the reduced risk associated with the specific intervention in comparison to those who received the alternative treatment. Depending on the outcome of interest, relative and absolute risk can also be thought of as "beneficial" (i.e., relative benefit increase; absolute benefit increase). This would be applicable for desirable outcomes in which the standard of care is improvement in functioning (e.g., maintenance of functional independence), as opposed to prevention of an adverse event (e.g., transition to assisted living). In the example study, if we were to utilize the event rates reported directly in the paper as being good outcomes (i.e., the percentage of individuals remaining at or above baseline at follow-up), the resulting event rates would lead to calculation of the relative benefit increase and absolute benefit increase.

The Number Needed to Treat (NTT) is the inverse of the ARR (i.e., dividing 1 by the ARR) and provides an indication of the number of people who would need to receive the treatment in order to prevent one additional harmful or undesirable outcome (Straus et al., 2011). The NNT is reported as a whole number and is expressed relative to the length of time represented by the study. In the ACTIVE trial, for example, the resulting NNT would reflect the number of individuals who would need to be treated in a 10-year period (as this was the length of follow-up) in order to prevent one additional undesirable outcome defined in terms of deterioration from baseline. The duration of intervention introduces an added calculation when comparing CAT analyses and NNTs between multiple interventions. Unless the studies were completed in the same amount of time, one of the two time intervals will need to be adjusted by using the shorter period as a scale factor in an effort to mathematically account for the difference in length. As shown in Straus et al. (2011; p. 84): NNT (hypothetical) = NNT (observed) x (observed time/hypothetical time). In general, smaller NTT values are preferable, though there is no universal standard for what is considered acceptable. Utilizing clinical expertise, individual costs and burdens associated with the treatment, and the severity of the outcome that is to be prevented are all factors that should be considered when evaluating NNTs, and doing so requires careful consideration.

As with most neuropsychological measures, the risk reduction statistics and NNT values calculated should not be considered precise estimates, but rather a foundation on which a confidence interval (CI) can be constructed that will contain the true value. CIs can and should be calculated for both event rates, as well as the NNT, for clinical decision-making. These are typically calculated as a 95% CI and interpreted much the same way as any other CI in clinical practice. When determining the significance of an effect, if the 95% CI built around RRR or ARR includes zero, it cannot be said with any certainty that the treatment is associated with any reliable reduction in risk over the control group. The formula for calculating the CI is long and complex, and it is advisable to use an online calculator or CAT maker (for example: www.cebm.net/catmaker-ebm-calculators) to calculate the CIs in order to reduce the possibility of calculation errors.

To calculate the relevant statistics for the ACTIVE trial, we will focus initially on the memory intervention training, as this is an intervention of primary interest for our hypothetical patient. As previously mentioned, the reporting of percentages by Rebok et al. facilitates CAT analysis, as the event rates for cognitive stability are reported directly. For our purposes, we are using cognitive decline as the outcome of interest to facilitate interpretation as a reduction in risk. Thus, we simply need to use the remaining percentage of participants as our event rates, which reflect the proportion of people with memory decline in the respective treatment and control groups.

Memory Training: Completers or Per-Protocol Analysis

Based on the values reported by Rebok and colleagues in their Table 2, we see that 35.9% of participants in the memory training group who were assessed at 10-year follow-up ($n = 300$: see their Figure 1) remained at or above baseline. We can therefore infer that the remaining 64.1% demonstrated cognitive decline, which would be our memory intervention EER for the completers (i.e., the people who stayed in the study until the 10-year follow-up). If we were to calculate the raw frequency outcomes by group, we can determine that 108 (35.9% of 300) people remained cognitively stable and 192 (64.1% of 300) declined, based on the reported number of completers in the memory-training group. Had raw frequency outcomes been reported, we would simply divide 192 by the analyzed sample size to calculate the same EER. In the control group, 31.0% of the assessed completers ($n = 285$: see their Figure 1) remained stable and 69.0% declined, which translates to 88 stable and 197 declined, respectively. The completed 2 x 2 matrix is presented in Table 12.2. Note that we are undertaking a completers analysis here. An example ITT analysis will be described below.

Using the event rates shown in Table 12.2, the ARR for the memory training is 5.1%, the RRR is 7.0%, and the NNT is 20 (i.e., 1/0.051 = 19.6, rounded). Note that it is always advisable to enter raw frequency data into the calculator to get the correct CIs (Straus et al., 2011). Using the Oxford CEBM calculator

Table 12.2 Completed 2 x 2 Matrix for 10-Year Follow-up on the Memory Outcome Measure for the ACTIVE Trial (from Rebok et al., 2014)

	Cognitive Stability	**Cognitive Decline**	**Completers Total**
Treatment Group	108	192	300
Control Group	88	197	285

referenced previously, estimating a 95% CI around the ARR, however, reveals a range from -0.03% to 12.7%. Because this range spans zero, we cannot say with certainty that there is any statistically significant benefit from memory treatment (Straus et al., 2011). The 95% CI for RRR also spans zero, leading to the same conclusion, that there is no statistically significant risk reduction. In these circumstances, further examination of the NNT is not necessary, because the risk reduction analysis does not allow us to reject the null hypothesis of no risk reduction. However, the 95% CI around the NNT probably would include infinity as one boundary, meaning that we would have to treat an infinite number of people to avoid one additional person with memory decline, obviously an ineffective treatment (Straus et al., 2011).

Speed Training: Completers Analysis

For comparison sake, calculating the same statistics for the processing-speed training intervention shows a more beneficial result. The CER of decline for completers in the processing-speed group is 52.2% (149 of 285 completers), and the EER is 29.3% (93 of 319 completers) at 10-year follow-up (see Rebok et al., 2014, their Figure 1). At this point, it is clear that the treatment resulted in a much lower rate of decline than the control group, which can be explored further. Again, using the CEBM CATmaker, the RRR is 43.7%, and the ARR is 22.9%, with a CI of 15.2%–30.6%. The NNT in this example is 4 (i.e., 1/.229 = 4.4, rounded), with a CI of 3–7. We can therefore say with 95% confidence that we would need to treat between three and seven individuals over a 10-year period in order to prevent one person from showing the specified decline in information-processing speed. Had we calculated the same set of statistics using cognitive stability as the outcome of interest rather than decline, the resulting 2 x 2 matrix would have been inverted and led to negative values for the ARR and RRR. Doing so is perfectly valid, and given the desirability of the outcome (i.e., cognitive stability), we would interpret these values as a relative and absolute *benefit increase* (Straus et al., 2011).

Speed Training: Intention-to-Treat Analysis

An alternative and recommended approach to the risk-reduction analysis is to undertake an ITT analysis. An ITT analysis is recommended as part of the CONSORT guidelines (Gupta, 2011). To undertake an ITT analysis, we need to calculate the event rate, not, as was done in the preceding sections, as a proportion of those who completed the study, but as a proportion of the people who were randomized at the commencement of the study. At the beginning of the study, 704 people were randomized to the control condition and 712 to the Speed Training condition (see Rebok et al., 2014, Figure 1). Therefore, an ITT analysis that assumed that all those lost to follow-up were treatment successes (stable) could estimate the CER as 149 declined out of 704 randomized to the control condition, or .212. The EER would be 93 declined out of 712 randomized to the Speed Training condition, or .131. These event rates lead to RRR = .38 (95% CI: .20 – .57), an ARR of .081 (95% CI: .042 – .120), and an NNT = 12 (95% CI: 8–24). Fortunately, the ITT analysis still leads to the inference of an effective treatment, although the NNT of 12 is not as impressive as the NNT of 4 reported from the Speed Training completers analysis in the previous section.

This approach is just one of several possible "imputation" methods for ITT, in the above example, where all missing data are assumed to have not experienced the event. In the case of the Rebok et al. study, this approach assumes that all missing cases were good outcomes (stable) in all conditions, including the control group. The Oxford CEBM CATmaker calculator estimates an ITT analysis in the same way. See Gupta (2011) and the Cochrane Handbook (http://handbook.cochrane.org/chapter_16/16_2_2_intention_to_treat_issues_for_dichotomous_data.htm) for discussion of pros and cons of various alternative approaches to ITT analysis.

TRANSLATING RESULTS TO THE INDIVIDUAL PATIENT

Once the event rates and NNT have been established for a given study, we next need to determine whether or not the valid, important results are applicable to our individual patient or population. When integrated with clinical expertise and individual patient values and preferences, the direct utilization of empirical evidence to guide clinical decisions forms the core of EBP. Clinical expertise comes from training and research-guided knowledge acquisition (Haynes, 2002), and the CAT method helps us identify and evaluate the best available evidence and translate it into meaningful metrics. How then, does this information get integrated with the individual values and preferences of our patient or population?

As a CAT analysis is completed, it is important to consider the extent to which the participants in the study are comparable to our patient or population of interest. Reviewing the demographic factors, as well as any injury or disease characteristics, is certainly important. It would be of little use to conduct a CAT on an intervention for survivors of traumatic brain injury if our population or patient of interest has suffered a stroke. Being mindful of whether or not the intervention is even feasible in the treatment setting and for the patient is also important. If not, it may be of little use to make a recommendation that cannot be realistically implemented. Weighing the costs of treatment against any potential benefits, in the context of the patient's expected outcomes and preferences, is also important. Bearing in mind availability of resources and the palatability of an intervention for a patient can readily influence adherence. Failure to do so may increase the odds of a poor outcome.

An important caveat of the NNT is that it does not account for individual patient factors affecting risk. The NNT reflects the probabilities of risk-reduction in a population similar to that included in the study subject to appraisal. To refine CAT analysis even further, the NNT can be custom-tailored to account for a patient's individual level of risk. This is done by comparing the individual patient to the control group on the basis of individual characteristics, which is expressed as the decimal f_t. A value of 1.0 implies that the patient has a chance of benefit from treatment comparable to that of the average control patient. A value of 2.0 would indicate double the chances of benefit, and a value of 0.5 signifies half the chance of benefit. Assigning f_t values is certainly not a precise science and draws heavily on clinical acumen and expertise. Dividing the study NNT by our patient's individual risk can be used as a more refined estimate of individual risk for a particular patient. The degree of individualization can only go so far, and there is no clear restriction on the size of the f_t value. However, if considerable adjustment is necessary, it raises the question of whether the reviewed study is appropriate. Unless the appraised study has previously been determined to be the absolute best available, if there are drastic differences between a patient and the control group, it may be best to try to find a study of more comparable participants.

In the case of our patient, he is of similar age and educational background to the average of the control group. However, recall that he has two first-degree relatives with dementia, which increases his risk at least twofold (Cupples, Farrer, Sadovnick, Relkin, Whitehouse, & Green, 2004). Although typically there would be no reason to calculate any additional CAT statistics for an intervention that is not associated with a significant risk reduction (in this case, the memory-training intervention), we will proceed with our example for continuity and illustration purposes.

By dividing the NNT from the memory-training group in our study by 2.0 (our patient's individual chance of benefit), we arrive at an individual NNT of 10. For the processing-speed training, the revised completers NNT is 2. Thus, we would need to treat 10 higher-risk people like our patient for 10 years with the study's memory-training intervention to prevent one of them from declining in memory. In other words, our patient has a 1 in 10 chance, or 10% likelihood, of benefitting from the memory treatment. Contrasted to the processing-speed intervention, where our patient has a 50% chance of maintaining his processing-speed ability should he undergo treatment, the odds that his memory will improve or remain stable are much, much lower. Our patient clearly has a preference for cognitive training, and implementation is feasible. Results from our CAT analysis suggest that there may be benefits for processing speed. However, our patient's expectation is to improve his memory functioning, where results from this study yield equivocal findings. Armed with these data from our complete CAT analysis, we can now provide our patient with information that is much more informative (e.g., percentages, odds, NNTs, etc.).

Using Completed CATs

Once a CAT has been completed in a specific study, it should certainly be saved for future reference. A single-page summary, documenting each of the aforementioned steps, presenting the quantitative outcomes and relevant event rates, and conclusions drawn should be prepared as part of the appraisal, and formatted worksheets are readily available to facilitate archiving (see Oxford CEBM site referenced previously). In addition to the event rates and NNT values, a succinct clinical conclusion should be stated, as well as any caveats. It is also important that the summary include the citation of the article and who completed the CAT analysis, as well as an expiration date. Specifying an expiration date will help ensure that only current evidence is used for clinical decision making. By archiving completed CATs, a repository of evidence will accumulate that can be quickly referenced when a similar clinical scenario is encountered, facilitating EBP.

While the current number of published CATs is limited, this is a remediable situation. With the simplicity of CAT analysis, updating reporting guidelines to require a completed CAT analysis with each published RCT is one feasible solution. Doing so would also move away from the limitations associated with using alpha levels below a minimum threshold and mean group differences. Creating a venue for publishing CATs is also warranted, as doing so would not only facilitate publication, it would simultaneously create a searchable repository of completed CATs that could be used by many clinicians, comparable to searching the empirical literature.

As an alternative to a repository of completed CATs, a collaborative knowledgebase of published categorical outcomes could be generated from current and future clinical trials that would allow individual CATs to be completed on the basis of patient parameters entered by clinicians. For example, a clinician could enter the demographic and clinical data for a given patient, and results returned would include several NNTs that are automatically generated. Individual risk factors could also be automatically accounted for, and adjusting for time differences between CATs (i.e., scaling the NNT) automated to facilitate comparison between interventions. Essentially, such an automated CAT maker would operate based on individual patient parameters, which could be used to custom-tailor evidence-based recommendations.

Limitations of CAT Analysis

While the critical appraisal has numerous strengths, it is not without limitations. Perhaps the most notable is that CAT analysis suffers considerably from the lack of generalizability to patients and populations beyond those in the particular study. With the sometimes highly stringent inclusion and exclusion criteria used in RCTs, it can be difficult to make the leap from the participants in the study to our individual patients, who are more often than not going to present with more complex clinical situations than the ideal patients studied. Use of individual risk adjustments can help with this problem of generalizability to some extent, but this method can only do so much. It goes without saying that continued research on new interventions and with diverse populations is one way to address this issue, but certainly it is not feasible to study every possible clinical presentation or intervention available. Improving reporting of current research, however, would at least allow greater application of CAT methods to more of the research that does get published.

Another limitation is that there is currently a very limited number of published CATs available. Although completing a CAT requires minimal time and effort, especially with the use of automated calculators, very few individual CATs have been formally published. This may be due in part to the lack of a publishing forum, but it is also likely to be related to their relatively low utilization, particularly among the behavioral sciences. Not only does this decrease awareness of critical appraisal methods, without regular dissemination or a searchable repository, when practitioners complete a CAT on a study that has already been appraised, they are engaging in redundant work.

SUMMARY AND CONCLUSIONS

The previous review of critical appraisal methods is intended to shed light on what can be a powerful clinical tool, and presents an additional method of evaluating the empirical literature. Viewing results in the form of specific event rates and translating them into the likelihood of a reduction in risk or increase in benefit places study findings in a very different light than standard significance testing for mean differences between groups. Even in studies in which statistically reliable mean differences are found between groups, critical appraisal using categorical outcomes and event rates can lead one to draw considerably different conclusions. When critical appraisal methods consistently serve as the basis for making treatment recommendations and are integrated with clinical expertise and the individual values, preferences, and expectations of patients, evidence-based practice becomes a routine component of clinical practice and, over time, and should lead to better patient outcomes.

REFERENCES

APA Presidential Task Force. (2006). Evidence-based practice in psychology. *American Psychologist, 61*(4), 271–285. doi:10.1037/0003-066x.61.4.271

Ball, K., Berch, D. B., Helmers, K. F., Jobe, J. B., Leveck, M. D., Marsiske, M., . . . Willis, S. L. (2002). Effects of cognitive training interventions with older adults: A randomized controlled trial. *Journal of the American Medical Association, 288*(18), 2271–2281.

Canese, K. (2006). PubMed celebrates its 10th anniversary! *NLM Tech Bulletin, Sep–Oct*(352), e5.

Chambless, D. L., & Hollon, S. D. (1998). Defining empirically supported therapies. *Journal of Consulting and Clinical Psychology, 66*(1), 7–18.

Cochrane Collaboration. (2014a, May 26, 2014). *Cochrane Database of Systematic Reviews in Numbers.* Retrieved June 20, 2015, from http://community.cochrane.org/cochrane-reviews/cochrane-database-systematic-reviews-numbers.

Cochrane Collaboration. (2014b, March 31, 2015). *Cochrane Organizational Policy Manual.* Retrieved June 20, 2015, from http://community.cochrane.org/organisational-policy-manual.

Cook, T. D., & Campbell, D. T. (1979). *Quasi-Experimentation: Design and Analysis for Field Settings.* Boston, MA: Houghton Mifflin.

Cupples, L. A., Farrer, L. A., Sadovnick, A. D., Relkin, N., Whitehouse, P., & Green, R. C. (2004). Estimating risk curves for first-degree relatives of patients with Alzheimer's disease: The REVEAL study. *Genetics in Medicine, 6*(4), 192–196. Retrieved from http://dx.doi.org/10.1097/01.GIM.0000132679.92238.58.

Gupta, S. K. (2011). Intention-to-treat concept: A review. *Perspectives on Clinical Research, 2*(3), 109–112.

Howick, J., Chalmers, I., Glasziou, P., Greenhalgh, T., Heneghan, C., Liberati, A., . . . Thornton, H. (2011). *The 2011 Oxford CEBM Evidence Levels of Evidence (Introductory Document).* Retrieved June 22, 2015, from http://www.cebm.net/ocebm-levels-of-evidence/.

National Library of Medicine. (2014a, June 18, 2015). *Fact Sheets: MeSH.* Retrieved June 20, 2015, from http://www.nlm.nih.gov/pubs/factsheets/mesh.html.

National Library of Medicine. (2014b, August 26, 2014). *Fact Sheets: PubMed.* Retrieved June 20, 2015, from http://www.nlm.nih.gov/pubs/factsheets/pubmed.html.

Masic, I., Miokovic, M., & Muhamedagic, B. (2008). Evidence based medicine—New approaches and challenges. *Acta Informatica Medica, 16*(4), 219–225. http://doi.org/10.5455/aim.

Miller, J. B., Schoenberg, M. R., & Bilder, R. M. (2014). Consolidated Standards of Reporting Trials (CONSORT): Considerations for neuropsychological research. *The Clinical Neuropsychologist, 28*(4), 575–599. doi:10.1080/13854046.2014.907445.

Moher, D., Liberati, A., Tetzlaff, J., & Altman, D. G. (2009). Preferred reporting items for systematic reviews and meta-analyses: The PRISMA statement. *Annals of Internal Medicine, 151*(4), 264–269, W264.

National Academy of Neuropsychology. (2001). Definition of a clinical neuropsychologist. *The Clinical Neuropsychologist, 3*(1), 22.

Rebok, G. W., Ball, K., Guey, L. T., Jones, R. N., Kim, H. Y., King, J. W., . . . Willis, S. L. (2014). Ten-year effects of the advanced cognitive training for independent and vital elderly cognitive training trial on cognition and everyday functioning in older adults. *Journal of the American Geriatric Society, 62*(1), 16–24. doi:10.1111/jgs.12607.

Sackett, D. L., Rosenberg, W. M., Gray, J. A., Haynes, R. B., & Richardson, W. S. (1996). Evidence based medicine: What it is and what it isn't. *British Medical Journal, 312*(7023), 71–72.

Sauve, S., Lee, H. N., Meade, M. O., Lang, J. D., Farkouh, M., Cook, D. J., & Sackett, D. L. (1995). The critically appraised topic: A practical approach to learning critical appraisal. *Annals of the Royal College of Physicians and Surgeons of Canada, 28*(7), 396–398.

Schulz, K. F., Altman, D. G., & Moher, D. (2010). CONSORT 2010 statement: Updated guidelines for reporting parallel group randomized trials. *Annals of Internal Medicine, 152*(11), 726–732. doi:10.7326/0003-4819-152-11-201006010-00232.

Straus, S. E., Glasziou, P., Richardson, W. S., & Haynes, R. B. (2011). *Evidence-Based Medicine: How to Practice and Teach It* (4th ed.). Edinburgh, UK: Churchill Livingston.

TRIP Database. (1997). Retrieved June 20, 2015, from https://www.tripdatabase.com/info/.

Wyer, P. C. (1997). The critically appraised topic: Closing the evidence-transfer gap. *Annals of Emergency Medicine, 30*(5), 639–640.

13

Key Skills for the Evidence-Based Practitioner

STEPHEN C. BOWDEN

Becoming an evidence-based clinical neuropsychologist requires an extensive skill set. A clinical neuropsychologist requires extensive knowledge of the structure and function of the central nervous system and knowledge of clinical neurosciences. Also, a clinical neuropsychologist requires understanding of the cognitive and psychosocial manifestations of neuropsychological disorders, both in terms of their impact on everyday behaviors and in terms of formal diagnostic criteria and relevant assessment methods, together with the burgeoning range of intervention techniques. Since psychopathology is a common, often treatable, primary or secondary diagnosis in patients with neuropsychological disorders, neuropsychologists need a broad skill set to effectively assess and care for their patients (see Alkemade, Bowden, & Salzman, 2015; Reynolds & Kamphaus, 2003; and Chapter 4 this volume).

With the changing nature of expertise (Haynes, Devereaux, & Guyatt, 2002), clinical neuropsychologists also need sophisticated skills in understanding rules of research evidence and test score interpretation (Straus, Richardson, Glasziou, & Haynes, 2011). As illustrated in many chapters in this volume, the principles of evidence-based practice provide a educational challenge for clinicians, namely, to acquire skills in finding and interpreting the best-quality evidence with the aim of enhancing the care of patients.

Although they may be challenging to those who have not encountered the ideas before, the skills of evidence-based practice are designed to be acquired and practiced in routine clinical work (Straus et al., 2011). Extensive educational resources are available to assist clinicians through the learning and skill-maintenance processes. Once they have acquired these skills, clinicians who are well-versed in evidence-based practice will never again approach the reading of a journal article in the uncritical way that a pre–evidence-based practitioner may do. Nor will the evidence-based practitioner listen to "experts" present their views on any topic without critically reflecting on the quality of evidence that underlies the experts' arguments and conclusions. As illustrated in this volume, an evidence-based practitioner learns to rank opinion and evidence in terms of what are now well-established, though evolving, criteria for quality. An evidence-based practitioner also learns to identify quality opinions. For example, an expert opinion on any area of actively researched clinical practice that does not reflect the conclusions from a well-conducted systematic review should immediately raise questions regarding the scientific status of that expert opinion. Critical reflection on quality of evidence is a set of skills readily acquired by practitioners and underlies the critical-appraisal techniques described in detail in Chapters 8, 11, and 12 in this volume. Effective critical-appraisal skills begin with scrutiny of individual diagnostic-validity or treatment studies (Chapters 11 and 12), then generalize to other forms of study and then to critical-appraisal of systematic reviews. Clinicians who use critical appraisal skills can be confident that they are using criteria to evaluate the quality of clinical evidence that have, in turn, been subject to some of the most intense scientific scrutiny and peer-review of any quality criteria in the history of health care, and have not been bettered (Greenhalgh, 2006).

THE IMPORTANCE OF THEORETICAL CONTEXT FOR EXPERTISE

Expertise requires a theoretical context, and critical-appraisal skills are only a focused extension and refinement of clinical-thinking skills that have been discussed in clinical psychology and clinical neuropsychology for several decades (e.g., Meehl, 1973, 1997). In particular, fundamental aspects of evidence-based practice dovetail with the principles of research design and of criterion-related validity that have been used in psychology for many years to establish the classification accuracy of clinical tests for identifying psychopathology or cognitive disability. The criterion-related-validity process is a subset of the broader construct-validity enterprise used by psychologists to advance theory and practice. A brief history and current description of the theoretical and applied endeavor of construct validity is in Chapter 2 by Riley and colleagues in this volume. Riley and colleagues argue that the long tradition of clinical test development though criterion-related-validity methods has been remarkably successful in providing practitioners with a variety of assessment methods to identify neuropsychological disorders. The success of the criterion-related-validity endeavor contrasts with the debate regarding the best models of cognitive function to motivate test development and a taxonomy of cognitive abilities. Riley and colleagues review some examples of assessment practices motivated by diverse theories of cognitive and broader psychological function, and conclude that criterion-related validity will be more successful if it is based on better theory.

> Accordingly, when an assessment measure of a neuropsychological construct predicts a form of cognitive functioning as it should, based on an existing theory, the matrix of empirical support for the validity of that predictive relationship includes, not only the successful prediction itself, but also the body of empirical evidence that underlies the theory. (Riley et al., p. 15 this volume)

In other words, construct validity in neuropsychology is enhanced through the converging lines of evidence derived from successful assessment practices, if those assessment practices can be grounded in theory and good models of disorders.

Following this line of argument, Chapters 3 and 4 in this volume review contemporary models of cognition and psychopathology, respectively, models designed to guide clinical assessment. Jewsbury and Bowden (Chapter 3) review some of the more prominent approaches to modelling cognition for theoretical refinement or diagnostic classification. These authors argue that, although various theoretical and empirical approaches have been advanced to describe human cognition, at the present time, the psychometric latent-variable approach provides the most practical value and comprehensive framework for describing individual differences relevant to clinical assessment and diagnosis. In addition, these authors show that, although the concept of executive function has achieved extraordinary prominence in neuropsychological practice, assessment of executive function relies on many tests that have a long history in clinical neuropsychology, known under other nomenclatures at different times during this history. Jewsbury and Bowden show that an impressive array of evidence is emerging that suggests strong measurement overlap between concepts of executive function and core latent variables in an expanded, contemporary psychometric model of cognitive abilities.

These authors tentatively propose that one model has the potential to provide a comprehensive taxonomy of cognitive abilities, in clinical, developmental, and non-clinical populations alike and, as theoretical integration, draws together the criterion-related-validity evidence from diverse assessment traditions under one construct-validity framework. This is the *Cattell-Horn-Carroll* model of cognitive abilities, now cited as the theoretical foundation for many contemporary cognitive ability batteries.

Turning to the assessment of psychopathology in neuropsychological and other populations, Lee and colleagues in Chapter 4 describe the challenges for effective assessment using the categorical classification systems that are prominent across disciplines in mental health care. Instead, Lee and colleagues note, evidence from large epidemiological studies indicates that the co-occurrence or "comorbidity amongst mental disorders is the rule (not the exception) for most mental disorders" (p. 66, this volume). As an alternative approach to assessment, Lee and colleagues identify the theoretical and empirical advantages of a dimensional approach to assessment of psychopathology. They describe what they term the *Multivariate Correlated Liabilities Model*—which distinguishes internalizing disorders from externalizing disorders. These authors also summarize research proposing extensions of this model to include the additional latent variables of psychosis and somatization, which together provides the theoretical basis for assessment of a wide array of mental health conditions. The potential conceptual power of the Multivariate Correlated Liabilities Model is shown through empirical integration with the five-factor model of personality, proposing that " it does not matter which personality model one examines, as they typically map onto each other and represent different levels of analyses within the broader personality hierarchy" (p. 75, this volume). Lee and colleagues conclude their chapter by showing that some of the best contemporary psychopathology-assessment instruments incorporate these theoretical innovations to provide clinicians with the kind of theoretically motivated tests that build on a strong history of criterion-related validity evidence. Together, these chapters suggest that neuropsychologists have access to robust models of cognition and psychopathology, models with an impressive array of explanatory power, to guide theoretical refinement and evidence-based assessment practices, to an extent not available before.

ASSESSMENT, CLINICAL INVESTIGATION, AND CLINICAL THINKING SKILLS

A change in focus to detailed assessment practice is reflected in the topic of Chapter 5, in which Bowden and Finch review fundamental concepts of test score reliability and the calculation of *confidence* or *prediction* intervals. These authors provide a non-technical introduction to the common ways to estimate the reliability of test scores and how to calculate confidence intervals for test scores. They note that, although interval estimation has become routine for the interpretation of sample means in clinical research studies, the same logic of interval estimation is sometimes ignored in clinical assessment. In addition, these authors show that calculation of confidence intervals leads to some surprising conclusions, for example, when using test scores with lower reliability, the appropriate confidence interval for the best estimate of the test score may not include the observed score. Formulae for calculation of confidence and prediction intervals are provided in this chapter. Although based on the cumulative foundation of psychometric principles, estimation of predicted true scores and the associated confidence intervals is one of the most neglected skills in psychological and neuropsychological assessment. Bowden and Finch also make the point that the concepts of reliability and precision in inference relates to any information that is used to make clinical decisions, not just formal test scores. These authors conclude their chapter by showing the impact of the principles of interval estimation for test scores on evidence-based practice.

In Chapter 6, Hinton-Bayre and Kwapil provide a detailed description of the use of reliable change indices (RCIs), a specific application of the concept of prediction intervals described in Chapter 5. RCIs provide objective criteria for detecting change in scores over time, either in response to a treatment or intervention, or in response to change in clinical condition, for example, recovery from brain injury or deterioration with a degenerative dementia. These authors highlight that one of the most useful applications of RCIs involves calculation of event rates for treatment studies. RCIs provide a psychometrically sound, and less arbitrary, method for establishing significant change after a treatment intervention, for the calculation of risk-reduction, or treatment–benefit analysis (see Chapter 12 by Miller in this volume). Hinton-Bayre and Kwapil indicate that, under conditions of high reliability, all recommended RCIs are likely to lead to similar clinical inferences. However, under conditions of lower reliability and, in particular circumstances regarding the observed baseline scores, some methods may be biased to detect change. These authors conclude that more work is required to identify the optimal application of RCIs.

In Chapter 7, Chelune then shifts the focus to the key skills for knowledge maintenance and professional development, when a clinician aims to achieve the highest level of clinical expertise. Chelune describes some of the historical origins of evidence-based practice, showing that effective evidence-based practice is a values-driven combination of best-evidence, expertise, and patient values. Chelune also highlights the distinction from traditional notions of expertise derived from experiential learning. He then describes the core skills in evidence-based practice, including the ability to ask answerable questions, find good study-evidence, then evaluate the quality of evidence for patient impact and relevance. The goal of finding and evaluating quality evidence with patient impact involves techniques that are described under critical-appraisal (Straus et al., 2011), a recurrent theme in this book, and described in detail in Chelune's chapter along with worked examples in Chapters 11 and 12. Chelune shows how the focus of expertise has shifted from the older notions of experiential learning in seasoned clinicians to the criterion of how well any clinician, younger or older, is able to access, identify, and interpret quality evidence. Chelune defines evidence-based clinical neuropsychological practice, "not as a discrete action or body of knowledge, but as a process—an ongoing 'pattern' of routine clinical practice" (Chapter 7, this volume, pp. 160).

One of the most dramatic technological developments over recent decades in clinical neuroscience has been modern neuroimaging. However, with dramatic developments in clinical *and* research techniques, the evidence-based practitioner faces the challenge of discriminating between established techniques with demonstrated clinical validity, versus techniques that are not yet ready for clinical application. In Chapter 8, Bigler describes the diversity of modalities currently available from clinical neuroimaging. Bigler shows the many ways in which clinical imaging modalities, particularly CT and MRI, measures of white matter integrity, gross morphology, and blood-product deposition, all provide alternative and complementary methods to quantify brain integrity. In addition, in this chapter, a range of inexpensive, accessible methods with established validity is highlighted that can be used to improve the objectivity of clinical interpretation of neuroimaging findings. Bigler concludes his chapter by describing the tremendous innovations in imaging together with newer techniques such as diffusion tensor imaging, noting that these and other research techniques are not yet the basis for generalizable clinical diagnostic methods.

Improving interpretation of the scientific importance, and patient relevance, of published clinical research findings would be of less benefit if there were not a related aspiration by many scientific journal editors to improve the standards of published studies. This initiative has been evolving for some years, initially known as the CONSORT consortium (www.equator-network.org/reporting-guidelines/

consort/). There is a now a unified endeavor to improve the quality and transparency of reporting standards in health care that falls under the rubric of the EQUATOR network, incorporating the CONSORT guidelines and many other publication guidelines besides. In Chapter 9 in this volume, Schoenberg and colleagues describe the relevance of these initiatives to the practice of evidence-based neuropsychology. Schoenberg and colleagues reiterate a point made by Chelune in Chapter 7, that these widely embraced publication guidelines are beneficial to both producers *and* consumers of research. The guidelines provide a comprehensive, though not necessarily exhaustive, checklist of criteria by which to design and report many types of clinical studies. The guidelines also provide checklists to guide peer review, as well as the broader framework in which the critical-appraisal process is nested. Readers familiar with the EQUATOR network guidelines will appreciate that the critical-appraisal methods (see Chapters 11 and 12, this volume) are partly derived from the quality-criteria incorporated within the guidelines for respective study designs, whether treatment-intervention or diagnostic validity.

The STARD criteria (www.equator-network.org/reporting-guidelines/stard/) for evaluating the validity of a test are one example of the guidelines highlighted by Schoenberg. The STARD criteria require a careful description of what have become the two most important classification accuracy statistics in clinical practice, namely, sensitivity and specificity. Without a good understanding of how to interpret these criterion-related validity statistics, any clinician is hampered in her or his ability to understand the scientific process of diagnosis. However, skillful interpretation of these statistics alone is not enough to be a skilled diagnostician. Instead, these statistics interact with a quantity that varies from one clinical setting to another. The latter quantity is known as the *local base-rate* (or prevalence, or the pre-test probability) of the condition to be diagnosed. In Chapter 10, Bunnage describes these statistics, methods of calculation, and online and graphical calculation aids. These aids make relatively easy the process of re-estimating the probability of the patient having the diagnosis after the test results are known. These skills are so fundamental to clinical practice that no clinician should be unfamiliar with these statistics. The accurate interpretation of sensitivity and specificity has profound implications for clinical judgement and constitutes a fundamental skill for a scientific clinician, providing the numerical content of evidence-based diagnosis.

CRITICAL-APPRAISAL SKILLS FOR NEUROPSYCHOLOGISTS

The two concluding exposition chapters in this volume (Chapters 11 and 12) draw together the principles of evidence-based practice, essential elements of the reporting guidelines, and the application of interpretive criteria to determine patient relevance. These two chapters are designed to provide demonstrations of the techniques of critical appraisal. In both chapters, the role of critical-appraisal is shown to be a variant of the concept of post-publication peer review (http://about.scienceopen.com/what-is-post-publication-peer-review/). However, the critical-appraisal approach is specifically designed to address health-care research and individual patient needs. Acquisition of critical-appraisal skills allows the skilled reader to interpret and discern the methods quality and patient relevance of any published study.

Berry and colleagues' Chapter 11 provides a detailed description of the critical appraisal of a diagnostic test, reported from a single validity study. In Chapter 12, Miller takes the reader through the process of formulating an answerable question, finding a suitable study, and interpreting the results for importance and patient relevance. Miller reiterates the demonstration of the critical-appraisal techniques with the evaluation of a published treatment study. Both of these critical-appraisal chapters contain rich details of educational value to all clinicians not familiar with the techniques. Following the critical-appraisal approach, any clinician can learn to quickly identify the quality of available knowledge with respect to a specific treatment or diagnostic question. The techniques also facilitate identification of gaps in our knowledge, when no useful or good-quality information can be identified. Under such circumstances, clinicians can clearly demarcate the limits of our scientific understanding, advise patients appropriately and, ideally, motivate new studies to fill the knowledge gaps.

CONCLUSION

In view of the rapidly evolving scientific basis of neuropsychological practice, neuropsychologists, like all other health care professionals, need to acquire skills for continuous learning (Straus et al., 2011). The methods of evidence-based practice have evolved to address these needs (Straus et al., 2011). As in other areas of professional expertise, the benefits of training and a good education have a finite shelf-life. Unless practitioners learn effective skills for maintaining and updating their knowledge, they are likely to become increasingly out of date. The need to update knowledge is one reason for mandating professional development activities in most professional organizations, as in psychology. As was shown in the first chapter of this volume, expertise in neuropsychology and in health care in general is no longer defined as a function of the number of patients seen or the number of years in clinical practice. It is possible to develop and maintain severe misunderstandings about patients and their clinical conditions, through many years of practice. This is because learning from experience may mislead the clinician, who may fail to correct these misapprehensions. The methods of evidence-based practice, elements of which are described in this volume, provide one of the most effective and widely accepted strategies for maintaining and updating clinical knowledge.

REFERENCES

Alkemade, N., Bowden, S. C., & Salzman, L. (2015). Scoring correction for MMPI-2 Hs scale in patients experiencing a Traumatic Brain Injury: A test of measurement invariance. *Archives of Clinical Neuropsychology, 2015*, 39–48.

Greenhalgh, T. (2006). *How to Read a Paper: The Basics of Evidence-Based Medicine (3rd ed.)*. Malden, MA: Blackwell Publishing.

Haynes, R. B., Devereaux, P. J., & Guyatt, G. H. (2002). Clinical expertise in the era of evidence-based medicine and patient choice. *Evidence Based Medicine, 7,* 36–38.

Meehl, P. E. (1973). Why I do not attend case conferences. In P. E. Meehl (Ed.), *Psychodiagnosis: Selected Papers* (pp. 225–302). Minneapolis, MN: University of Minnesota Press.

Meehl, P. E. (1997). Credentialed persons, credentialed knowledge. *Clinical Psychology: Science and Practice, 4,* 91–98.

Reynolds, C. R., & Kamphaus, R. W. (Eds.). (2003). *Handbook of psychological and educational assessment of children: Personality, Behaviors, and Context (2nd ed.)*. New York, NY: The Guilford Press.

Straus, S., Richardson, W. S., Glasziou, P., & Haynes, R. B. (2011). *Evidence-Based Medicine: How to Practice and Teach EBM* (4th ed.). Edinburgh, UK: Churchill Livingstone.

Index

Tables and figures are represented by an italicized *t* or *f*, respectively.

Printed in the USA/Agawam, MA
February 23, 2018

670299.020